TOXICOLOGY SECRETS

TOXICOLOGY SECRETS

Louis J. Ling, MD, FACEP, FACMT
Medical Director, Hennepin Regional Poison Center
Associate Medical Director for Medical Education
Hennepin County Medical Center
Professor and Director, Emergency Medicine Program
University of Minnesota Medical School
Minneapolis, Minnesota

Richard F. Clark, MD, FACEP, FACMT
Associate Professor of Medicine
Division of Medical Toxicology
Department of Emergency Medicine
University of California, San Diego, School of Medicine
Attending Physician, UCSD Medical Center
San Diego, California

Timothy B. Erickson, MD, FACEP, FACMT
Associate Professor, Department of Emergency Medicine
University of Illinois College of Medicine
Director, Division of Clinical Toxicology
Residency Director, Program in Emergency Medicine
Consultant, Illinois Poison Center
Chicago, Illinois

John H. Trestrail III, RPh, FAACT, DABAT
Managing Director
DeVos Children's Hospital Regional Poison Center
Grand Rapids, Michigan

HANLEY & BELFUS, INC./Philadelphia

Publisher: HANLEY & BELFUS, INC.
                Medical Publishers
                210 South 13th Street
                Philadelphia, PA 19107
                (215) 546-7293; 800-962-1892
                FAX (215) 790-9330
                Web site: http://www.hanleyandbelfus.com

Note to the reader: Although the information in this book has been carefully reviewed for correctness of dosage and indications, neither the authors nor the editors nor the publisher can accept any legal responsibility for any errors or omissions that may be made. Neither the publisher nor the editors make any warranty, expressed or implied, with respect to the material contained herein. Before prescribing any drug, the reader must review the manufacturer's current product information (package inserts) for accepted indications, absolute dosage recommendations, and other information pertinent to the safe and effective use of the product described. This is especially important when drugs are given in combination or as an adjunct to other forms of therapy.

Library of Congress Cataloging-in-Publication Data

Toxicology secrets / edited by Louis Ling . . . |et al.|
      p. ; cm.—(The Secrets Series®)
    Includes index.
    ISBN 1-56053-410-9 (alk. paper)
      1. Toxicology—Miscellanea. 2. Drugs—Toxicology—Miscellanea. I. Ling, Louis, 1954–
II. Series.
    |DNLM: 1. Toxicology—Examination Questions. QV 18.2 T755 2000|
RA1211.T638 2000
615.9—dc21

                                                      00-058093

TOXICOLOGY SECRETS   ISBN 1-56053-410-9

Last digit is the print number: 9 8 7 6 5 4 3 2 1

DEDICATION

To Beth, Ali, Amanda, and Eric, who make everything worthwhile
To the staff of the Hennepin Regional Poison Center who care for
poisoned patients every minute of every day
To the students devoted to learning toxicology by reading this book

LJL

To my students, who provide me with an audience
To Alex, Ben, and Cate, who make it Christmas morning every day
To Therese, who comprises everything else

RFC

To Valerie, Camille, Isabelle, Celeste, and Julian, and all those who
love toxicology, history, humor, and trivia

TE

To my parents, John Harris Trestrail and Edith (McClay) Trestrail,
my wife, Mary, and our children, John and Amanda

JHT

CONTENTS

V. CARDIAC DRUGS

VI. PSYCHOPHARMACOLOGIC MEDICATIONS

VII. DRUGS OF ABUSE

XII. FOOD POISONING

XIII. BOTANICALS

XIV. ENVENOMATIONS

XV. TOXIC TERRORIST THREATS

CONTRIBUTORS

Steven E. Aks, D.O., FACMT, FACEP
Clinical Associate Professor, Department of Emergency Medicine, University of Illinois College of Medicine; Fellowship Director, Toxikon Consortium, Cook County Hospital; Attending Physician, Department of Emergency Medicine, Mercy Hospital and Medical Center, Chicago, Illinois

Timothy E. Albertson, M.D., Ph.D.
Professor of Medicine, Medical Pharmacology and Toxicology, and Anesthesiology, Department of Medicine, University of California, Davis, School of Medicine, Davis, California; University of California, Davis, Medical Center, California Poison Control System-Sacramento Division, Sacramento, California; Veterans Administration Northern California Health Care, Mather, California

John Alexis, M.D.
Clinical Instructor, Department of Emergency Medicine, University of Illinois College of Medicine; Attending Physician, MacNeal Hospital, Chicago, Illinois

Linda G. Allison, M.D., M.P.H.
Clinical Assistant Professor, Department of Emergency Medicine, West Virginia University School of Medicine, Morgantown, West Virginia

Ilene B. Anderson, Pharm.D.
Associate Clinical Professor of Pharmacy, University of California, San Francisco; Senior Toxicology Management Specialist, California Poison Control System-San Francisco Division, San Francisco, California

John G. Benitez, M.D., M.P.H., FACMT, FACEP
Associate Professor, Departments of Emergency Medicine and Environmental Medicine, University of Rochester School of Medicine, Rochester, New York

Paul Bolger, M.D.
Clinical Instructor, Department of Emergency Medicine, University of Illinois College of Medicine, Chicago, Illinois; Attending Physician, Ottawa Hospital, Ottawa, Illinois

G. Randall Bond, M.D.
Professor, Departments of Pediatrics and Emergency Medicine, University of Cincinnati College of Medicine; Medical Director, Drug and Poison Information Center, Cincinnati, Ohio

Lynn D. Bui, M.D.
Assistant Clinical Professor of Medicine, University of California, San Francisco, School of Medicine; San Francisco General Hospital, San Francisco, California

Anthony Burda, R.Ph., DABAT
Associate Director, Illinois Poison Center, Chicago, Illinois

Andrea G. Carlson, M.D.
Senior Toxicology Fellow, Department of Emergency Medicine, University of Illinois College of Medicine; Toxikon Consortium, Cook County Hospital, Chicago, Illinois

Helen Choi, M.D.
Department of Emergency Medicine, Christ Hospital and Medical Center, Oak Lawn, Illinois

Summon Chomchai, M.D.
Faculty, Department of Preventive and Social Medicine, Mahidol University, Siriraj Hospital, Bangkok, Thailand

Jason Chu, M.D.
New York Poison Control Center, New York, New York

Kent Clark, M.D.
Department of Emergency Medicine, North Shore University Hospital, Manhasset, New York

Richard F. Clark, M.D., FACEP, FACMT
Associate Professor of Medicine, Division of Medical Toxicology, Department of Emergency Medicine, University of California, San Diego, School of Medicine; Attending Physician, UCSD Medical Center, San Diego, California

Kirk L. Cumpston, D.O.
Department of Emergency Medicine, University of Illinois College of Medicine, Chicago, Illinois

Samuel Dorevitch, M.D.
Division of Occupational Medicine, Cook County Hospital, Chicago, Illinois

Suzanne Doyon, M.D.
Medical Director, Maryland Poison Center, University of Maryland School of Pharmacy; Attending Physician, Mercy Hospital Center, Baltimore, Maryland

K. Sophia Dyer, M.D.
Assistant Professor, Department of Emergency Medicine, Boston University School of Medicine; Boston Medical Center, Boston, Massachusetts

Bernard H. Eisenga, Ph.D., M.D.
Medical Director, DeVos Children's Hospital Regional Poison Center; Staff Attending, Department of Internal Medicine, Spectrum Health, Grand Rapids, Michigan

Timothy B. Erickson, M.D., FACEP, FACMT
Associate Professor, Department of Emergency Medicine, University of Illinois College of Medicine; Director, Division of Clinical Toxicology; Residency Director, Program in Emergency Medicine; Consultant, Illinois Poison Center, Chicago, Illinois

Susan E. Farrell, M.D.
Instructor, Division of Emergency Medicine, Harvard Medical School; Beth Israel Deaconess Medical Center, Boston, Massachusetts

Thomas J. Ferguson, M.D., Ph.D.
Associate Clinical Professor, Department of Pulmonary and Critical Care Medicine, University of California, Davis, School of Medicine, Davis, California; University of California, Davis, Medical Center, Sacramento, California

Bryan Finke, M.D.
Department of Emergency Medicine, University of Illinois College of Medicine; Toxikon Consortium, Cook County Hospital, Chicago, Illinois

Susan S. Fish, Pharm.D., M.P.H.
Associate Professor, Department of Epidemiology and Biostatistics, Boston University School of Public Health, Boston, Massachusetts; Director of Regulatory Affairs, CareStat, Inc., Chestnut Hill, Massachusetts

Christofer Fore, M.D.
Department of Emergency Medicine, University of Pittsburgh School of Medicine, Pittsburgh, Pennsylvania

Rotem Friede, M.D.
Department of Emergency Medicine, University of Illinois College of Medicine, Chicago, Illinois

Frederick Fung, M.D., M.S.
Clinical Professor, Department of Occupational Medicine, University of California, Irvine, School of Medicine, Irvine, California; Sharp Rees-Stealy Medical Group, San Diego, California

Richard J. Geller, M.D., M.P.H.
Assistant Clinical Professor, Department of Emergency Medicine, University of California, San Francisco, School of Medicine, San Francisco, California; Medical Director, California Poison Control System-Fresno Division; Fresno Community Hospital and Medical Center, Fresno, California

Richard D. Gerkin, Jr., M.D.
Clinical Adjunct Professor, Division of Emergency Medicine, Department of Surgery, University of Arizona College of Medicine, Tucson, Arizona; Associate Director, Samaritan Regional Poison Center, Good Samaritan Regional Medical Center, Phoenix, Arizona

Chulathida Greethong, M.D.
Junior Faculty, Department of Pediatrics, Mahidol University, Siriraj Hospital, Bangkok, Thailand

David D. Gummin, M.D.
Division of Medical Toxicology, Department of Emergency Medicine, University of Illinois College of Medicine; Toxikon Consortium, Cook County Hospital, Chicago, Illinois

Leon M. Gussow, M.D., ABMT
Senior Attending Physician, Department of Emergency Medicine, Cook County Hospital, Chicago, Illinois

Christine A. Haller, M.D.
Adjunct Assistant Professor, Division of Clinical Pharmacology and Experimental Therapeutics, Department of Medicine, University of California, San Francisco, School of Medicine; California Poison Control System-San Francisco Division, San Francisco General Hospital, San Francisco, California

Fred P. Harchelroad, M.D.
Director, Medical Toxicology Treatment Center, Allegheny General Hospital, Pittsburgh, Pennsylvania

Carson R. Harris, M.D.
Assistant Professor, Clinical Emergency Medicine Program, University of Minnesota Medical School, Minneapolis, Minnesota; Senior Staff, Department of Emergency Medicine, Regions Hospital, St. Paul, Minnesota

Robert J. Hoffman, M.D.
Clinical Instructor, Division of Emergency Medicine, New York University Medical Center; Bellevue Hospital, New York Poison Control Center, New York, New York

Marianne Ingels, M.D.
Department of Emergency Medicine, Integris Baptist Medical Center, Oklahoma City, Oklahoma

Evan L. Kahn, M.D.
Department of Emergency Medicine, University of Illinois College of Medicine; University of Illinois Hospital, Chicago, Illinois

David C. Lee, M.D.
Director of Research, Department of Emergency Medicine, North Shore University Hospital, Manhasset, New York

Maerry L. Lee, M.D.
Clinical Instructor, Department of Emergency Medicine, University of Illinois College of Medicine; Attending Physician, St. Elizabeth Hospital, Chicago, Illinois

Louis J. Ling, M.D., FACEP, FACMT
Professor of Clinical Emergency Medicine and Pharmacy; Director, Emergency Medicine Program, University of Minnesota Medical School; Medical Director, Hennepin Regional Poison Center; Associate Medical Director for Education, Hennepin County Medical Center, Minneapolis, Minnesota

Binh T. Ly, M.D.
California Poison Control System–San Diego Division, UCSD Medical Center, San Diego, California

Anthony S. Manoguerra, Pharm.D., DABAT, FAACT
Professor, Departments of Clinical Pharmacy, Pediatrics, and Pharmacology, University of California, San Diego, School of Medicine; Director, California Poison Control System–San Diego Division, San Diego, California

Jean L. Martinucci, M.D.
Department of Emergency Medicine, Cook County Hospital, Chicago, Illinois

Stephen W. Munday, M.D., M.P.H., M.S.
Division of Medical Toxicology, Department of Emergency Medicine, University of California, San Diego, School of Medicine, San Diego, California

Mark B. Mycyk, M.D.
Department of Toxicology, Toxikon Consortium, Cook County Hospital, Chicago, Illinois

Sean Patrick Nordt, Pharm.D., DABAT
University College, Dublin, School of Medicine, Dublin, Ireland

Jennifer M. Owens, M.D.
Department of Emergency Medicine, Cook County Hospital, Chicago, Illinois

Frank P. Paloucek, Pharm.D., DABAT
Clinical Associate Professor, Department of Pharmacy Practice, University of Illinois; Director, Residency Programs in Department of Pharmacy, University of Illinois Hospital, Chicago, Illinois

Manish M. Patel, M.D.
Department of Emergency Medicine, University of California, San Francisco, School of Medicine, San Francisco, California

Shahrzad Rafiee, M.D.
Clinical Instructor, Department of Emergency Medicine, University of Illinois College of Medicine; Attending Physician, Resurrection Hospital, Chicago, Illinois

Cyrus Rangan, M.D., FAAP
Clinical Instructor, Department of Pediatrics, Children's Hospital of Los Angeles; Assistant Medical Director, California Poison Control System-Los Angeles Division, Los Angeles, California

Joseph B. Reuben, M.D.
Department of Emergency Medicine, University of Illinois College of Medicine; Toxikon Consortium, Cook County Hospital, Chicago, Illinois

Anne-Michelle Ruha, M.D.
Department of Medical Toxicology, Good Samaritan Regional Medical Center, Phoenix, Arizona

Adhi N. Sharma, M.D.
Clinical Instructor, Division of Emergency Medicine, Department of Surgery, New York University School of Medicine; New York Poison Control Center; Bellevue Hospital, New York, New York

Shu Shum, M.B., B.S., FAAP, FACMT
Clinical Associate Professor, Department of Pediatrics, Texas Tech University Health Sciences Center; Medical Director, Texas Panhandle Poison Center, Northwest Texas Hospital, Amarillo, Texas

Mark Su, M.D.
Medical Toxicology Fellow, New York Poison Control Center, New York, New York

David A. Tanen, M.D.
Department of Emergency Medicine, Naval Medical Center, San Diego, California

Andrew Topliff, M.D.
Associate Medical Director, Hennepin Regional Poison Center, Minneapolis, Minnesota

John H. Trestrail III, R.Ph., FAACT, DABAT
Managing Director, DeVos Children's Hospital Regional Poison Center, Grand Rapids, Michigan

Michael Wahl, M.D.
Assistant Professor, Department of Emergency Medicine, University of Illinois College of Medicine; Medical Director, Illinois Poison Center; Illinois Masonic Medical Center, Chicago, Illinois

Kevin L. Wallace, M.D.
Clinical Associate Professor, Section of Medical Toxicology, University of Arizona College of Medicine, Tucson, Arizona; Good Samaritan Regional Medical Center, Phoenix Children's Hospital, Phoenix, Arizona

Saralyn R. Williams, M.D.
Assistant Clinical Professor of Medicine, Division of Medical Toxicology, University of California, San Diego, School of Medicine, San Diego, California

Michele Zell-Kanter, Pharm.D., ABAT
Coordinator, Toxikon Consortium, Division of Occupational Medicine, Cook County Hospital, Chicago, Illinois

PREFACE

We are surrounded by poisons and toxins everywhere. Learning about all of this toxicology can be an intense and laborious undertaking. However, a thorough knowledge of the basic concepts and common exposures can be accomplished with just a little planning and organization and the right tools. This book is one of those tools.

Keeping true to The Secrets Series® format, this book does not attempt to cover every detail about every toxin. This book *does* cover the important ideas and the common poisons that a physician or other health care professional may encounter. It addresses the important questions that you would ask yourself and gives you the concise answers that you need to manage the poisoned patient. *Toxicology Secrets* is just the right length for a short course or clinical rotation and is very suitable for self study. Thus, this text is perfect for medical students and emergency medicine residents, but it is also useful for pharmacy, nursing, and physician assistant students. It is the ideal first reference for new poison center staff members and toxicology fellows. *Toxicology Secrets* does not replace any of the fine comprehensive textbooks on the subject, but if you know all of the answers in this book, you know a lot of toxicology.

To prevent these lessons from becoming dry and tedious, and to challenge the more advanced and curious students of toxicology, there are extra-credit trivia questions scattered throughout the book. This allows every reader to stump their teachers, sound amazingly erudite on rounds, and bask in the center of attention at cocktail parties. This special feature, is only possible through the contributions of the incomparable John Trestrail. John is the undisputed King of Toxicology Trivia and is the Master of Ceremonies at the Annual Toxicology Trivia Bowl of the American Association of Poison Control Centers.

Of course, we would like to thank all of the authors, who shared their experience and wisdom, and all of our patients, who inspire us to learn more.

Louis J. Ling, MD
Richard F. Clark, MD
Timothy D. Erickson, MD
John H. Trestrail III, RPh

I. General Principles

1. HISTORY OF TOXICOLOGY

John H. Trestrail III, R.Ph.

1. What is the origin of the word *toxicology*?

Of course, the word means the study of poisons. The origin of words containing the prefix "toxic-" comes from *tox*, the ancient Greek word for bow. This is thought to be associated with their use of poisoned arrows in warfare.

2. What are the earliest writings on toxicology?

The writings found in the Egyptian *Papyrus Ebers* (1552 B.C.) provide the most complete information on the medicine and pharmacy of ancient Egypt. This work contains many recipes for poisons and mentions antimony, copper, lead, hyoscyamus, opium, turpentine, and verdigris. Writings from India (600–100 B.C.) include the *Charaka Samhita*, which mentions copper, gold, iron, lead, silver, and tin, and the *Susruta Samhita*, which describes the toxicology of food, vegetable and animal poisons, and the treatment of snake bites and insect stings.

3. Who were the great ancient Greek and Roman toxicologists?

The Greek physician Hippocrates (460–370 B.C.), the Father of Medicine, separated medicine from religion and philosophy to make it an independent subject. He wrote on snake bites and described severe colic in men who extracted metals. His writings show that the ancient Greeks had a knowledge of treating poisons by influencing absorption. Theophrastus (370–286 B.C.) wrote *De Historia Plantarum*, which covered the subject of toxic plants. Nicander of Colophon (185–135 B.C.), a physician to Attalus III, King of Pergamum, experimented with poisons on condemned criminals and compiled the first poison pharmacopoeia. He also wrote poetic treatises on poisons and antidotes: *Alexipharmica* (consisting of 600 lines dealing with antidotes) and *Theriaca* (consisting of 1000 lines dealing with poisonous animals). Mithridates, King of Pontus (~100 B.C.), had a reputation of knowing more about poisons and their antidotes than any other man of his time. He invented mithridatum, a "universal" antidote against poisons, that was popular up until the end of the 1600s. Pendacious Dioscorides (A.D. 50), called the Father of Materia Medica, was a Greek army surgeon who traveled with the Roman legions and was considered the greatest of the medical botanists. In his work, *Materia Medica*, he classified poisons as animal, vegetable, or mineral. The Roman scholar Pliny the Elder (A.D. 23–79) wrote of mercury poisoning among the slaves working the quicksilver mines of Almaden, Spain. The Greek physician Claudius Galen (A.D. 130–200) undertook the task of reforming medicine. He developed nut theriac as an antidote for stings and poisons.

4. Who were some contributors to the science of toxicology between 800 and 1300?

Avicenna (980–1037) was one of the most famous scientists of the Islamic world. He developed an electuary against all bites. Moses Maimonides (1135–1204), who compiled a list of remedies for drawing out poisons, wrote the treatise *Poisons and Their Antidotes*. In China, Wang in Hoai (~1250) wrote *Collected Excerpts Concerning Injustice Eliminated*, a text dealing with forensic medicine. He also wrote books on poisoning cases and first aid.

5. What happened in the world of toxicology during the Middle Ages?

During the 1000-year period known as the Middle Ages or "Dark Ages" (~ 500–1500), there were few developments in the science of toxicology. During this time, diseases were regarded as a chastisement from God or a visitation from the Devil. Many monks held to the principle of *similia similibus*, or treating like with like. It was during the end of this period, in the late 1400s, that members of the infamous Borgia family in Italy were applying their skills as poisoners to consolidate their power and wealth.

6. Which toxicologist has the longest name?

During the Age of Enlightenment, one of the premier toxicologic scientists of the time was Paracelsus, the pseudonym of Philippus Aureolus Theophrastus Bombast von Hohenheim (1493–1541). It was Paracelsus who first stated one of the basic concepts of toxicology when he wrote: "What is it that is not poison? All things are poison and nothing is without poison. It is the dose only that makes a thing not a poison." He also authored the first monograph on the occupational diseases of miners and smelters, which was published posthumously in 1567. Unfortunately, he died at age 48 from wounds he suffered in a tavern brawl in Salzburg.

7. Who contributed most to the science of toxicology between 1400 and 1700?

Georgius Agricola (1494–1555) was a physician in Joachimsthal, in the Erzgebirge Mountains on the German-Czechoslovakian border. He observed the toxicologic effects that result from mining and smelting gold and silver and compiled his findings in *De Re Metallica*. Ambroise Paré (1517–1590) wrote *Reports to Court* in 1575, and the chapter on poisoning was thought to be superior to the views of most of his contemporaries. He discussed accidental death by "coal-gas" (carbon monoxide) as well as the intestinal changes caused by corrosive poisons. Rodrigo a Castro (1545–1627), a Jewish refugee doctor from Portugal, published *Medicus Politicus* (The Political Doctor) with a chapter on the signs of poisoning. Paul Zacchias (1584–1659), considered the Father of Legal Medicine, published *Questiones Medico-legales* (Medicolegal Problems) in 1621. Because of the undeveloped science of chemistry, he identified poisons chiefly through smell, taste, and response of experimental animals that were fed poisons. In the late 1600s, under the reign of the French king Louis XIV, there were many homicidal poisonings, involving such infamous poisoners as Marie Madeleine Marchioness de Brinvilliers, St. Croix, and Catherine Deshayes (La Voisin). Their nefarious crimes led to the formation of the judiciary trial body known as the "Chambre Ardente" (1679–1682), and their many crimes became known as the "l'Affaire des Poisons."

8. Who is the Father of Occupational Medicine?

Bernardino Ramazzini (1633–1714) specialized in epidemiology and authored the work *De Morbis Artificum Diatriba*, describing the diseases of tradesmen. He wrote a basic tenet for the occupational toxicologist when he stated, "when a doctor visits a working-class home, he should be content to sit on a three-legged stool if there isn't a gilded chair, and he should take time for his examination; and to the questions recommended by Hippocrates, he should add one more— what is your occupation?"

9. Name some of the contributors to the science of toxicology in more modern times.

The most well-known is Matthieu Joseph Bonaventura Orfila (1787–1853); he will be discussed in another question. Francois Magendie (1783–1855) studied arrow poisons, strychnine, and emetine. Claude Bernard (1813–1878), who was a student of Magendie, first identified the site of action of curare. He also discovered that carbon monoxide plus hemoglobin yields carboxyhemoglobin. In his writings, he stated that "the physiological analysis of organic systems . . . can be done with the aid of toxic agents." Louis Lewin (1854–1929), the famous German pharmacologist, wrote a toxicologist's view of world history in his *Die Gifte in der Weltgeschichte* (Poison in World History), published in 1920.

Jean-Servais Stas (1813–1891), a Belgian chemist, developed a method of extracting alkaloids from cadavers. This became the first effective method of extraction of organic poisons from biological materials. His isolation of nicotine played an important role in the famous Belgian murder trial of Compte Hippolyte De Bocarme (1851).

10. Which historical figures helped to give us a better understanding of the popular poison arsenic?

Sir Robert Christison (1797–1882), an English physician who studied under Orfila in Paris, devoted much time to the detection of arsenic and was the expert witness at the then-famous trial of Madeleine Smith. In 1829, he published *A Treatise on Poisons*, which divided poisons into three groups: irritants, narcoticoacids, and narcotics. Hugo Reinsch developed a test for arsenic by deposition on copper (1842). In 1836, James Marsh (1794–1846) published his method for arsenic testing. The Marsh test standardized testing for the presence of arsenic in body tissue and fluids. By converting arsenic to arsine gas and then depositing the arsine gas as a metallic mirror on porcelain, it became possible to detect as little as 0.02 mg of arsenic. This accurate test for the popular homicidal poison revolutionized the investigation of poisonings and was used in the celebrated Marie LaFarge poisoning case in 1840. Sir Rudolph Peters studied the mechanism of action of arsenical war gases and developed the antidote British antilewisite (BAL) or dimercaprol.

11. Who was the first American to write a book on toxicology?

In 1868, Theodore George Wormley (1826–1897) published the *Micro-Chemistry of Poisons*, the first American book devoted entirely to toxicology. It contained many original techniques resulting from his own investigations. The series of plates on the crystalline structure of various poisons for identification purposes was a milestone in the development of toxicologic techniques.

12. Who is considered the Father of Toxicology?

Professor Matthieu Joseph Bonaventura Orfila is considered by most to be the Father of General Toxicology. He was the leading medicolegal expert of his time. Orfila was born in Minorca, Spain, studied in Valencia, Barcelona, and Paris, and was one of the founders of the Academie de Medecine. He held the chair of legal medicine at the Sorbonne in Paris, where he was a popular teacher who is remembered particularly for his writings on toxicology. Orfila played an important role in the LaFarge case in Paris by adopting the new Marsh test for arsenic (see question 10). In 1814, he published his two-volume work, *Traite des poisons*, which was the first work on general toxicology. In this work, he divided poisons into six classifications: corrosives, astringents, acrids, stupefying or narcotics, narcoticoacids, and septica or putreficants. An English translation of his pioneering work first appeared in Britain in 1816, and the first American-translated edition was published in 1817.

13. When were antidote and decontamination procedures first used?

Gastric lavage to treat poisoning was first proposed by two physicians, an American named Philip Physik (in 1805) and a Frenchman named Baron Guillaume Dupuytren. In 1813, another Frenchman, M. Bertrand, mixed 5 gm of arsenic trioxide with charcoal and ingested it publicly to prove the efficacy of adsorption of poisons. This exhibition was repeated in 1831 by the French pharmacist P. F. Touery, who swallowed ten lethal doses of strychnine mixed with charcoal and survived, much to the amazement of the French Academy of Medicine.

14. Where were the first poison centers established?

In 1949, specialized medical units devoted to poisoned patients were established in the cities of Copenhagen and Budapest. The first poison information service was begun in 1949 in the Netherlands.

15. When did the first poison centers appear in the United States?

The first pilot poison information center was begun in 1953 in Chicago. By 1957, there were seventeen operating poison centers in the United States; by 1962, 462 poison centers were in operation; and by 1978, the number had mushroomed to over 661. With the advent of the regional poison center movement in the 1970s and the certification of poison centers, the number of centers has decreased to 75–100 centers, with approximately 50 of them certified by the American Association of Poison Control Centers.

16. How have poisons been used in warfare?

During ancient times, poisons and biologicals were used during military campaigns. At the siege of Plataea (428 B.C.), one of the earliest recorded uses of chemicals in a military operation, the Spartans used gas as an offensive weapon against the Athenians. They burned wood saturated with pitch and sulfur under the walls of the city. They repeated this technique at the siege of Delium (423 B.C.) with even greater success. Around 360 B.C., the Greeks placed a suffocating, incendiary mixture of pitch, sulfur, town, and resinous wood chips into clay pots and threw them from the walls of besieged towns onto their attackers. At the siege of Caffa (1347), the Tartars spread bubonic plague by hurling their dead from catapults into the Genoese city. During the China War (1860), at the battle of North Taku Fort, the Chinese defenders threw pots filled with caustic soda (sodium hydroxide) on the British troops.

The beginning of chemical and biological warfare started in earnest during World War I (1914–1918) at the Battle of Ypres in Belgium (April 22, 1915), where the Germans released 6000 cylinders of chlorine gas in an attack. The use of this gas produced 5000 casualties in minutes. This event could be called the birthday of modern chemical warfare. At the Battle of Loos (September 1915), the British used chlorine gas on the Germans. Phosgene was first used on December 11, 1915, and mustard gas on July 12, 1917. An analysis of epidemiologic statistics after the Great War revealed that 120,000 tons of chemicals had been used, producing 1,250,000 casualties. The use of chemical agents produced 27% of the battle casualties in the U.S. Army. During World War II (1939–1945), the explosion of the American merchantman *SS John Harvey* (Bari, Italy, July 2, 1943) released 100 tons of mustard gas contained in 2000 M47A1 aerial bombs. The infamous Japanese research unit 731, located at Harbin, China, used biological weapons on the Chinese in Manchuria and also conducted experiments on prisoners of war.

17. When were the first clinical toxicologic organizations established?

The American Association of Poison Control Centers (AAPCC) was established in 1958. The American Academy of Clinical Toxicology (AACT) was established in 1968. The American Board of Medical Toxicology (ABMT) was established in 1974 to set standards for physician toxicologists. The American Board of Applied Toxicology (ABAT) was established to set standards for nonphysician toxicologists in 1985. The European Association of Poison Centers and Clinical Toxicologists (EAPCCT) was established in 1964.

18. How do I become a medical toxicologist?

Physicians are first residency trained in emergency medicine, occupational medicine, or pediatrics for 3 years. Then, future toxicologists take a 2-year fellowship in medical toxicology, where they learn about taking care of inpatients, hospitalized patients, poison center operations, and research methods. The official subspecialty of medical toxicology offered its first board examination in 1994.

19. What is the Toxicological History Society (THiS)?

Founded in 1990, THiS is an international group interested in preserving the history of poisons and the poisons of history. Their main activities include presenting and publishing research papers on historical events in toxicology and on toxicologic events in history; holding an annual meeting with the North American Congress of Clinical Toxicology; publishing the semiannual newsletter *Mithridata*; and maintaining the *Index Toxicologicum*, a bibliographical list of known toxicology books printed before 1960. Information on THiS can be obtained by writing to the society at 5757 Hall Street, SE, Grand Rapids, MI 49546-3845, USA.

20. Who wrote the first book dealing totally with the subject of poisons used as weapons for murder?

The book *Criminal Poisoning: Investigational Guide for Law Enforcement, Toxicologists, Forensic Scientists, and Attorneys*, published in 2000, is authored by toxicologist and author of this chapter John H. Trestrail III. It was designed as a manual to assist law enforcement personnel and toxicologists in dealing with the various forensic aspects of murder by poison.

BIBLIOGRAPHY

1. de Maleissye J: Histoire de poison [History of Poison]. Paris, Editions Francois Bourin, 1991.
2. Martinetz D, Lohs K: Poison: Sorcery and Science, Friend and Foe. Leipzig, Germany, Editions Leipzig, 1987.
3. Thompson CJS: Poison Mysteries in History, Romance, and Crime. Philadelphia, J.B. Lippincott, 1924.
4. Trestrail JH 3d: Criminal Poisoning: Investigational Guide for Law Enforcement, Toxicologists, Forensic Scientists, and Attorneys. Totowa, NJ, Humana Press, 2000.
5. Villenueve R: Le Poison et les empoisonneurs celebres [Poison and Famous Poisoners]. Paris, La Palatine, 1960.
6. Wax PM: History. In Goldfrank LR, Flomenbaum NE, Lewin NA, et al (eds): Goldfrank's Toxicologic Emergencies, 6th ed. Norwalk, CT, Appleton & Lange, 1998, pp 1–14.

2. GENERAL MANAGEMENT OF POISONINGS

Louis J. Ling, M.D.

1. What is the first priority in poisoned patients?

The airway, of course. As with other patients, supportive care to stabilize the airway breathing, and circulation (ABCs) is still the most important. This may entail intubation in comatose patients or those with other airway difficulties.

2. Is there any other special treatment for comatose patients?

After stabilizing the comatose patient, a "coma cocktail" should be considered. This includes naloxone, either dextrose or a rapid bedside glucose determination, and 100 mg of thiamine. Flumazenil is not a standard item in the coma cocktail but may be given to patients with a benzodiazepine overdose or with respiratory depression without risk for seizures. Tricyclic antidepressant overdose would be a contraindication for using flumazenil.

3. How do I make the diagnosis in poisoned patients?

History is still the most important factor. However, be aware that patients may not supply a completely accurate history because they may not be sure themselves. You should always consider chemicals and medications available to a patient. Having the actual bottles may decrease the chance for misidentification.

4. What do I look for on the physical examination?

The examination should concentrate on cardiovascular and central nervous system (CNS) signs, because the most dangerous effects will occur there. Efforts should be made to identify toxidromes, syndromes caused by a toxin, which may suggest specific toxins (see Chapter 3).

5. What type of intervention can I make for poisoned patients?

The majority of poisoned patients recover with good, careful, supportive care. Specific antidotes exist for a few toxins, and practitioners should be aware of these specific toxins (see Table), even though you may not recall the antidote name or specific dose.

TOXIN	ANTIDOTE
Acetaminophen	*N*-Acetylcysteine
Anticholinergics	Physostigmine
Arsenic and mercury	Dimercaprol, D-penicillamine
Benzodiazepines	Flumazenil
Beta-blockers	Glucagon
Black widow spider bite	*Latrodectus* antivenin
Botulism	*Botulinum* antitoxin
Brown recluse spider bite	*Loxosceles* antivenin
Calcium channel blockers	Calcium, glucagon
Chlorine gas	Sodium bicarbonate
Coral snake bite	Elapid antivenin
Cyanide	Amyl nitrite, sodium nitrite, thiosulfate
Digitalis glycosides	Digoxin-specific FAB
Ethylene glycol	Ethanol, fomepizole, pyridoxine
Heparin	Protamine
Hydrogen sulfide	Sodium nitrite
Hypoglycemic agents and insulin	Dextrose

(Table continued on next page.)

TOXIN	ANTIDOTE
Iron	Deferoxamine
Isoniazid, monomethylhydrazine	Pyridoxine
Lead	Calcium EDTA, dimercaprol, DMSA
Methanol	Ethanol, fomepizole, folate, leucovorin
Methemoglobin-forming agents	Methylene blue
Methotrexate	Folate, leucovorin
Opiates	Naloxone, nalmefene
Organophosphates and carbamates	Atropine, pralidoxime
Rattlesnake bite	*Crotalidae* antivenin
Scorpion sting (*Centruroides* spp.)	Antivenin
Serotonin syndrome	Cyproheptadine
Tricyclics	Sodium bicarbonate
Warfarin anticoagulants	Vitamin K

FAB = fragment, antigen-binding [of immunoglobulins]; EDTA = ethylenediamine tetraacetic acid; DMSA = dimercaptosuccinic acid

6. *Extra credit:* **What word do we use in toxicology that comes from the Greek words for "against" and "to give"?**

Antidote, from the Greek *anti-* + *didonai.*

7. Describe the best treatment for decreasing the absorption of poisons.

Activated charcoal is the best method for decreasing the amount of drug absorbed by the patient. Try to get a 10:1 ratio of activated charcoal to poison, on a weight basis, to maximize its effect. Typically, a dose of charcoal given 1 hour after ingestion can absorb about 50% of that poison.

8. How does activated charcoal work?

Activated charcoal has a large surface area: between 1000 and 2000 m^2 (the size of a tennis court) for every gram of activated charcoal. The charcoal particles have many pores and holes where chemical and drug molecules can get lost and are held in by weak van der Waal's forces (remember those?). This means that charcoal absorption is not permanent and that drugs and chemicals can certainly desorb from the charcoal at some later time.

9. What is the role of a cathartic?

The theory behind cathartics is that they will speed up transit time of the charcoal, allowing the charcoal to catch up with pills already in the bowel and also rid the body of the charcoal before desorption of the drug can take place. The cathartic has never been proven to be of benefit, but a single dose of a cathartic such as magnesium sulfate or sorbitol is unlikely to be harmful and may be of some benefit.

10. Does charcoal work for all poisons?

No. Although it works for many drugs and poisons, charcoal is not universal and does not bind (1) small ions such as lithium and potassium, (2) acids and alkalis, (3) metals such as iron and lead, or (4) hydrocarbons.

11. When do I get to "pump the stomach"?

Gastric lavage, or pumping the stomach, and other gastric emptying methods were very popular, but several studies have proven them to be of no clinical benefit. Although it is shown to remove up to about 40% of poisons and drugs an hour after ingestion, in general, it has not been demonstrated to alter the clinical course. In addition, gastric lavage is uncomfortable and exposes the patient to aspiration and other complications.

12. Is there any role for gastric lavage?

Lavage may be beneficial in patients who ingest a chemical or drug that is not effectively absorbed by charcoal, especially if it occurs very quickly after the overdose. Because small red rubber nasogastric (NG) tubes are too small to remove pills or pill fragments, a large-bore 36–40 French tube in adults should be used through the mouth when gastric lavage is done.

13. Is there any role for syrup of ipecac?

Vomiting after ingestion of syrup of ipecac usually occurs within 20–30 minutes, and this delay usually makes it ineffective for hospital treatment. It also delays administration of activated charcoal, which is the most effective treatment. Syrup of ipecac is still useful for home treatment with the advice of a poison control center because it can be administered almost immediately after the ingestion.

14. *Extra credit:* The untimely death from bulimia of what famous singer almost jeopardized the nonprescription sales of syrup of ipecac?

Karen Carpenter.

15. What is whole bowel irrigation in the treatment of acute poisonings?

Whole bowel irrigation uses polyethylene glycol (Golytely, Colyte) to flush the drug or chemical rapidly through the bowel. This has been most useful, again, with drugs that are not absorbed by activated charcoal, such as iron and lithium. It may also be useful in ridding the body of sustained-release preparations or when packets of street drugs such as cocaine or heroin have been ingested.

16. What is the dose for whole bowel irrigation?

In adults, whole bowel irrigation can be started at 2 L/hour and slowed down if the patient has bloating or vomiting. Five hours has been suggested empirically as an adequate length of treatment or until the bowel effluents are clear.

17. If one dose of charcoal is good, are multiple doses of charcoal better?

In some cases, yes. According to the theory called **gastrointestinal dialysis**, chemicals and drugs in the blood can be drawn into the gut where large amounts of activated charcoal serve as a sink for these drugs. It is important to remember that the majority of drugs and chemicals probably do not benefit from multiple doses of charcoal.

18. What are the most common potential toxins that people come in contact with?

The most common exposures are cleaning substances, analgesics, cosmetics, and personal products. These are most frequently accidental ingestions by children. Often, the small amount and nontoxic nature allow these patients to be treated at home with the advice of a poison center.

19. What are the most common causes of death in poisonings?

Consistently, analgesics, antidepressants, stimulants, and street drugs are the most common cause of deaths reported to poison centers across the country. Most deaths are in adults who are suicidal.

20. What about chemicals in the eyes?

Irrigation of the eyes is the universal treatment for all serious eye exposures. This should be done as soon as possible, even before medical treatment. Irrigation may be performed in a drinking fountain, in a shower, or by having the patient blink in a sink full of water. Many household chemicals are nontoxic, but the cornea should be examined for abrasions and burns.

21. Are acids or alkalis worse for the eyes?

Alkalis disrupt cell membranes, which allows penetration much deeper into the tissue whereas acids tend to coagulate the tissue and form eschar, which tends to block penetration. With irrigation, alkali injuries take longer to return to a neutral pH than acid injuries.

22. Describe the clinical signs of severe globe injury.

Erythema and swelling of the conjunctiva are common, but if the conjunctiva is burned and loses its vascular supply, it becomes difficult to heal. Corneal clouding and elevated intraocular pressure occur with more serious injuries.

23. What is the role of a regional poison center in caring for poisoned patients?

Poison centers throughout the country are available to help teach awareness of poison prevention and to answer calls from the public. Over 80% of the exposures reported to the poison center can be treated safely at home in an efficient and cost-effective manner. High-risk poisonings can be identified and referred for treatment to the most appropriate facility.

24. How can poison centers help me as a health care provider?

You should work with your poison center to have quick access to drug and treatment information, to help identify potential signs and symptoms for various poisons, and to assist you with the most optimal management and treatment. You should also notify poison centers, even if you already know how to manage the patient, so that they can accurately report the poisoning to the Toxic Exposure Surveillance System, a national database that tracks and reports on all human exposures in the country.

25. When should I refer poisoned patients?

Although most patients do well with general supportive care, some patients benefit from specialized centers that have dialysis, critical care, on-site toxicology laboratory, hyperbaric oxygen, liver transplant, and medical toxicology specialists.

BIBLIOGRAPHY

1. Cooney DO: Activated Charcoal in Medical Applications. New York, Marcel Dekker, 1995.
2. Ford M, Delaney KA: Initial approaches to the poison patient. In Ford M, Delaney KA, Ling L, Erickson T (eds): Clinical Toxicology. Philadelphia, Harcourt, 2000, pp 1–4.
3. Goldfrank LR, Flomenbaum NA, Lewin NA, et al: Principles of managing the poisoned or overdosed patient: An overview. In Goldfrank LR, Flomenbaum NA, Lewin NA, et al (eds): Goldfrank's Toxicologic Emergencies, 6th ed. Stamford, CT, Appleton & Lange, 1998, pp 31–34.
4. Hoffman RS, Goldfrank LR: The poisoned patient with unconsciousness: Controversies in the use of a coma cocktail. JAMA 274:562–569, 1995.
5. Litovitz TL, Kleinschwartz W, Caravati EM, et al: 1998 Annual report of the American Association of Poison Control Centers Toxic Exposure Surveillance System. Am J Emerg Med 17:435–480, 1999.

3. TOXIDROMES AND VITAL SIGNS

Adhi N. Sharma, M.D., John G. Benitez, M.D., M.P.H., Christofer Fore, M.D., and Linda G. Allison, M.D., M.P.H.

1. What is a toxidrome?
Toxidrome is a commonly used term that combines two Greek roots: *toxikon*, which means "bow" (arrows shot from bows often had poison tips), and *dromos*, "race course." Thus, toxidrome is the course that a poison runs, or in more modern terms, the syndrome caused by a specific toxin.

2. How are toxidromes helpful?
The history usually points to what a patient ingests, but when a reliable history is not available, the symptom complex may suggest the drug involved. Alternatively, a toxidrome can confirm or cast doubt on a suspicious history. When multiple drugs are involved, however, the manifestations of one drug may mask the other, preventing identification of an obvious syndrome or supplying a mixed picture.

3. Name the five most common toxidromes.
1. Anticholinergic
2. Sympathomimetic
3. Cholinergic
4. Opioid
5. Benzodiazepine

4. Describe the anticholinergic toxidrome.
Patients who are anticholinergic present with dry mucous membranes, flushed skin, urinary retention, decreased bowel sounds, altered mental status, dilated pupils, and cyclopegia (inability to accommodate for near vision). Most of these symptoms are described in the mnemonic **blind as a bat, hot as hades, red as a beet, dry as a bone, and mad as a hatter**. Agents that commonly cause this are antihistamines, tricyclic antidepressants, antipsychotic drugs, skeletal muscle relaxants, antiparkinson medications, amantadine, jimson weed, and *Amanita muscaria*. These drugs exert their affect by blocking muscarinic acetylcholine receptor sites.

5. "Coma with stable vital signs" is the hallmark of which toxidrome?
Classic **benzodiazepine** overdose. The level of consciousness of patients who overdose on oral benzodiazepines ranges from mildly sedate to unresponsive. However, in the absence of a mixed ingestion (e.g., ethanol), serious vital sign aberrations are rare, and patients will not require intubation or pressors. Intravenous benzodiazepine administration can result in transient hypotension and respiratory depression.

6. List the features of the sympathomimetic toxidrome.

Psychomotor agitation	Dilated pupils
Hypertension	Tremor
Tachycardia	Seizures (in severe cases)
Hyperpyrexia	Hypotension (in severe cases)
Agitation	Dysrhythmias (in severe cases)
Diaphoresis	

Agents that have pure alpha or beta activity will not produce all of the symptoms (e.g., reflex bradycardia may be present if the agent is a pure alpha-adrenergic agonist).

7. Name some common sympathomimetics.

- Cocaine
- Theophylline
- Amphetamines
- Caffeine
- Over-the-counter decongestants (e.g., phenylpropanolamine, ephedrine, pseudoephedrine).

8. What causes the sympathomimetic toxidrome?

Increased release of catecholamines (amphetamines)
Inhibition of reuptake (cocaine)
Interference with metabolism (monoamine oxidase inhibitors [MAOIs])
Direct stimulation at the receptor site (epinephrine)

9. How can the anticholinergic and sympathomimetic toxidromes be distinguished from one another?

Although both syndromes are very similar, anticholinergics tend to completely inhibit gastrointestinal motility and to cause dry skin. Diaphoresis, hyperactive bowel sounds, reactive pupils, and lack of urinary retention are subtle clues that suggest a sympathomimetic toxidrome. Frequently, symptoms do not indicate clearly one toxidrome or the other, and the differential diagnosis for both classes of drugs needs to be considered.

10. What is the cholinergic toxidrome?

This toxidrome is also known as the SLUDGE syndrome, an acronym for this toxidrome's symptoms: *s*ialorrhea (drooling), *l*acrimation, *u*rination, *d*iaphoresis, and *g*astric *e*mptying (diarrhea and vomiting). The more clinically relevant symptoms of seizures and bradycardia, bronchorrhea (pulmonary edema), and bronchospasm (BBB) are not included in this acronym. Cholinergic symptoms are caused by excess acetylcholine activity; however, the symptoms vary depending on whether stimulation is at a muscarinic, nicotinic, or central cholinergic receptor (see Table).

Cholinergic Symptoms

MUSCARINIC SYMPTOMS	NICOTINIC SYMPTOMS	CENTRAL SYMPTOMS
Miosis	Mydriasis	Agitation
Bradycardia	Tachycardia	Confusion
Bronchorrhea, bronchospasm	Bronchodilation	Lethargy
Vomiting, diarrhea	Hypertension	Coma
Sialorrhea, lacrimation	Diaphoresis	Seizure
Urinary incontinence	Weakness	Death

11. What are the main causes of the cholinergic toxidrome?

Organophosphates (pesticides such as malathion or diazinon), carbamates (physostigmine, carbaryl), and certain mushrooms (clitocybes, inocybes) can elicit any or all of the symptoms listed in the table in question 9. Agricultural workers are at the highest risk for exposure, but anyone using pesticides at home or at work may be exposed. Military and antiterrorist groups worry about nerve gases, including sarin. Physostigmine, neostigmine, and edrophonium are used in neuromuscular diseases, although overt cholinergic symptoms from these drugs are rare.

12. Which of the features of the cholinergic toxidrome cause the greatest harm?

Muscle weakness (can lead to respiratory arrest)
BBB
Intractable seizures

13. Describe the clinical presentation of the opioid toxidrome.

An opioid is a class of drug that is either a naturally occurring opiate (morphine) or a synthetic analogue (meperidine). These drugs bind to central opioid receptors and result in central nervous system (CNS) depression, pinpoint pupils (miosis), and respiratory depression. Peripheral effects include bradycardia, hypotension, and decreased gastrointestinal motility. Opioids are reversible with naloxone.

14. What class of nonopioid drug can mimic the opioid toxidrome?

The **imidazolines** (e.g., clonidine, tetrahydrozoline, oxymetazoline) can cause symptoms of somnolence, respiratory depression, bradycardia, and hypotension. The CNS effects usually can be reversed with naloxone.

15. What is the serotonin syndrome?

The serotonin syndrome, which is caused by excessive 5-hydroxytryptamine stimulation, comprises three symptoms:
1. **Altered mental status** (agitation, delirium, and coma)
2. **Autonomic dysfunction** (mydriasis, diaphoresis, hyperthermia, tachycardia, and fluctuating blood pressure)
3. **Abnormal neuromuscular activity** (tremor, rigidity, and seizures)

16. What are the main etiologies of the serotonin syndrome?

The trend to use selective serotonin reuptake inhibitors (SSRIs) instead of tricyclic antidepressants has led to an increased incidence of this syndrome, especially when SSRIs are taken with other medications with serotonin properties.

17. What is a "packidrome"?

Packidrome is an unofficial term that describes the mixed toxidromes apparent in patients with multi-ingredient drug ingestions. This is seen commonly with cold and flu preparations that contain antihistamines, analgesics, antipyretics, and decongestants in one package.

18. *Extra credit:* There are several less common toxidromes for specific drugs and medications. Ingestion of what particular acid may cause a dermal rash that has sometimes been called the "boiled lobster syndrome."

Boric acid.

19. *Extra credit:* The gray baby syndrome is the most serious form of toxicity from what drug?

Chloramphenicol.

20. List several toxidromic causes of hyperthermia.

A drug that results in one or more of these effects can raise a patient's core temperature to lethal levels:
- Agitation or seizures (sympathomimetics, phencyclidine [PCP], hallucinogens)
- Inability to sweat (anticholinergics)
- Uncoupling of oxidative phosphorylation (aspirin, dinitrophenol)
- Conditions that increase muscle tone (neuroleptic malignant syndrome, serotonin syndrome)

21. What are common toxidromic causes of hypothermia?
- Drugs that cause CNS depression (sedative-hypnotics, ethanol, opioids, imidazolines)
- Drugs that reduce total body glucose (insulin, oral hypoglycemics)

22. Drugs that cause hypertension often cause tachycardia. Name two drugs that raise blood pressure but cause bradycardia.

The alpha agonists **phenylpropanolamine** and **phenylephrine** can result in profound hypertension with a resultant reflex bradycardia.

22. What is a widened pulse pressure?

Pulse pressure = systolic blood pressure – diastolic blood pressure

Normal pulse pressure is $\cong$ 40 mmHg (120 – 80 = 40). Any pulse pressure > 50 mmHg is considered widened.

23. What drugs widen pulse pressure?

Beta agonists typically widen the pulse pressure. Beta stimulation of the heart results in tachycardia with an increase in cardiac output, thus raising the systolic pressure. However beta$_2$ stimulation results in vasodilatation and a drop in the diastolic blood pressure. The net effect is to widen the pulse pressure. Nonspecific beta agonists such as theophylline, caffeine, and albuterol can have this effect.

24. When can a normal pulse oximetry reading be misleading?

Pulse oximeters may show 100% oxygen saturation in the blood despite profound tissue hypoxia. Carbon monoxide (CO), cyanide (CN), and hydrogen sulfide (HS) affect oxygenation at several levels, including alteration of the hemoglobin molecule, impairing its ability to bind to oxygen and to dissociate with O_2 to deliver it to tissues. Additionally, these agents impair respiration at the cellular level; that is, they inhibit oxidative phosphorylation, resulting in tissue hypoxia.

25. What class of drugs can cause significant hypotension with normal mental status?

Significant hypotension results in impaired perfusion of the CNS with resultant change in mental status. However, **calcium channel blocker** overdose often results in significant hypotension with preservation of mental status.

26. Which toxins cause tachypnea?

- Agents that cause CNS stimulation can result in tachypnea.
- Aspirin induces tachypnea through an unclear central mechanism.
- Beta agonists can directly increase respiratory rate.
- Agents that cause hypoxia (e.g., CO, CN, HS, methane, CO_2) or pulmonary edema (e.g., chlorine gas, aspirin, organophosphates) can increase respiratory rate as a response to hypoxia.
- Agents that cause a metabolic acidosis (e.g., ethylene glycol, methanol, metformin) can result in hyperventilation as a compensatory mechanism.

BIBLIOGRAPHY

1. Barker SJ, Tremper KK, Hyatt J: Effects of methemoglobinemia on pulse oximetry and mixed venous oximetry. Anesthesiology 70:112–117, 1989.
2. Bravo EL: Phenylpropanolamine and other over-the-counter vasoactive compounds. Hypertension 11(Suppl II):II.7-II.10, 1988.
3. Ellenhorn MJ: The clinical approach. In Ellenhorn MJ (ed): Ellenhorn's Medical Toxicology: Diagnosis and Treatment of Human Poisoning, 2nd ed. Baltimore, Williams & Wilkins, 1997, pp 3–46.
4. Fredriksen A: Systemic reaction to subarachnoid injection of phenylephrine. Br J Anaesth 54:1337–1338, 1982.
5. Kulig K: General management principals. In Rosen P, Barkin R (eds): Emergency Medicine: Concepts and Clinical Practice, 4th ed. Philadelphia, Mosby, 1998, pp 1244–1250.
6. Kulig K: Initial management of ingestions of toxic substances. N Engl J Med 326:1678–1682, 1992.
7. Martin TG: Serotonin syndrome. Ann Emerg Med 28:520–526, 1996.
8. Olson KR: Comprehensive evaluation and treatment of poisoning and overdose. In Olson KR (ed): Poisoning and Drug Overdose. East Norwalk, CT, Appleton & Lange, 1994, pp 2–58.

4. LABORATORY PRINCIPLES

Bernard H. Eisenga, Ph.D., M.D.

1. Of what benefit is the toxicology laboratory?

The toxicology laboratory analyzes biological specimens for the presence of drugs. Often, the toxicology laboratory can do substance analysis as well. Most laboratories are capable of both qualitative and quantitative analysis. These functions may be essential for the optimal management of the poisoned patient.

2. Which drugs require quantitative analysis for optimal patient management?

Although the old adage "treat the patient, not the poison" is sound, a number of drugs require quantitative analysis for optimal patient care:

Analgesics (acetaminophen, aspirin)
Alcohols (ethylene glycol, methanol, ethanol)
Theophylline
Iron and other metal poisons
Lithium
Carboxyhemoglobin
Digoxin

3. What techniques are used for drug analysis?

Routine quantitative measurement of drugs is accomplished by enzymatic, spectrophotometric, and chromatographic techniques. The most common immunoassays are enzyme-multiplied and fluorescence polarization. Spectrophotometric analysis is accomplished by measuring color change or color development. Chromatographic techniques include high-performance liquid chromatography, gas chromatography, gas chromatography and mass spectrometry, and thin-layer chromatography.

4. Define sensitivity and specificity.

Sensitivity is the ability of the assay to measure the quantity of drug present in the sample. Specificity is the ability of the assay to identify the presence of drug.

5. What are the advantages and disadvantages of techniques used for drug analysis?

The three major variables used to assess these techniques are the speed of sample turnover, the sensitivity of the assay, and the specificity of the assay. **Spectrophotometric** analysis by colorimetric means is simple and rapid but lacks both sensitivity and specificity. Often, compounds interfere with colorimetric analysis, and the measurement of color change in samples that have extremely low concentrations of drug is neither practical nor reliable.

Immunoassays are extremely rapid and generally quite sensitive but often lack the specificity of chromatographic techniques. Cross-reactivity of opiate, phencyclidine, and amphetamine antibodies with other common drugs has been reported.

Both liquid and gas **chromatographic** techniques are extremely sensitive and specific. Unfortunately, these techniques have a slow processing time. To analyze a specimen using one of the chromatographic techniques, the sample must be prepared and the drug extracted. This step, together with the direct analysis, delays the results.

6. How do liquid and gas chromatography work?

Both techniques require expensive instruments and well-trained technicians for operation. The instruments used for each of these techniques consist of an injector port, a column, and a detector. After preparation and concentration of the sample, a known volume is injected onto the column. For gas chromatography, the sample is vaporized at the injector and is eluded from the column by an inert gas, usually nitrogen. The drug moves down the column based on its affinity for the column under the given conditions. This permits separation from other drugs in the sample. Liquid chromatography differs in that it requires high-pressure pumps to push a solvent through the column. Again, the drug is separated from other compounds based on the specific conditions of the column and solvent. Detection of the drug occurs as it elutes from the column at the detector. Identification is made by comparing the retention time of the sample drug to retention times of known drugs.

7. What is involved in mass spectrophotometry?

Mass spectrophotometry uses either liquid or gas chromatography (most commonly) for drug separation. Once the drug is separated from other drugs, it is "hit" with an electrical charge in the detector. This charge fractures the drug into smaller fractions called **mass spectra**. The spectra are detected and identified by comparing them to known drug spectral data. Mass spectrophotometry provides the chemical "fingerprint" of the drug and excludes all other drugs and compounds.

8. How does thin-layer chromatography provide drug analysis?

Thin-layer chromatography is a simple but time-consuming technique for drug separation. This technique also can be used for drug identification by color reactions. The sample is plated and dried in a specific column of a multichanneled silica plate. The other channels contain standards of known drugs. The plate is placed in a solvent solution and the drug elutes up the plate. After sufficient elution, the plate is dried, sprayed with chemicals, and placed under ultraviolet light. Analysis is made by comparing the sample to the standards, and a tentative identification is made.

9. When is a toxicology screen indicated?

As with other laboratory data, the drug screen aids in the diagnosis, although history and clinical findings remain the mainstay of medical diagnosis. Coma or acute delirium, anion gap metabolic acidosis, active seizures, and hypoventilation are conditions in which a comprehensive toxicology screen may be beneficial. The clinician must use good judgment in ordering a toxicology screen because the tests are expensive and time consuming.

10. What drugs are not routinely detected on toxicology screens?

The answer to this question will depend on the laboratory service that you are using for the toxicology testing. Many toxicology services offer comprehensive testing, but there are some common drugs and toxins that are not routinely identified. Drugs or compounds with high polarity (highly water soluble) such as antibiotics, diuretics, ethylene glycol, and lithium and those with high volatility such as hydrocarbons or nitrous oxide require special assays for analysis. These compounds elute from the gas chromatography column as such a rapid rate that they are lost in the solvent phase. Other compounds such as steroids, digoxin, colchicine, and other plant derivatives are either too non-polar or non-volatile for routine analysis by gas chromatography.

Toxic anions such as thiocyanate, cyanide, fluoride, and bromine are not seen on routine drug screens. Drugs or compounds that exist in low concentrations in the plasma or urine owing to high potency or large volumes of distribution may be difficult to find on routine drug screens. These include gamma hydroxybutyrate (GHB), LSD, colchicine, ergot alkaloids, and nitraflurazepam (Rohypnol). Other drugs and compounds not routinely detected include theophylline, vitamins, pesticides, radioactive compounds, iron, and other metals. It is imperative that the physician communicate with the toxicology laboratory when there are questions about certain drugs. It is also often helpful to include a list of suspected toxins with any drug screen to provide the technician some indication of the potential compounds.

11. How long can a toxicology screen detect drugs after a person stops using the drug?

The answer to this question depends on a number of variables and usually depends on the drug in question. The amount of drug ingested, the chronicity of drug use, the lipid solubility of the drug, and volume of distribution of the drug are important factors in metabolic clearance.

In an acute overdose, toxic amounts of most drugs will prolong the drug half-life and drug clearance owing to saturation kinetics.

Drugs with high lipid solubility will accumulate in adipose tissue. Even after discontinuation of the drug, amounts may be leached into the circulation for a number of days and thus may be seen on a drug screen. This is the case for marijuana; tetrahydrocannabinol (THC) may be seen for a number of weeks after discontinuation of the drug in heavy users who have chronically abused the substance. Measurement of the urinary clearance of THC relative to creatinine clearance may help to identify acute exposure.

Other drugs such as the rapid-acting barbiturates, which have a high volume of distribution and high degree of lipid solubility, also may be found on a drug screen many days after discontinuation of the drug.

12. If a patient has a positive drug screen but denies using the drug, should I believe him?

This is a problem encountered by many physicians, the answer to which may be extremely complicated. Many drug rehabilitation programs require constant monitoring to ensure patient compliance. Issues related to employment or continued employment may also be dependent on the results of drug testing.

Drugs such as marijuana (THC) are highly lipid soluble and possess high volumes of distribution. There may be continued leaching of the drug from the adipose store over a period of many weeks after cessation of drug use. This makes it difficult to determine an acute exposure. Some experimental evidence suggests that comparison of the urinary excretion of THC to creatinine provides a means of assessing an acute exposure. This is based on the belief that urinary creatinine clearance is relatively stable over time. The effect of oral creatine supplementation or other compounds on the urinary clearance of creatinine has not yet been determined.

Also casual exposure via inhalation may in fact be enough to cause positive findings for many of the illicit compounds such as cocaine and marijuana. Testing laboratories have attempted to limit the problem of casual exposure by setting higher cut-off limits for these compounds.

Drug cross reactivity also may occur, and this is a problem that may be seen with certain immunoassays. General screening tests are usually enzyme-mediated immunoassays. This technique is extremely sensitive and generally specific, yet a number of compounds can cause false-positive results. Over-the-counter cold preparations containing dextromethorphan, phenylephrine, and pseudoephedrine have been known to cross react with the opiate, amphetamine, and phencyclidine antibody immunoassays. If there are questions, contact the specific laboratory to determine how the testing was performed and possible causes for false-positive results.

13. Are ethanol levels helpful?

Most states will not permit an individual with a blood ethanol that is 100 mg/dL to drive. Releasing a patient with an ethanol level that is within this range places the physician at great liability, especially if the patient is hurt or becomes involved in an accident after release. Clinical assessment often does not reveal the extent of intoxication and is often fraught with error. Also, do not assume that ethanol is the only depressant involved.

14. How reliable are breathalyzers?

The breathalyzer uses an infra-red source to measure breath ethanol concentration. In theory at equilibrium, ethanol, a volatile substance, exerts a vapor pressure in the alveolus gas proportional to its concentration in the alveolar capillary blood. This blood-to-breath ratio has been estimated to be 2280 and is generally rounded off to 2300. An important fact is that equilibrium is not reached after oral intake of ethanol but becomes fairly constant in the postabsorptive or elimination phase. Experimentally observed ranges for the blood-to-breath ratio has been determined to be 1700–3100. Obviously, this wide range of ratios can cast doubt on the accuracy of the breathalyzer for any given individual.

Generally, if the instrument is well maintained and the test performed by trained personnel, the results are usually reasonably accurate and admissible in court. Yet, there is some evidence that the intrabreath variability range may be high. Also experimentally, the relationship between breath and blood ethanol measurements has been shown to be variable. Furthermore, the presence of ethanol in the mouth may falsely elevate the breathalyzer measurement. Measurements must be performed in the postabsorptive state (hence the delay of 20–30 minutes after stopping the individual), because the ratio of alveolar air ethanol concentrations to venous blood ethanol concentrations is not constant in the preabsorptive phase.

15. What is an osmolar gap?

Measurable ions and glucose contribute to the tonicity of the serum. Other substances, particularly the alcohols, will also contribute to the osmolarity of the serum when ingested. When an unmeasured solute is present in the serum, there will be a gap between the measured osmoles and the calculated osmoles. This difference is called the osmolar gap. To determine the calculated osmolarity of the serum the following formula is used:

$$(2 \times Na) + (BUN/2.8) + glucose/18$$

This value is subtracted from the measured osmolarity to determine the osmolar gap. The normal gap is less than 10, and the contribution from each individual alcohol can be determined mathematically once the individual alcohol has been measured. Similarly, one may calculate the approximate blood level for a specific alcohol by using the molecular weight of the alcohol.

16. Does a normal osmolar gap rule out anything?

There are generally two accepted methods for measuring osmolar gaps: vaporization and freezing point depression. You must know which method is used by your laboratory. Determining an osmolar gap using the vaporization technique will underestimate the presence of an unmeasured solute and should not be used. Errors have been made, and patients have suffered. Also, there have been case reports of intoxication with ethylene glycol and methanol, even when there was no measured osmolar gap by freezing point depression (the acceptable method). A normal osmolar gap does not rule out intoxication with ethylene glycol or methanol, particularly in a patient with an anion gap acidosis.

17. Can a patient get a positive cocaine test if his roommate smokes a lot of crack?

Yes, although it is not likely. The enzyme immunoassays are extremely sensitive to the presence of cocaine metabolites, and a positive test can result in a person who is exposed to large amounts of second hand smoke. In fact, there have been reports of positive test results in bank tellers who have handled a large number of one hundred dollar bills during normal work conditions. Laboratories have raised the cut-off values for positive results to limit this problem, but it still does occur.

BIBLIOGRAPHY

1. Ellenhorn MJ, Schonwald S, Ordog G, et al (eds): Ellenhorn's Medical Toxicology: Diagnosis and Treatment of Human Poisoning, 2nd ed. Baltimore, Williams & Wilkins, 1996.
2. Goldfrank LR, Flomenbaum NE, Lewin NA, et al (eds): Goldfrank's Toxicologic Emergencies, 6th ed. Stamford, CT, Appleton & Lange, 1998.
3. Hardman JG, Limbird LE, Molinoff PB, et al (eds): Goodman and Gilman's The Pharmacological Basis of Therapeutics, 9th ed. New York, McGraw-Hill, 1996.

5. PHARMACOKINETIC PRINCIPLES

Bernard H. Eisenga, Ph.D., M.D.

1. What is drug pharmacokinetics?

Pharmacokinetics is the study of the mechanisms involved in drug accumulation and elimination by body tissues. These mechanisms are dynamic and include drug absorption, distribution, metabolism, and excretion. Rate constants for these processes are determined experimentally. These rate constants are used to estimate peak blood levels, drug half-lives, and other useful parameters to help predict the actions of the drug.

2. What is drug absorption?

Absorption is the process of a drug being taken into the circulation for distribution to other body tissues. To gain access to the circulation, the drug must cross cell membranes. Sometimes, active processes facilitate drug absorption, but most often drug absorption is a passive process that occurs down a concentration gradient—from areas of higher drug concentration to areas of lower drug concentration. Drug absorption may be affected by a number of conditions including site of administration, disease process, concomitant drugs, foods, and pH.

3. Does drug absorption occur just in the gastrointestinal tract?

No. Drugs are administered a number of ways: transcutaneously, intradermally, subcutaneously, intravenously, orally, sublingually, and inhalationally. Although each route has advantages and disadvantages, intravenous drug administration provides complete and instantaneous drug absorption, whereas the other sites allow incomplete and delayed drug absorption.

4. How does drug absorption change patient management after an overdose?

Drugs such as aspirin, digoxin, and iron are notoriously slow absorbers. Repeat drug levels are necessary to ensure that patients do not continue absorbing the drug and develop unanticipated, delayed symptoms.

5. What is drug bioavailability?

The fraction of drug that is completely absorbed is termed the bioavailability of the drug. This measure is important since only drugs that are administered intravenously are completely absorbed. Many factors increase or decrease the portion of drug that is absorbed including disease states, coadministration of other drugs, and certain foods.

6. Does drug bioavailability matter to the poisoned patient?

One of the important treatments in toxicology is preventing absorption of the poison. Toxin removal prevents toxicity, but methods such as gastric lavage and syrup of ipecac have limited utility. Activated charcoal, on the other hand, has a high affinity for a number of substances and limits the bioavailability of the compound. Activated charcoal is inert and possesses no known toxicity, but it may cause serious consequences if aspirated. The surface area of activated charcoal is large, and, after administering activated charcoal, toxins become "coated" and adsorbed. This process prevents the toxin from being absorbed and helps to limit toxicity. Activated charcoal should be given early after oral exposure and repeated for drugs that have an extended enterohepatic circulation. Administration of activated charcoal before and after gastric lavage is recommended.

7. What is drug distribution?

The process of drug movement through the body is termed drug distribution. Drug movement may be affected by many factors. Drugs that are highly bound to plasma proteins are restricted from movement from the plasma. Other factors involved in drug distribution include lipid solubility of the drug and degree of drug ionization. Drugs that are highly lipid soluble have a high distribution, whereas drugs with low lipid solubility have a low distribution. In order to pass the lipid bilayer membrane of a cell, the drug must be nonionized. Ionized drug is restricted to the compartment in which it resides.

8. What is the volume of distribution of a drug?

The volume of distribution is a hypothetical value of the amount of body fluid required for complete dissolution of a known amount of drug to achieve a specific blood concentration. These volumes of distribution are determined experimentally and are based on drug dosage, drug bioavailability, and measured blood drug concentrations. Many factors affect the volume of distribution including disease states, blood flow rates, lipid solubility of the drug, tissue type, plasma protein binding, and pH.

9. How does the volume of distribution affect the poisoned patient?

Although the volume of distribution is determined experimentally, it provides an indication of the persistence of the drug in a patient. Drugs with high volumes of distribution and values > 1 L/kg are widely distributed in the patient. This means that only a small portion of the drug is present in the plasma. Under these circumstances, only a small amount would be removed by hemodialysis. Amitriptyline, for example, has a volume of distribution of over 8 L/kg under therapeutic conditions. Practically, for a 60-kg person, less than 1% of the total dose would be accessible for hemodialysis, and hemodialysis would not remove enough to have much impact on the toxicity. Aspirin, on the other hand, has a volume of distribution of 0.2 L/kg under therapeutic conditions (a value 40 times smaller than amitriptyline). In this scenario, more than 40% of a given dose is present in the plasma and is, therefore, readily accessible for removal by hemodialysis.

10. What is the Henderson-Hasselbach equation?

Drugs may exist as highly charged ions, uncharged molecules (steroids and large sugars), or partially charged molecules. Most drugs act as either acids or bases. The pK_a of the drug determines whether the drug is an acid or a base. Drugs with low pK_as act as strong acids, whereas drugs with high pK_as act as bases in solution. The Henderson-Hasselbach equation determines the degree of ionization (charge) of a drug at a given pH and known drug pK_a. Because only nonionized drug can cross cell membranes, the percentages of ionized and nonionized drug at a given pH can be calculated using the Henderson-Hasselbach equation.

11. What impact does the Henderson-Hasselbach equation have on the poisoned patient?

The classic example of the use of the Henderson-Hasselbach equation in toxicology is the patient poisoned with aspirin. Aspirin toxicity is manifested by an early respiratory alkalosis followed by a profound anion gap metabolic acidosis. The metabolic acidosis is caused by a number of factors including uncoupling of oxidative phosphorylation, production of ketoacids by the liver, utilization of amino acids, and the direct effect of the drug itself. Aspirin has a low pK_a and acts as a strong organic acid.

Early in aspirin toxicity, the patient attempts to buffer the effect of the salicylate in the serum by generating bicarbonate through the elimination of acid as carbon dioxide through the lungs. The patient breathes more deeply and rapidly. As the toxicity continues, the patient becomes less able to maintain this breathing pattern and becomes physically exhausted. No longer able to generate sufficient quantities of bicarbonate to buffer the strong organic acids, more of the salicylate exists in the nonionized form. In this form, it is able to cross cell membranes and exert a more toxic effect on cells. In effect, the aspirin has increased its own volume of distribution and permitted distribution to more tissues with higher amounts of toxic salicylate. Because of this effect, patients die from aspirin toxicity at levels that are generally considered only moderately toxic.

To prevent serious aspirin toxicity, removal of the toxic salicylate ion is imperative. This is accomplished by alkalization of the urine through sodium bicarbonate administration or by hemodialysis. Because aspirin is a strong acid with a low pK_a, the addition of bicarbonate causes the salicylate to be ionized and thus trapped in the renal tubules and eliminated in the urine.

12. Where does drug metabolism occur?

The principal organ of metabolism is the liver, although other organ sites also participate in drug metabolism. Both the kidneys and the intestine have high metabolic rates. The purpose of metabolism is: (1) to terminate the effect of the drug, (2) to make the drug more polar, and (3) to eliminate the drug from the body. Drug administered orally is absorbed from the intestine into the venous portal circulation. This circulation perfuses through the liver and eventually into the heart and remainder of the body. Drug can be metabolized by intestinal tissue or by the liver prior to delivery to the remainder of the body. Metabolism prior to delivery to the general circulation is called **first-pass metabolism**. Some drugs such as propranolol and diphenhydramine have a high first-pass metabolism. Although metabolism generally helps to terminate the drug effect, occasionally metabolism initiates the drug effect or produces a toxic metabolite. An example of the formation of a toxic metabolite is the toxic consequences of an acetaminophen overdose.

13. What happens during drug metabolism?

Drugs are made more polar so that they may be eliminated through the kidneys or the gastrointestinal tract. Polarity is achieved by conjugating the drug with sugar residues, acetic acid (acetylation), inorganic ions such as sulfate, or oxidation. Conjugation reactions are called **phase-two reactions**. Another means of making the drug more polar is the addition of oxygen; this is a **phase-one reaction**. Phase-one reactions involve iron-containing enzymes called monooxygenases or cytochrome P450 and require the reducing agent reduced nicotinamide adenine dinucleotide phosphate (NADPH) to function. There are at least ten families of cytochrome P450s. The addition of molecular oxygen creates a reactive by-product that may then be conjugated in a phase-two reaction. Regardless of the reaction, these processes produce a more polar drug. Polarity is important because it makes the drug metabolite more water soluble and thus easily eliminated by the intestine or kidney.

14. Does everyone metabolize drugs the same?

There appears to be a genetic predisposition to certain drug metabolizing capabilities. Alternations in the type and amount of certain hepatic monooxygenases have been identified, and there appears to be a genetic variant of the ability to acetylate drugs. Drug metabolism varies with the age of the individual. The neonate has a low ability to metabolize drugs evident for both conjugation and oxygenation reactions. Generally, the elderly have decreased ability to metabolize drugs and may suffer from drug toxicity. Poor nutrition and liver disease also may affect metabolic capability.

15. What clinical impact does this have?

One of the families of P450 that has recently received much attention is 3A4. This complex is involved in the metabolism of a number of drugs. Prescribing a combination of drugs that use this system, most notably erythromycin, ketoconazole, terfenadine, and cisapride, has been shown to cause widened QTc and episodes of fatal torsades de pointes. This finding has led to the removal of terfenadine (Seldane) and cisapride (Propulsid) from the market. Other drugs use this oxidation system, and caution should be used when prescribing two drugs that are each principally metabolized by cytochrome P450 3A4.

For some drugs (toxins), there is no known method for enhancing elimination. The toxic effect ends when the compound is cleared metabolically. In these instances, patient care should be supportive until metabolism has occurred.

16. Describe drug elimination.

Intestinal elimination involves biliary secretion of the drug metabolite into the gut. Some of the metabolite may be reabsorbed in transit through the gut or eliminated in the feces. Generally, this route of elimination is small, but for some drugs there is a high degree of biliary secretion. In this enterohepatic circulation, some of these metabolites may be active, and enhancement of decontamination may be achieved by the use of multiple doses of activated charcoal, which impedes reabsorption. For drugs such as theophylline, hemodialysis may be required in addition to repeated doses of activated charcoal to maximize drug removal.

Through urine, the kidneys provide the major route of elimination. Urinary excretion of some drugs can be enhanced by varying the pH of the urine, as is the case with salicylate. Hemodialysis, which acts as an artificial kidney, also is effective at enhancing the clearance of certain drugs. Some drugs are eliminated through the lungs exclusively (nitrous oxide) or through sweat, saliva, and tears. Drug elimination through these routes is negligible compared with the other routes of elimination.

17. What is drug clearance?

Clearance, a measure of the ability to eliminate a drug, is the sum total of drug removed through renal, hepatic, and other routes. Clearance is useful in determining dosing rates at steady-state drug concentrations and in determining the single dose of a drug.

18. What is drug half-life?

The half-life of a drug is the time it takes for the drug concentration to decrease by 50%. If it takes 4 hours for an acetaminophen level to drop from 200 µg/ml to 100 µg/ml, then the half-life is 4 hours. The half-life can be used to calculate disappearance of a drug, because it requires 4 half-lives to eliminate about 94% of a drug. Using the above acetaminophen example, it would take 16 hours to eliminate about 94% of the ingested acetaminophen dose. Half-life is determined by the amount of drug ingested and the mechanism of clearance. In a toxic situation, many drugs exhibit zero-order kinetics because of saturated clearance sites that result in prolonged half-life. Under these circumstances, the toxic effect usually is also prolonged.

19. Explain zero-order kinetics.

In most toxic situations, the drug elimination process reaches a saturation point and only a fixed amount of drug can be removed from the system. **Zero-order kinetics** refers to the situation when, regardless of the drug concentration, only a fixed amount will be removed. Typically, if an enzyme is saturated and the drug is already metabolized at the maximum rate, any increase in the drug causes the drug to build up. This build-up is the cause of most drug toxicity.

20. What is first-order kinetics?

Generally, drug clearance is constant over a wide range of drug blood concentrations, and the rate of elimination is proportional to the drug concentration. **First-order kinetics** occurs when an increase of drug in the system causes an increase in drug elimination.

21. What is Michaelis-Menton kinetics?

Michaelis-Menton kinetics is a hybrid of zero-order kinetics and first-order kinetics whereby the linear or first-order kinetics occurs at low drug concentrations, and zero-order kinetics occurs at higher drug concentrations. Drugs that exhibit Michaelis-Menton kinetics include phenytoin, aspirin, and ethyl alcohol. These are all linear at low concentrations, but occasionally small dosage changes may result in toxicity secondary to a large overshoot in drug concentration from zero-order, saturation kinetics.

22. *Extra credit:* After how many half-lives is a substance essentially 99% eliminated from the body?

Seven.

BIBLIOGRAPHY

1. Evans WE, Schentag JJ, Jusko WJ (eds): Applied Pharmacokinetics: Principles of Therapeutic Drug Monitoring, 2nd ed. Vancouver, WA, Applied Therapeutics, 1986.

2. Ferner RE: Forensic Pharmacology: Medicine, Mayhem, and Malpractice. New York, Oxford University Press, 1996.
3. Howland MA: Pharmacokinetics and toxicokinetics. In Goldfrank LR, Flomenbaum NE, Lewin NA, et al (eds): Goldfrank's Toxicologic Emergencies, 6th ed. Stamford, CT, Appleton & Lange, 1998, pp 173–194.
4. Platt D: Pharmacokinetics of drug overdose. Clin Lab Med 10:261–269, 1990.
5. Ritschel WA, Kearns GL: Handbook of Basic Pharmacokinetics. Washington, DC, American Pharmaceutical Association, 1999.
6. Watson WA, Rose SR: Pharmacokinetics and toxicokinetics. In Ford MD, Delaney KA, Ling L, Erickson T (eds): Clinical Toxicology. Philadelphia, W.B. Saunders, 2000, pp 73–78.

II. Over-the-Counter Drugs

6. ACETAMINOPHEN

Susan E. Farrell, M.D.

1. Why is it important to know about acetaminophen toxicity?

Acetaminophen is contained in more than 100 over-the-counter drug preparations and, as such, is routinely reported by the American Association of Poison Control Centers Toxic Exposure Surveillance System as the most common pharmaceutical agent involved in overdose. Fulminant hepatic failure due to acetaminophen overdose is the number one cause of liver failure requiring transplantation in the United Kingdom and the second most common cause of liver failure requiring transplantation in the United States.

2. *Extra credit:* We call it acetaminophen in the United States, but what is it called in Europe?

Paracetamol, derived from *para*-aminophenol. It is commonly abbreviated APAP.

3. How does acetaminophen cause toxicity?

Under normal metabolic conditions and recommended acetaminophen doses, 90–93% of acetaminophen is conjugated in the liver to glucuronide and sulfate conjugates, which are eliminated in the urine. About 2% of acetaminophen is eliminated unchanged by the kidneys and 5% of acetaminophen is metabolized oxidatively by the cytochrome P450 mixed-function oxidase system in the liver, specifically by cyp2E1 and cyp1A2 enzymes. This route of metabolism creates a reactive intermediate, *N*-acetyl-*para*-benzoquinoneimine (NAPQI), which is rapidly bound to glutathione and detoxified. When glutathione levels fall to less than 30% of normal, NAPQI is free to bind to hepatocyte membranes and cause cell death and liver necrosis.

4. What happens in an acetaminophen overdose?

If too much acetaminophen is around, the conjugation and sulfation metabolic routes are saturated. This means more of the parent acetaminophen compound is metabolized by the P450 system, which forms more of the toxic metabolite NAPQI.

5. What dose of acetaminophen causes toxicity?

The recommended therapeutic dose of acetaminophen over a 24-hour period is 4 gm in adults and 90 mg/kg in children. A dose of 150 mg/kg or 7.5 gm in adults can cause toxicity (see exceptions in question 20).

6. How long after an overdose ingestion does toxicity from acetaminophen occur?

In general, there is a delay of approximately 24 hours to the onset of clinical symptoms of hepatotoxicity. A subclinical rise in transaminases occurs as early as 12 hours postingestion. This phase is followed by the development of right upper quadrant pain and tenderness, nausea, vomiting, and jaundice and, in severe cases, can progress to fulminant hepatic failure with coagulopathy and encephalopathy with cerebral edema and death.

7. What is the time course of acetaminophen toxicity?

Four Phases of Acetaminophen Toxicity

PHASE	TIME	CHARACTERISTICS
Phase 1	Up to about 24 hours	Patient has anorexia, nausea, or vomiting; transaminases are rising
Phase 2	24–72 hours	Right upper quadrant pain develops; trans-aminases are peaking; bilirubin and prothrombin time (PT) are elevated
Phase 3	72–96 hours	Hepatic necrosis is characterized by jaundice, coagulopathy, encephalopathy, acute renal failure, and death
Phase 4	96 hours–14 days	Resolution of liver dysfunction and healing of the pathologic liver damage

8. When do laboratory abnormalities suggestive of toxicity become evident?

Transaminases peak at about 72 hours postingestion. Hepatic dysfunction with coagulopathy indicated by prolonged prothrombin time (PT) occurs at this time also. Resolution occurs over several days to 2 weeks after ingestion.

9. How do you decide if your patient is at risk for hepatotoxicity?

The Rumack-Matthew nomogram was developed in 1975 and is based on clinical data collected by Prescott in the United Kingdom in 1971 (see Figure, next page). Patients with a single acetaminophen overdose at a known time were grouped based on their measured acetaminophen level and the development of hepatotoxicity. A nomogram was created that predicts the risk of subsequent toxicity in patients who have an acetaminophen level drawn 4 or more hours postingestion. This nomogram assumes that acetaminophen absorption is complete by 4 hours and that elimination occurs with a half-life of 4 hours. The original nomogram consists of a line drawn from the serum level of 300 mg/L at 4 hours to 45 mg/L at 15 hours, above which the patient is considered at definite risk of hepatotoxicity. A line drawn from the serum level of 200 mg/L at 4 hours to 15 mg/L at 15 hours is predictive of probable risk. The authors added a "conservative" line drawn from the level of 150 mg/L at 4 hours to 12 mg/L at 15 hours to define possible risk to account for outlined inaccuracy in data and time reporting. By comparing a patient's serum acetaminophen level drawn at least 4 hours postingestion to the nomogram, the patient's risk of toxicity can be estimated. In the United States, the current practice is to treat all patients who have acetaminophen levels above the "possible risk" line.

10. *Extra credit:* In October 1982, there was a national panic when seven people died in Chicago from cyanide-laced acetaminophen capsules. Who was eventually found to be responsible for this tampering incident?

The perpetrator was never found.

11. Is there an antidote for patients with potential acetaminophen hepatotoxicity?

Yes. The antidote is *N*-acetylcysteine (Mucomyst), but most toxicologists just call it NAC.

12. How does NAC work?

NAC is hypothesized to work in several ways. It acts as a precursor to cysteine, and then to glutathione. By repleting glutathione stores, it provides sulfhydryl donors to which NAPQI can bind and be detoxified. It may also enhance the innate sulfation of any remaining acetaminophen and, therefore, reduce the amount of NAPQI that is produced. It has also been shown to improve survival in patients with fulminant hepatic failure presumably by acting as a free radical scavenger, by enhancing oxygen uptake and utilization in peripheral tissues, including the brain, and by improving microcirculation.

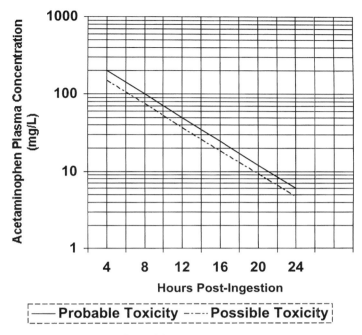

Rumack-Matthew nomogram.

13. When should NAC be administered?

When NAC is administered anytime within 8 hours of ingestion, it is nearly 100% protective against hepatotoxicity. Therefore, NAC should be given whenever a potentially toxic acetaminophen level is measured above the line on the nomogram. However, if a patient presents close to 8 hours postingestion, and a level will not be available before the 8-hour time occurs, the loading dose of NAC should be administered immediately while serum measurements are taking place. The efficacy of NAC decreases after 8 hours, so, if a patient presents more than 8 hours postingestion, NAC should be administered as soon as the history of ingestion is obtained. Delay in NAC treatment correlates with increased morbidity and mortality. Although there is some controversy over its use in "late presenters," NAC therapy may be beneficial even 24 hours postingestion.

14. What is the dose of NAC?

The current NAC protocol that is approved by the U.S. Food and Drug Administration (FDA) is 140 mg/kg loading dose, followed by 17 doses of 70 mg/kg administered every 4 hours, for a total of 1330 mg/kg over 72 hours. Recently, some centers are only treating for 24–36 hours in healthy patients without preexisting liver disease and in the setting of chronic ingestion without evidence of hepatic damage.

15. How is NAC administered?

NAC solution should be diluted from the 20% solution to a 5% solution in juice or a carbonated beverage to maximize palatability. It still smells and tastes pretty bad. Vomiting frequently complicates oral NAC administration, and antiemetics such as high-dose metoclopramide, up to 1–2 mg/kg, and ondansetron may be necessary to help the patient retain the NAC. Slow instillation through a nasogastric tube may also aid in NAC retention.

16. Can NAC be administered along with activated charcoal (AC) ?

Yes. Although the in vitro studies that confirmed NAC is adsorbed to AC caused some concerns, this reduction in bioavailability of NAC for treatment of liver toxicity is probably inconsequential. In fact, one study showed that patients who received AC and NAC in the usual recommended dose had decreased morbidity. If a patient presents within 1–2 hours postingestion, AC should be administered and the 4-hour acetaminophen level measured. If the level is within the potentially toxic range or above, the patient should be given the loading dose of NAC. If the patient presents near 8 hours postingestion, you can skip the AC and just give the loading dose of NAC. If the patient requires multiple-dose AC for a mixed overdose and NAC, these doses may be staggered, but the usual recommended doses of NAC are still sufficient to protect the patient from hepatotoxicity.

17. When is intravenous NAC indicated?

Outside of the United States, NAC is administered intravenously by two protocols. The 20-hour protocol begins with 150 mg/kg of intravenous NAC over 15 minutes; this is followed by 50 mg/kg IV over 4 hours, which in turn is followed by 100 mg/kg IV over 16 hours. The second protocol consists of a loading dose of 140 mg/kg IV over 1 hour followed by 12 doses of 70 mg/kg administered every 4 hours. There does not appear to be any difference in efficacy between these two protocols. IV NAC is not approved by the FDA, but quite a few reports indicate it is generally safe. Indications for its use include any case where oral NAC is not tolerated by the patient or cannot be administered for medical reasons (e.g., uncontrollable vomiting, gastrointestinal bleeding or obstruction, encephalopathy, or cases in which coingestion of another substance requires ongoing gastrointestinal decontamination).

18. How should IV NAC be administered?

The IV NAC solution is prepared in a similar fashion to oral NAC but is labeled as "pyrogen-free." Oral NAC has been administered intravenously for the treatment of acetaminophen overdose. The oral preparation is diluted from a 20% solution to a 3% solution in 5% dextrose solution and infused through a 0.2-μm millipore filter. This is an off-label use of NAC and therefore should be considered in cases when oral NAC truly cannot be used and the patient has provided consent to IV NAC administration or when its use is necessary to save the patient's life. Practitioners should consult their pharmacy for guidelines.

19. What adverse events may occur from IV NAC administration?

The rate of adverse drug reactions associated with IV NAC averages 5–6% and ranges from less than 1% to up to 20%, depending on the report. The most common side effects of IV NAC are anaphylactoid in nature and consist of flushing, urticaria, and angioedema. These reactions seem to be dose related, occurring during the initial 15-minute infusion of NAC. They resolve spontaneously or with the administration of diphenhydramine and a reduction of the infusion rate. There are rare case reports of more serious adverse events related to IV NAC, including status epilepticus, hypotension, and death. These seem to have occurred due to overdose of NAC.

20. Are any patients at increased risk of hepatotoxicity from acetaminophen?

Any patients who might have an enhanced ability to make NAPQI or the reduced ability to detoxify it are considered to be at increased risk of toxicity. Induction of the P450 enzymes responsible for NAPQI formation may occur in patients who are taking anticonvulsants or rifampin or patients who chronically abuse ethanol. Reduced glutathione stores can occur in patients with a history of chronic ethanol abuse, fasting, malnutrition, or HIV infection.

21. Should the chronic alcoholic patient with acute acetaminophen ingestion be treated differently?

Although animal and human reports of ethanol-treated acetaminophen exposures differ in their results, most toxicologists agree that chronic alcoholics may be at increased risk for acetaminophen hepatotoxicity due to induction of the P450 isoenzymes. Therefore, an added note of caution should be applied to these patients. In the United Kingdom, some have advocated lowering the nomogram treatment line to a 4-hour level of 100 mg/L when assessing alcoholic patients with acetaminophen overdose.

22. Are there any special considerations for a pregnant patient with acute acetaminophen ingestion?

Acetaminophen has been shown to cross the placenta and to cause hepatotoxicity in a fetus, which has functioning mixed-function oxidase liver enzymes. This begins at about 14–16 weeks' gestation. The fetus also appears to be at an increased risk for cardiotoxicity due to acetaminophen toxicity in the mother. Therefore, any pregnant patient with acetaminophen ingestion should receive NAC as soon as the history is taken without waiting for confirmatory laboratory evaluation. Delay in NAC treatment in this case is associated with fetal demise. The fetus should be closely monitored while the mother is treated and resuscitated and obstetric consultation obtained in the event of fetal distress and decisions regarding emergency cesarean section.

23. Should children with acute acetaminophen ingestion be treated differently?

There is some evidence that children may fare better after ingestion of acetaminophen, perhaps because of an enhanced capacity for sulfation in their livers. Some recent studies are looking at the use of 2-hour acetaminophen levels to predict toxicity risk after the ingestion of liquid APAP formulas. Some have suggested that NAC is unnecessary under ingestion of 200 mg/kg, whereas conservative experts still use 150 mg/kg.

24. What should I do with a patient with a "chronic" ingestion of acetaminophen over several days?

The nomogram is meant just for single acute overdose and does not apply in the setting of multiple supra-therapeutic doses of acetaminophen. Evaluation of these patients includes assessment of hepatotoxicity (elevated aspartate aminotransferase [AST], alanine aminotransferase [ALT], PT, and international normalized ration [INR]), as well as the presence of any unmetabolized acetaminophen. NAC treatment should be instituted if acetaminophen is still measurable or there is evidence of hepatotoxicity and should be continued until at least 24 hours after the last dose of acetaminophen or until the patient is improved.

25. Should the patient with an ingestion of an extended-relief acetaminophen product be treated differently?

Extended-relief acetaminophen is composed of a layer of 325 mg of acetaminophen for immediate release and a central matrix of 325 mg of acetaminophen for continued, slow release for up to 8 hours. The recommended dose is not to exceed two caplets every 8 hours or 3900 mg/24 hours. The elimination half-life of the extended-relief product approximates that of immediate-release acetaminophen but may be delayed in onset. Because this was released in 1995, there is not much data in predicting toxicity, but patients with an overdose of this product should have an initial acetaminophen level measured at 4 hours postingestion, followed by a second level obtained 4 hours later. If either of these levels is above the nomogram line for potential toxicity, the patient should be treated with NAC. Alternatively, an initial level at 4 hours may be followed by repeat levels at 6 and 8 hours postingestion. If the second level is greater than the first, or if either of the subsequent levels is greater than half the possible toxicity line, then the patient should receive NAC therapy. These patients may require continued observation and repeat levels if they have also ingested other agents that might delay gastric emptying and acetaminophen absorption.

26. What findings indicate a poor prognosis after acetaminophen overdose?

King's College Hospital in London has developed predictors of death and, therefore, the need for liver transplantation in patients with acetaminophen hepatotoxicity.

- Patients with a serum pH < 7.3 that corrects after resuscitation have a mortality rate of 52%.
- Patients with a normal serum pH but with a PT > 100 seconds and creatinine > 3.4 mg/dl, with grade III or IV encephalopathy, have a mortality rate of 81%.
- Patients with a serum pH < 7.3 that does not correct with resuscitation have a mortality rate of 90%.

Other predictors of mortality, such as factor V concentrations and factor VIII:factor V ratios, have not been proved reliable. Delay in time to NAC treatment and coagulopathy are predictive of hepatic encephalopathy.

27. Can acetaminophen toxicity be characterized by any other pathology?

There are case reports of early development of metabolic acidosis and coma after massive acetaminophen ingestion. Acute tubular necrosis has been reported (rarely) to occur in the absence of hepatotoxicity.

28. Why should I order acetaminophen levels on patients who deny taking acetaminophen?

The initial symptoms of toxicity are very nonspecific, and occasionally a patient with impending toxicity may be missed. Unfortunately, if the patient returns later, the window for using NAC may have passed.

BIBLIOGRAPHY

1. Bizovi KE, Aks SE, Paloucek F, et al: Late increase in acetaminophen concentration after overdose of Tylenol extended relief. Ann Emerg Med 28:549–551, 1996.
2. Bradberry SM, Hart M, Bareford D, et al: Factor V and factor VIII:V ratio as prognostic indicators in paracetamol poisoning. Lancet 346:646–647, 1995.
3. Cetaruk EW, Dart RC, Hurlbut KM, et al: Tylenol extended relief overdose. Ann Emerg Med 30:104–108, 1997.
4. Clark RF, Chen R, Williams SR, et al: The use of ondansetron in the treatment of nausea and vomiting associated with acetaminophen poisoning. J Toxicol Clin Toxicol 34:163–167, 1996.
5. Hershkovitz E, Shorer Z, Levitas A, Tal A: Status epilepticus following intravenous N-acetylcysteine therapy. Isr J Med Sci 32:1102–1104, 1996.
6. Izumi S, Langley PG, Wendon J, et al: Coagulation factor V levels as a prognostic indicator in fulminant hepatic failure. Hepatology 23:1507–1511, 1996.
7. Johnston SC, Pelletier LL: Enhanced hepatotoxicity of acetaminophen in the alcoholic patient: Two case reports and a review of the literature. Medicine 76:185–191, 1997.
8. Jones AL: Mechanism of action and value of N-acetylcysteine in the treatment of early and late acetaminophen poisoning: A critical review. J Toxicol Clin Toxicol 36:277–285, 1998.
9. Makin AJ, Wendon J, Williams R: A 7-year experience of severe acetaminophen-induced hepatotoxicity (1987–1993). Gastroenterology 109:1907–1916, 1995.
10. Perry H, Shannon MW: Acetaminophen. In Haddad LM, Shannon MW, Winchester JF (eds): Clinical Management of Poisoning and Drug Overdose, 3rd ed. Philadelphia, W.B. Saunders, 1998, pp 664–674.
11. Roth B, Woo O, Blanc P: Early metabolic acidosis and coma after acetaminophen ingestion. Ann Emerg Med 33:452–456, 1999.
12. Stork CM, Rees S, Howland MA, et al: Pharmacokinetics of extended relief vs. regular release Tylenol in simulated human overdose. J Toxicol Clin Toxicol 34:157–162, 1996
13. Tucker JR: Late-presenting acute acetaminophen toxicity and the role of N-acetylcysteine. Pediatr Emerg Care 14:424–426, 1998.
14. Wang PH, Yang MJ, Lee WL, et al: Acetaminophen poisoning in late pregnancy: A case report. J Reprod Med 42:367–371, 1997.
15. Woo OF, Mueller PD, Olson KR, et al: Shorter duration of oral N-acetylcysteine therapy for acute acetaminophen overdose. Ann Emerg Med 35:363–368, 2000.
16. Yip L, Dart RC, Hurlbut KM: Intravenous administration of oral N-acetylcysteine. Crit Care Med 26:40–43, 1998.

7. SALICYLATES

Susan S. Fish, PharmD, M.P.H.

1. *Extra credit:* **In 1915, aspirin production began in the United States. The drug became popular with the public, despite toxicity in high doses. What was unique about the formulation of this drug?**

It was the first drug to be manufactured in the U.S. in tablet form.

2. *Extra credit:* **After World War I, what forced the Germans to relinquish their remedy for fever and rheumatism (aspirin)?**

The Treaty of Versailles.

3. Does anyone overdose on aspirin any more?

Other drugs with antipyretic or analgesic properties have replaced aspirin in popularity, packaging laws have decreased pediatric access to quantities of aspirin, and pediatric use has declined because of aspirin's association with Reye's syndrome. Nonetheless, aspirin continues to be a significant source of poisoning for both unintentional and intentional overdose, with about 18,000 poisonings a year.

4. Aspirin is an over-the-counter drug. It can't be too toxic, can it?

That is the belief of much of the lay public. Unfortunately, aspirin (salicylic acid) can produce substantial toxicity and even death. Some patients intentionally ingest substances in an attempt to get help from the medical or psychiatric communities or to get attention from loved ones. However, these so-called suicide gestures involve ingestions of large quantities of over-the-counter drugs that can lead to unintended death.

5. How much aspirin is too much?

Acute ingestions and chronic ingestions (those that occur over 1–2 days) have different levels of toxicity. Acute ingestions of 150–200 mg/kg (one-half to one 325-mg tablet per kg) produce mild symptoms, whereas 300–400 mg/kg produce serious toxicity. On the other hand, 100 mg/kg/day for 2 days or more will produce symptoms of chronic toxicity.

6. What products other than aspirin contain salicylate?

More than 200 aspirin-containing products are available in the U.S.:
- Aspirin is often combined with **antihistamines**, **decongestants**, and other **cold and cough** and **arthritis preparations**.
- **Oil of wintergreen**, available in 1-ounce bottles and in products such as BenGay, contains methyl salicylate (530 mg/ml). Eight milliliters of oil of wintergreen is equivalent to thirteen adult (325-mg) aspirin tablets. A 4-ml dose of oil of wintergreen has caused death in children. Thus, ingestion of even small amounts of methyl salicylate produces salicylate poisoning, and absorption is quite rapid.
- Topical salicylic acid (Compound W) is used as a **keratolytic**.
- **Pepto-Bismol** (bismuth subsalicylate) contains 8.8 mg/ml. The 240-ml dose commonly used for traveler's diarrhea contains the equivalent of eight 325-mg tablets.

7. How does salicylate cause acid-base disorders?

The mechanism of toxicity begins with central stimulation of the respiratory center, which produces hyperventilation. This leads to respiratory alkalosis, compensatory metabolic acidosis, and dehydration. Inhibition of the Krebs cycle results in lactic acidosis. Because salicylate is really acetyl salicylic acid, the elevated serum level directly causes a metabolic acidosis as more is absorbed.

8. As an antipyretic, aspirin decreases body temperature. How can it increase temperature in an overdose?

Salicylate uncouples oxidative phosphorylation, which increases oxygen consumption, glucose use, and heat production. This results in fever, tachypnea, tachycardia, and hypoglycemia.

9. How does aspirin affect the blood?

Salicylate alters platelet function and bleeding time and may cause hypoprothrombinemia.

10. What is a toxic level of salicylate?

Classification of Acute Salicylate Poisoning (3-6 Hours Postingestion)

	SERUM SALICYLATE LEVEL
Moderate	50 mg/dl
Severe	75 mg/dl
Potentially lethal	100 mg/dl (correlates with seizures)

11. Who was Done and what is his nomogram?

Alan Done, one of the fathers of modern clinical toxicology, published a salicylate nomogram in 1960 to correlate salicylate levels at different times after ingestion of a single acute overdose to determine the severity of the poisoning. Because of the delay in absorption, the nomogram is not used to determine treatment, unlike the acetaminophen nomogram. Treatment decisions should be based on clinical symptoms and laboratory findings rather than on the nomogram.

12. Explain the difference between acute poisoning and chronic poisoning.

Not only is the amount ingested that produces toxicity different between acute and chronic poisonings (see question 7), but the symptoms are distinctly different, the pharmacokinetics (both elimination half-life and the protein binding) are different, and the treatment is different.

13. What are the symptoms of salicylate toxicity?

Acute poisoning produces vomiting, gastrointestinal (GI) irritation and bleeding, hyperpnea, tinnitus, and lethargy. Respiratory alkalosis and metabolic acidosis follow. Severe poisoning can result in restlessness, irritability, seizures, coma, hyperthermia, hypoglycemia (or occasionally hyperglycemia), and pulmonary edema. Death is usually due to cardiovascular collapse, respiratory failure, or central nervous system (CNS) failure.

Chronic poisoning is more likely to produce nonspecific symptoms such as lethargy, confusion, hallucinations, metabolic acidosis, and dehydration. However, death, usually from pulmonary or cerebral edema, is more common in patients with chronic poisoning than with acute poisoning and occurs at lower salicylate levels.

14. Why is chronic poisoning dangerous at lower serum levels?

Acetyl salicylic acid is polar and very slow at crossing the blood-brain barrier. With chronic poisoning, there is more time for the brain level to keep up with the serum level and keep in equilibrium.

15. Do symptoms correlate with serum level?

Symptoms of severe toxicity correlate more closely with CNS salicylate levels than with serum salicylate levels. This is true for both acute and chronic poisonings and helps explain why symptoms occur at lower serum levels with chronic ingestions. Consequently, treatment decisions must be based on clinical symptoms and laboratory test abnormalities rather than on serum levels alone.

16. What is the time course of salicylate toxicity?

Symptoms can begin within 1–2 hours after an acute ingestion or may be delayed for more than 4–6 hours. Absorption usually occurs over a few hours but can be delayed after the ingestion of sustained-release or enteric-coated preparations. In addition, salicylate can form concretions in the stomach; these concretions can continue to release drug slowly, producing rising serum levels for up to 12 hours.

Severity of symptoms sometimes does not peak until 12–24 hours. However, if there are no symptoms within 6 hours, it is unlikely that the patient will experience severe toxicity, unless a sustained-release preparation was ingested.

17. Does it take a long time for the body to eliminate salicylate?

It depends. After therapeutic doses of aspirin, the elimination half-life of salicylate is about 3–4 hours. After higher doses, such as those used to treat arthritis, or after overdose, the elimination half-life can exceed 24 hours. Chronic ingestion of salicylate also produces an elimination half-life of > 24 hours. At these higher blood levels, there is a shift from first-order elimination to zero-order elimination.

18. What laboratory tests are useful with salicylate toxicity?

Serum salicylate levels should be drawn if aspirin or other salicylate poisoning is suspected. In cases where levels are positive and there is suspicion of a substantial ingestion, serial levels should be noted every 3–4 hours until levels drop by about 10% from the previous result. Because of concretion formation, levels can continue to rise, and severe poisoning can result even if the initial level was not worrisome.

Other useful laboratory parameters to monitor include arterial blood gases, electrolytes (especially potassium), complete blood count (CBC), glucose, blood urea nitrogen (BUN), creatinine, liver function tests, and prothrombin time. An anion gap can suggest an etiology to a metabolic acidosis. In addition, urine pH and specific gravity are helpful.

19. What is the differential diagnosis of a metabolic acidosis with an increased anion gap?

Remember the mnemonic A MUDPILES:

Alcohol
Methanol
Uremia
Diabetic ketoacidosis
Paraldehyde
Isoniazid and **i**ron
Lactic acidosis
Ethylene glycol
Salicylate and **s**tarvation

20. Are x-rays useful?

Abdominal x-rays may be helpful if they reveal enteric-coated or sustained-release formulations of aspirin or a concretion. Negative abdominal x-rays are not helpful.

21. If a patient vomits from salicylate poisoning, does that get rid of the salicylate and decrease the chance of toxicity?

A patient vomiting after salicylate ingestion indicates at least mild to moderate poisoning. Vomiting does not remove the entire GI contents, so toxicity can continue. In addition, if vomiting was induced using syrup of ipecac (which is rarely used in the hospital but may be used at home), a substantial amount of salicylate may remain in the GI tract, available for absorption and thus toxicity.

22. Does activated charcoal bind salicylate?

Activated charcoal binds salicylate quite well and should be used for treatment of salicylate poisoning. In addition, repeat doses may be recommended if a sustained-release preparation was ingested or if a concretion has formed. However, salicylate is not bound permanently to activated charcoal, and the drug can desorb from the bound complex. Thus, it is important to ensure that the activated charcoal-drug complex is eliminated from the GI tract.

23. Do lab tests need to be repeated?

As indicated above, serum salicylate levels should be repeated regularly to ensure that they are not continuing to rise. If levels drawn 3–4 hours apart are similar, keep taking repeat levels until they decrease by at least 10%. It is possible that levels can be stable for 9–12 hours and then begin to rise.

Serial blood gases are used to monitor the metabolic state of the patient and must be repeated frequently once metabolic derangements are identified. In severe poisonings, watch for pulmonary edema using blood gases and chest x-rays.

Dehydration is common and electrolyte derangements should be monitored by repeat laboratory tests.

24. Is there an antidote for salicylate poisoning?

No.

25. What is the treatment for salicylate poisoning?

- Always begin with supportive care (maintain airway, assist ventilation as needed).
- Treat coma, seizures, pulmonary edema, and hyperthermia as you would from any cause.
- Metabolic acidosis should be treated with sodium bicarbonate. Severe acidemia should be avoided because it can increase CNS salicylate levels. Bicarbonate also helps alkalize the urine and enhance elimination of the salicylate. With bicarbonate treatment, monitor to avoid alkalemia and sodium overload.
- Treat fluid and electrolyte imbalances as you would from any cause. Remember to rehydrate patients adequately but cautiously, while monitoring for pulmonary and cerebral edema.
- Give vitamin K as needed for coagulopathy.
- Except in cases where there are severe symptoms that need to be treated first, activated charcoal is usually the first intervention.

26. When is enhanced elimination indicated? How is it done?

Urinary alkalization helps eliminate salicylate from the body. Salicylic acid, which is eliminated renally, is trapped in an alkaline urine, and reabsorption in the renal tubule is prevented. Alkalization of the urine can be accomplished by adding 50–100 mEq of sodium bicarbonate to D_5W and infusing it at 150–200 ml/hr. Serum potassium must be normalized with supplemental potassium in order for the urine pH to reach ≥ 7.5. Monitor urine pH frequently while administering bicarbonate to alkalinize the urine. Be careful to monitor for pulmonary and cerebral edema and avoid overhydration. Elimination also can be enhanced using repeat doses of activated charcoal. Monitor fluid imbalances.

27. When is hemodialysis indicated?

Hemodialysis may be used in:

- Severely ill patients to rapidly remove salicylate from the blood while correcting fluid and acid-base imbalances
- Patients with serum salicylate levels > 100 mg/dl or severe acidosis after an acute ingestion
- After chronic ingestion, patients with levels of 60 mg/dl and lethargy or confusion
- Patients with severe symptoms such as coma or seizures, regardless of serum salicylate level

28. Is death from salicylate poisoning possible?

Absolutely! Death may be secondary to cardiovascular collapse, CNS overstimulation that causes seizures and hyperthermia, or pulmonary edema. Poison centers report about 35 deaths per year across the country.

BIBLIOGRAPHY

1. Abdel-Magid EH, el-Awad Ahmed FR: Salicylate intoxication in an infant with ichthyosis transmitted through skin ointment: A case report. Pediatrics 94:939–940, 1994.
2. Chan TY: Risk of severe salicylate poisoning following the ingestion of topical medicaments or aspirin. Postgrad Med J 72:109–112, 1996.
3. Ellenhorn MJ, Barceloux DG: Salicylates. In Ellenhorn MJ (ed): Medical Toxicology: Diagnosis and Treatment of Human Poisoning. New York, Elsevier, 1988, pp 562–572.
4. Gittelman DK: Chronic salicylate intoxication. So Med J 86:683–685, 1993.
5. Hofman M, Diaz JE, Martella C: Oil of wintergreen overdose. Ann Emerg Med 31:793–794, 1998.
6. Krenzelok EP, Kerr F, Proudfoot AT: Salicylate toxicity. In Haddad LM, Shannon MW, Winchester JF (eds): Clinical Management of Poisoning and Drug Overdose, 3rd ed. Philadelphia, W.B. Saunders, 1998, pp 675–687.
7. Liebelt EL, Shannon MW: Small doses, big problems: A selected review of highly toxic common medications. Pediatr Emerg Care 9:292–297, 1993.
8. Linden CH: Salicylate poisoning. In Harwood-Nuss AL, Linden CH, Luten RC, et al (eds): Clinical Practice of Emergency Medicine, 2nd ed. Philadelphia, Lippincott-Raven, 1996, pp 1408–1412.
9. Pierce RP, Gazewood J, Blake RL Jr: Salicylate poisoning from enteric-coated aspirin: Delayed absorption may complicate management. Postgrad Med 89:61–62, 1991.
10. Sporer KA, Khayam-Bashi H: Acetaminophen and salicylate serum levels in patients with suicidal ingestion or altered mental status. Am J Emerg Med 14:442–446, 1996.
11. Vernace MA, Bellucci AG, Wilkes BM: Chronic salicylate toxicity due to consumption of over-the-counter bismuth subsalicylate. Am J Med 97:308–309, 1994.

8. CAFFEINE

Shu Shum, M.B., B.S.

1. What type of over-the-counter (OTC) medications contain caffeine?

The following *may* contain caffeine:

Analgesics
Decongestants
Antihistamines
Diet pills
Cough and cold preparations
Energizers (stimulants)

Each group presents different clinical challenges. In addition, chemicals such as caffeine are added to many foods and can cause or add to symptoms.

2. How much caffeine is dangerous?

Acute ingestion of caffeine of more than 10 mg/kg of body weight is potentially toxic. The normal volume of distribution of caffeine is 0.5–0.7 L/kg in an adult, so a dose of 10 mg/kg will give a peak level of 20 µg/ml (using 0.5 L/kg as a denominator), which is considered above the upper limit of the therapeutic range. Thus, patients who ingest more than 10 mg/kg may develop life-threatening symptoms such as dysrhythmias or seizures.

Reported Caffeine Fatality Levels

AGE	DOSE (gm)	BLOOD LEVEL (µg/ml)
15 months	18	104
5 years	3	15.85
19 years	18	18.1
15 years	16	108
32 years	20	30

3. What if I just drink a lot of coffee but never overdose?

Chronic overuse of caffeine has been associated with increased risks of coronary heart diseases; cancer of the pancreas, ovary, and breast; and elevation of serum cholesterol. However, no dose-response curve has been established for these chronic conditions, and it remains controversial.

4. How is acute caffeine overdose managed?

A patient with a history of ingestion of a large amount of medication-grade caffeine, even if there are no other symptoms than anxiety and tachycardia, should be taken seriously. Dysrhythmias and seizures may occur without much warning. If the patient ingested more than 1 gm of caffeine or has an estimated peak serum caffeine level more than 20 µg/ml, intravenous access should be established.

The patient should be monitored carefully with serial blood pressure, electrocardiogram (ECG), and close bedside observation. Some of these patients are suicidal, and appropriate precautionary measures should be taken. Then proceed to the normal gastrointestinal decontamination with charcoal.

If ventricular tachyrhythmia occurs, consider the use of a short-acting beta-adrenergic blocker, such as esmolol, with a loading dose of 500 µg/kg over 1 minute, followed by a continuous infusion of 50–200 µg/kg/min with continuous ECG and blood pressure monitoring in an intensive care setting. If beta-adrenergic blockade fails, one should consider using 0.2 mg/kg of adenosine intravenously over 1–2 seconds.

When seizures occur, secure the airway and provide artificial ventilation. Consider the use of an ultra quick-acting benzodiazepine such as midazolam, with a loading dose of 0.2 mg/kg followed by a continuous infusion of 5 µg/kg/min. Repeating the loading dose a few times may be necessary. If this fails to stop the seizures, consider IV adenosine, as in tachyarrhythmias, or use pentobarbital anesthesia with continuous electroencephalogram (EEG) monitoring.

Another methylxanthine, theophylline, shares similar properties with caffeine. In particular, the acute or chronic ingestion situation may be more toxic, and the patient may be sicker. Thus, judicious use of seizure prophylaxis as well as hemodialysis and charcoal hemoperfusion should be borne in mind.

5. How does caffeine cause its effects?

Caffeine, like other methylxanthines, selectively blocks adenosine effect by acting as a competitive antagonist at the adenosine receptors. Blockade of the adenosine A_1 receptors by caffeine causes seizures, and typically this type of seizure fails to terminate spontaneously. In addition, blockade of the adenosine A_2 receptors prevents vasodilation, contributing to the insult to the central nervous system. This may explain the high mortality of caffeine-induced seizures. Furthermore, caffeine interferes with the uptake and storage of calcium ion by the sarcoplasmic reticulum in striated muscle and the myocardium. This may be the reason that caffeine can increase the strength and duration of contractions in both skeletal muscle and the myocardium. Caffeine elevates levels of intracellular cyclic adenosine monophosphate (cAMP) through the blockade of cyclic nucleotide phosphodiesterase, thus relaxing bronchiolar and vascular smooth muscles, causing bronchial dilation and hypotension.

6. Why are some people more affected by caffeine than others?

Caffeine is demethylated and oxidized by the microsomal cytochrome P450 mono-oxygenases system, primarily by the CYP1A2 and by cytosolic arylamine N-acetyltransferase, NAT2 to 5-(N-formylmethylamino)-6-amino-1,3-dimethyluracil. Thus, caffeine metabolism is under double pharmacogenetic regulation, both through the microsomal cytochrome P450 super family and the N-acetyltransferase system. Additionally, both of these enzyme systems mature in an age-dependent manner, which is probably why the elimination half-life is 60–100 hours in premature infants and neonates compared with an adult's 3–6 hours.

7. Does coffee have more caffeine than diet cola?

Typically, a cup of brewed coffee contains 100 mg/cup (6 oz) and a can of caffeinated soda contains 45 mg/can (12 oz). However, the amount of caffeine in a cup of coffee depends on the coffee bean used, time of harvest, species of bean, and method of brewing. Similarly, the amount of caffeine varies greatly among the different commercial preparation of the sodas.

Caffeine Content of Some Common Foods and Beverages

SUBSTANCE	AMOUNT
Coffee, brewed	100 mg/cup
Coffee, instant	70 mg/cup
Decaffeinated coffee	4 mg/cup
Tea	30-50 mg/cup
Caffeinated soda	35–72 mg/can
Cocoa beverage	2–20 mg/cup
Chocolate milk	2–7 mg/cup

(*Table continued on next page.*)

Caffeine Content of Some Common Foods and Beverages (Cont.)

SUBSTANCE	AMOUNT
Dark chocolate	20–25 mg/oz
Milk chocolate	6 mg/oz
Caffeine-containing cold drugs	30–75 mg/tablet
Caffeine-containing analgesics	25–65 mg/tablet
Stimulants	100–350 mg/tablet
Weight-loss aids	75–200 mg/tablet

Cup = 6 oz, can = 12 oz.

8. Is there such thing as caffeine withdrawal?

Yes. When a chronic caffeine user stops drinking coffee, the initial symptoms include fatigue, anxiety, and craving for a cup of coffee, followed by an intense headache and agitation. In addition, caffeine withdrawal seizure has been reported. Other characteristics of withdrawal include depression and use of analgesics to relieve discomfort.

The intense headache that is characteristic of caffeine withdrawal occurs in about 50% of coffee drinkers who stop drinking coffee abruptly. Withdrawal symptoms usually begin within 12–24 hours after cessation of caffeine consumption and may last up to 1 week. Infants born to mothers who drink coffee heavily may show signs of caffeine withdrawal. Typically, their symptoms start on the second day of life, but symptoms may be delayed for many days because of the long elimination half-life of caffeine in this age group.

9. Describe the symptoms of cold medication overdose.

Cough and cold preparations, depending on the ingredients, cause a combination of symptomatology, such as acute sympathetic syndrome, anticholinergic syndrome, and a narcotic-like syndrome with altered mental status, which may be resistant to even large doses of naloxone. This may be caused by dextromethorphan hydrobromide. Large doses of naloxone may overcome some of the effects of dextromethorphan; however, the bromide effect will persist, maintaining the altered mental status state.

Decongestant overdose may result in acute sympathetic syndrome, which is characterized by anxiety, palpitation, hypertension, hyperpyrexia, headache, and seizures. Particularly with phenylpropanolamine, reflex bradycardia secondary to the systolic hypertension as well as intracranial hemorrhage may occur. These symptoms may appear without warning, even after the usual therapeutic dose.

Antihistamine overdose typically results in acute anticholinergic syndrome, which manifests with flushing, increased temperature, anxiety, dry mucous membranes, and dilated pupils. Patients, especially children, may be delirious and agitated.

Cold medications often contain **caffeine**, which can increase symptoms when combined with other sources of caffeine such as beverages.

10. Can a person overdose on topical medications?

Nicotine patches are currently available over the counter to help nicotine addicts quit smoking. However, if a toddler accidentally ingests a used patch, he or she may develop symptoms of acute nicotinic syndrome including hypertension, hyperpyrexia, hyperreflexia, seizure, tachycardia, tremor, vomiting, and diarrhea. These sympathomimetic symptoms may mimic those of caffeine overdose.

11. Do OTC medications interact with any prescription drugs?

It depends on the prescription drugs and the OTC medications involved. Unfortunately, many patients do not consider OTC medications as drugs, so they don't mention them to their health care providers. A specific drug history should be obtained from patients, including OTC drugs, dietary supplements, and herbal products.

12. What type of drug interactions occur with caffeine or OTC drugs?

Caffeine may increase the diuretic effects of some drugs. Sympathomimetics may nullify the effects of antihypertensives. In addition, sympathomimetics may react violently with beta blockers because of the unopposed alpha effect, increasing the blood pressure, tachycardia, and agitation.

BIBLIOGRAPHY

1. Ellenhorn MJ, Schonwald S, Ordog G, et al: Ellenhorn's Medical Toxicology: Diagnosis and Treatment of Human Poisoning, 2nd ed. Baltimore, Williams & Wilkins, 1996.
2. Goldfrank LR, Flomenbaum NE, Lewin NA, et al (eds): Goldfrank's Toxicologic Emergencies, 6th ed. Stamford, CT, Appleton & Lange, 1998.
3. Haddad LM, Shannon MW, Winchester JF: Clinical Management of Poisoning and Drug Overdose, 3rd ed. Philadelphia, W.B. Saunders, 1998.
4. Jeffery EH: Human Drug Metabolism: From Molecular Biology to Man. Boca Raton, FL, CRC Press, 1993.
5. Price Evans DA: Genetic Factors in Drug Therapy: Clinical and Molecular Pharmacogenetics. New York, Cambridge University Press, 1993.
6. Shum S, Seale C, Hathaway D, et al: Acute caffeine ingestion fatalities: Management issues. Vet Human Toxicol 39:228–230, 1997.
7. Strain EC, Griffiths RR: Caffeine dependency: Fact or fiction. J Roy Soc Med 88:437–440, 1995.

9. VITAMINS

Suzanne Doyon, M.D.

1. Define RDA.

The Food and Nutrition Board of the Institute of Medicine of the National Academy of Sciences periodically reviews the scientific evidence and publishes the recommended daily allowance (RDA) of vitamins and other nutrients. Their standard is usually set two to six times higher than the minimum daily requirement, which is the amount of vitamins required to protect healthy, normal people from vitamin deficiency.

2. Why do so many healthy adults consume high-dose vitamins?

People take megadoses of vitamins to enhance their appearance, live longer, enhance athletic performance, and prevent or ameliorate nondeficiency-specific diseased states. The practice of taking megadoses of vitamins gained popularity in the early 1970s when Linus Pauling published a monograph entitled *Vitamin C and the Common Cold.* However, clinical trials of vitamin supplementation have demonstrated negative or equivocal results.

3. How many vitamins are there and why is their classification important?

There are 13 vitamins.

Water soluble:	*Fat soluble:*
Ascorbate	Vitamin A
Thiamine	Vitamin D
Riboflavin	Vitamin E
Niacin	Vitamin K
Pyridoxine	
Biotin	
Pantothenic acid	
Folate	
B_{12}	

Fat soluble vitamins are stored in tissues and are more likely to result in toxicity.

4. What happens when vitamin A builds up?

The primary food sources of vitamin A are fish livers, which contain retinol esters, and carrots, which contain the less toxic carotenoids. When the liver becomes saturated with vitamin A, due to excessive consumption, hepatic disease, or both, retinyl esters appear in the blood and cause membrane lipoprotein damage and altered gene expression.

Absorption of carotenoids is less complete, and they are not converted to retinol very rapidly. Excessive consumption of carotenoids is mostly associated with hyperpigmentation of the skin that can be differentiated from jaundice by the absence of scleral icterus.

5. How does vitamin A toxicity manifest?

The target organs usually affected by retinol toxicity are the central nervous system (CNS), liver, bone, skin, and mucous membranes. Typical early features are primarily neurologic and include irritability, fatigue, increased sleep, anorexia, vomiting, and increased intracranial pressure that may manifest as a bulging fontanelle in infants or signs of acute pseudotumor cerebri in older children and adults. Hepatomegaly, hair loss, and cheilitis (inflammation of the lips) follow the neurologic symptoms.

6. Do the manifestations of vitamin A excess differ based on the length of poisoning?

The clinical manifestations of chronic hypervitaminosis A are much the same with predominance of increased intracranial pressure, changes in the skin including scaliness, peeling, hair loss, cheilitis, and stomatitis. Hepatosplenomegaly is often present and may be accompanied by abdominal pain, ascites, and esophageal varices. Chronic hypervitaminosis A has been associated with hepatic cirrhosis. The skeletal system is also frequently affected, particularly in children, where complaints of bone pain and unexplained painful swelling of the extremities are common. Radiologic findings include osteoporosis or hypermineralization, periosteal calcifications, and cortical hyperostosis of the cranium and long bones.

7. Are laboratory tests helpful in the diagnosis of retinol toxicity?

Yes. Serum retinol and serum retinol esters should be assayed. Serum retinol levels in excess of 100 µg/dl are highly suggestive of retinol toxicity. Serum levels of retinol esters in excess of 7 µg/dl or greater than 5–8% of serum retinol are equally suggestive of toxicity. Routine chemistries and liver function tests are usually normal or only marginally elevated despite clinical evidence of hepatomegaly or, in some cases, the presence of ascites. Hypercalcemia can occur as can hypoprothrombinemia. Radiologic findings are described in question 6.

8. What is a toxic amount of vitamin A?

Acute ingestions in excess of 25,000 IU/kg are considered toxic. Daily intake of 4000 IU/kg for 6–15 months or more will result in chronic toxicity.

9. Is vitamin A teratogenic?

Yes. Typical manifestations include hydrocephalus, micrognatia, cleft palate, microtia, transposition of the great vessels, and tetralogy of Fallot. The calculated relative risk is 26% in women who used isotretinoin. The critical period of usage seems to be somewhere between the second and fifth week postconception.

10. How is hypervitaminosis A treated?

Prompt withdrawal of vitamin A supplements is critical. Following this measure alone, most symptoms resolve within weeks to months. Occasionally, repeated lumbar punctures, diuretic administration, or steroid use is required to treat the increased intracranial pressure; close monitoring by an experienced neurologist is advised in these cases.

11. What are the clinical signs of vitamin D toxicity?

Fatigue
Nausea
Vomiting
Hypertension
Polyuria
Polydipsia
Nephrocalcinosis

12. Are laboratory tests helpful in the diagnosis of vitamin D toxicity?

Hypercalcemia with variable phosphate levels is usually present as are elevated levels of 25-hydroxyvitamin D (25-OH-D). Ectopic calcifications in the kidneys, myocardium, and major vessels may be seen on x-rays.

13. How is hypervitaminosis D treated?

Prompt withdrawal of vitamin D supplements is necessary. Implementation of a diet low in calcium is also indicated. Renal failure may respond to short-term hemodialysis. Other more experimental agents include glutethimide and the biphosphonates clodronate and pamidronate.

14. Which vitamins are associated with hypercalcemia?

Hypercalcemia is often found in cases of hypervitaminosis A and D, though it is much more common in cases of excessive consumption of vitamin D than vitamin A.

15. Vitamin K is essential to the formation of which clotting factors?

Vitamin K is essential to the formation of factors II, VII, IX, and X. Other vitamin K-dependent proteins include anticoagulant protein C and S and osteocalcin.

16. Why are cases of hypervitaminosis K so rare?

Vitamin K is not available as an over-the-counter dietary supplement.

17. What happens with pyridoxine (vitamin B_6) toxicity?

Pyridoxine toxicity has been associated with sensory axonal neuropathy, without motor or CNS deficits. Findings include ataxia, severely impaired position and vibration sense, and a less dramatic loss of light touch, temperature, and pain sensations. Diminished deep tendon reflexes are also present.

18. I often administer intravenous thiamine (vitamin B_1) to my patients with chronic alcoholism. Are there any risks?

It is considered safe to administer thiamine intravenously. Few severe anaphylactoid reactions have been documented following IV administration of thiamine. In a large case series, however, the incidence of adverse events was 0.1% and consisted of one patient who developed pruritus.

19. *Extra credit:* We have often heard of vitamins such as B_1 and B_6, but what is vitamin B_{17}?

Laetrile, which is commonly found in pits of peaches, apricots, apple seeds, and other fruit.

20. What are the clinical manifestations of vitamin C toxicity?

Vitamin C toxicity is associated with gastrointestinal disturbances, poor wound healing, urinary calculi, and hemolysis in G6PD-deficient individuals. It usually responds to withdrawal of vitamin C. Abrupt withdrawal of vitamin C has been associated with rebound scurvy and should be closely monitored.

21. What is the niacin flush?

Nicotinic acid (niacin) is used extensively to treat hyperlipidemia. In therapeutic doses, nicotinic acid can cause flushing, vasodilation, headache, and pruritus. These effects are prostaglandin-related, and premedication with aspirin alleviates most of the symptoms. Nicotinic acid can induce hepatitis in large doses, unrelated to any hypersensitivity reaction.

BIBLIOGRAPHY

1. British Pediatric Association: Hypercalcemia in infants and vitamin D. Br Med J 2:149, 1956.
2. Feldman M, Schlezinger N: Benign intracranial hypertension associated with hypervitaminosis A. Arch Neurol 22:1–7, 1979.
3. Guebel AP, de Galocsy C, Alves N, et al: Liver damage caused by therapeutic vitamin A administration: Estimate of dose-related toxicity in 41 cases. Gastroenterology 100:1701–1709, 1991.
4. Moertel CG, Fleming TR, Creagan ET, et al: High dose vitamin C versus placebo in the treatment of patients who have no prior chemotherapy: A randomized, double-blind comparison. N Engl J Med 312:137–141, 1985.
5. Shaumburg H, Kaplan J, Windebank A, et al: Sensory neuropathy from pyridoxine abuse: A new megavitamin syndrome. N Engl J Med 309:445–448, 1983.
6. Stern RH, Spence JD, Freeman DJ, Parbtani A: Tolerance to nicotinic acid flushing. Clin Pharmacol Ther 50:66–70, 1991.
7. Stimson W: Vitamin A intoxication in adults. N Engl J Med 265:369–373, 1961.

10. ANTICHOLINERGIC POISONING

K. *Sophia Dyer*, M.D.

1. What is the mechanism of action of anticholinergic agents?
Pharmaceuticals and plant products that have anticholinergic effects work by competitively antagonizing the neurotransmitter **acetylcholine**. Acetylcholine acts on central receptors as well as muscarinic and nicotinic receptors peripherally. Many anticholinergic drugs cause their effects by blocking the muscarinic and central cholinergic receptors.

2. Where are muscarinic receptors found?
Muscarinic receptors exist as postganglionic receptors (sympathetic) on sweat glands and as postganglionic central nervous system (CNS) receptors in the parasympathetic nervous system. Muscarinic receptors work on a transmembrane protein called the G protein.

3. Where are nicotinic receptors located?
- As part of the autonomic ganglia
- On skeletal muscle motor end plates
- In the spinal cord

4. How is acetylcholine metabolized?
Acetylcholine is metabolized by the enzyme acetylcholinesterase, which is present at synaptic clefts. Organophosphate and carbamate insecticides inhibit this enzyme and result in excess cholinergic effect.

5. What mnemonic describes the common manifestations of an anticholinergic poison?
Mad as a hatter
Red as a beet
Dry as a bone
Blind as a bat
Hot as a hare

6. What signs and symptoms can be seen with central anticholinergic poisoning?
Visual and auditory hallucinations
Confusion
Psychosis
Coma
Seizures
Ataxia
Respiratory failure
Extrapyramidal effects

7. What is the most sensitive sign of toxicity?
Sinus tachycardia.

8. According to the American Association of Poison Control Centers (AAPCC), cough and cold products represent what percent of all ingestions in children 6 years and younger?
In the 1998 data published by the AAPCC, cough and cold preparations represented 5.5% of the most frequently involved substances—over 60,000 exposures. Most of these cough and cold preparations have antihistamines with some anticholinergic manifestations.

9. **Name some plants with anticholinergic properties.**
   Deadly nightshade (*Atropa belladonna*)
   Jimsonweed (*Datura stramonium*)
   Mandrake (*Mandragora officinarum*)
   Henbane (*Hyoscyamus niger*)

10. *Extra credit:* **The common name jimsonweed (*Datura stramonium*) is derived from a Virginia location. What is the location, and why did that town become associated with the plant?**
    Jimsonweed is an alteration of "Jamestown weed." In Jamestown, Virginia, advancing British soldiers ate the plant and suffered anticholinergic poisoning during Bacon's Rebellion in 1676.
    The seeds of the plant have the highest concentration of anticholinergic toxins. A hardy weed that can grow in both rural and urban environments, jimsonweed is used intentionally for its hallucinogenic effects.

11. *Extra credit:* **What was the commercial name of the over-the-counter form of *Datura stramonium*, which was once smoked by asthmatics to alleviate some of their symptoms?**
    Asthmador cigarettes.

12. **What drug groups have anticholinergic properties?**
    Antihistamines
    Antipsychotics
    Cyclic antidepressants
    Anti-Parkinson's medications (e.g., benzotropine mesylate)
    Atropine and atropine-related products (scopolamine)

13. **What mushroom is associated with anticholinergic properties? Hint: the family is frequently associated with hepatotoxic mushrooms.**
    Amanita muscaria (fly agaric).

14. **What is the most common cardiovascular side effect of anticholinergic drugs?**
    Sinus tachycardia. Conduction abnormalities are possible especially with the drugs that inhibit sodium channels. Cyclic antidepressants or large doses of diphenhydramine can widen the QRS complex. Sodium bicarbonate is used to improve those conduction disturbances.

15. **What drug is used as an antidote to anticholinergic poisoning?**
    Physostigmine (Antilirium) is a reversible cholinesterase inhibitor that works at both central and peripheral cholinergic receptors. It is most commonly used in its intravenous form.

16. **What are the potential benefits of physostigmine?**
    Physostigmine can ameliorate coma, delirium, and potentially seizures. It can clear up a patient's mental status long enough to confirm a history and obviate other procedures. It was once a routine part of the "coma cocktail" until reports about the negative effect of the drug surfaced.

17. **What are some of the complications associated with the use of physostigmine?**
    Seizures, cholinergic crisis, bradyarrhythmias, asystole, hypotension, and hypersalivation have all been associated with physostigmine use. In two small case series (N = 20–26), use of physostigmine was associated the seizure activity, although some patients had ingested tricyclic antidepressants. Physostigmine should be used with full understanding of these complications. Physostigmine should never be used for the anticholinergic effects from tricyclic antidepressant overdose because cases have resulted in asystole and death. Relative contraindications include asthma, vascular disease, and gastrointestinal or urinary mechanical obstruction.

18. What is an alternative to physostigmine?

Benzodiazepines should be considered for the treatment of less extreme cases of anticholinergic CNS toxicity.

BIBLIOGRAPHY

1. Burns MJ, Linden CH, Graudins A, et al: A comparison of physostigmine and benzodiazepines for the treatment of anticholinergic poisoning. Ann Emerg Med 35:374–381, 2000.
2. Kirk MA: Anticholinergics and antihistamines. In Haddad LM, Shannon MW, Winchester JF (eds): Clinical Management of Poisoning and Drug Overdose, 3rd ed. Philadelphia, W.B. Saunders, 1998, pp 641–649.
3. Litovitz TL, Klein-Schwartz W, Caravati EM, et al: 1998 Annual report of the American Association of Poison Control Centers Toxic Exposure Surveillance Systems. Am J Emerg Med 17:435–487, 1999.
4. Newton RW: Physostigmine salicylate in the treatment of tricyclic antidepressant overdosage. JAMA 231:941–943, 1975.
5. Shih RD, Goldfrank LR: Plants. In Goldfrank LR, Flomenbaum NE, Lewin NA, et al (eds): Goldfrank's Toxicologic Emergencies, 6th ed. Stamford, CT, Appleton & Lange, 1998, pp 1227–1257.
6. Taylor P: Anticholinesterase agents. In Hardman JG, Limbird LE (eds): Goodman and Gilman's The Pharmacological Basis of Therapeutics, 9th ed. New York, McGraw-Hill, 1996, pp 161–175.
7. Walker WE, Levy RC, Hanenson IB: Physostigmine: Its use and abuse. J Am Coll Emerg Physicians 5:436–439, 1976.

III. Prescription Medications

11. ORAL HYPOGLYCEMICS

Susan E. Farrell, M.D.

1. *Extra credit:* **The first oral hypoglycemic agent, marketed around 1955, was discovered while investigating its antibacterial effects. What was this compound?**
Tolbutamide.

2. What oral agents are available for the treatment of non–insulin-dependent diabetes mellitus (NIDDM)?
The most widely prescribed oral agents for the treatment of hyperglycemia are the sulfonylureas, substituted aryl-sulfonamides. These drugs are true hypoglycemic agents that stimulate insulin release from pancreatic beta cells. The biguanides are antihyperglycemic drugs that work in the presence of insulin to maintain euglycemia. The thizolidinediones, such as troglitazone, also work in the presence of insulin to improve peripheral cell responsiveness to insulin and improve glucose uptake and use by peripheral cells while decreasing hepatic glucose production. Troglitazone has been removed from the U.S. market because of its associated hepatotoxicity. Alpha-glucosidase inhibitors, such as acarbose, decrease gastrointestinal absorption of carbohydrates to lower postprandial systemic glucose concentrations.

3. How do the sulfonylureas work?
Sulfonylureas are the number one cause of drug-induced hypoglycemia. Their primary mechanism of action is the inhibition of adenosine triphosphate (ATP)–sensitive potassium channels on the membrane of pancreatic beta cells, augmenting depolarization of the cell and enhancing the release of endogenous insulin. They also increase peripheral tissue sensitivity to insulin, perhaps by increasing insulin receptors on tissues and by increasing glucose transporters on cell membranes. In addition, they decrease hepatic gluconeogenesis.

4. What are some sulfonylurea agents?
Tolbutamide
Acetohexamide
Chlorpropamide
Gliclazide (Canada)
Glipizide
Glyburide
Tolazamide

5. What is a dangerous dose of a sulfonylurea?
As little as one tablet of a sulfonylurea can cause hypoglycemia in a child.

6. How soon after ingestion of a sulfonylurea can hypoglycemia occur?
Hypoglycemia has been reported to occur anywhere from 30 minutes to many hours post ingestion. There are case reports of hypoglycemia developing 16–24 hours after ingestion, but these patients were being treated with IV dextrose solutions, which may have masked the true onset of hypoglycemia. In one review of accidental pediatric ingestions of sulfonylureas, 98% of patients developed hypoglycemia within 8 hours after ingestion.

7. How long do I have to watch for the onset of hypoglycemia?

Accidental pediatric ingestion of a sulfonylurea should be observed for at least 8 hours. However, because of the rare cases of very delayed hypoglycemia, 24 hours of observation is recommended.

8. What is the treatment for hypoglycemia?

The immediate treatment of hypoglycemia is the administration of glucose. In the patient who is awake and able to eat, a carbohydrate-rich meal will reverse hypoglycemia. In the hypoglycemic patient with altered mental status, emergent intravenous administration of dextrose solution is necessary, initially in bolus doses of 50% dextrose. Glucagon, a polypeptide secreted by the pancreatic alpha cells, increases hepatic gluconeogenesis and glycogenolysis. It has only a transient, inadequate effect in the treatment of hypoglycemia, and adequate glycogen stores are necessary for its glycemic effect. One milligram may be administered intravenously, intramuscularly, or subcutaneously.

9. Besides glucose, is there any other treatment for recurrent refractory hypoglycemia after sulfonylurea ingestion?

Sulfonylurea-induced hypoglycemia has been treated with both diazoxide (Hyperstat) and sandostatin (Octreotide).

Diazoxide is an antihypertensive drug that inhibits insulin release from beta cells by opening potassium channels and preventing beta cell depolarization. Complications include hypotension and sodium and fluid retention. The dose is 200 mg orally or 300 mg IV over 30 minutes.

Sandostatin is an analogue of somatostatin, which inhibits the secretion from both endocrine and exocrine glands. It also inhibits insulin secretion but does not exhibit the side effects of diazoxide. Sandostatin has a longer duration of action in the treatment of sulfonylurea-induced hypoglycemia and reduces the requirement for exogenous dextrose. The dose is 50–100 µg subcutaneously or intravenously.

10. How long does sulfonylurea-induced hypoglycemia persist?

Sulfonylurea-induced hypoglycemia can last for hours, depending on the duration of action of the particular agent. In general, the sulfonylureas are classified as first or second generation. The first-generation agents include acetohexamide, chlorpropamide, tolazamide, and tolbutamide. Their duration of action ranges from 6 hours up to 72 hours for chlorpropamide. The second-generation agents include glipizide and glyburide. Their duration of action ranges from 16 to 24 hours.

11. Who is at particular risk of hypoglycemia after sulfonylurea ingestion?

Children and the elderly who have renal or hepatic dysfunction are at greater risk for hypoglycemia.

12. Is their any other adjunctive treatment for sulfonylurea overdose?

Multiple-dose activated charcoal may be of benefit in enhancing the elimination of glipizide by interrupting its enterohepatic circulation. Urinary alkalization may enhance the elimination of chlorpropamide by ion-trapping of this renally excreted acidic drug. Extracorporeal drug removal by hemodialysis or hemoperfusion has been reported but is not of proven benefit because of the degree of protein binding of these agents.

13. What is the mechanism of action of the biguanides?

Metformin is the only biguanide currently approved for the treatment of NIDDM in the United States. It is usually used in combination with insulin or a sulfonylurea. Biguanides exert their antihyperglycemic effect by increasing glucose uptake, particularly into muscle cells, by increasing glucose metabolism to lactate in the intestine, by decreasing hepatic gluconeogenesis, and by decreasing glucose absorption from the intestine.

14. Why is there only one biguanide agent?

Phenformin was another biguanide but was withdrawn from the U.S. in 1976 because of an unacceptably high rate of refractory lactic acidosis. Metformin also causes lactic acidosis but at a much lower rate.

15. Do biguanides cause hypoglycemia?

No. In and of themselves, biguanides do not cause hypoglycemia in overdose or in therapeutic doses. That is why they are more correctly referred to as **antihyperglycemics**.

16. What toxicity can I expect from the biguanides?

The primary toxicity of the biguanide agents is the development of a type B lactic acidosis. Because they increase the nonoxidative use of glucose and production of lactate, they can cause systemic lactic acidosis when they accumulate in the body. Phenformin, the prototypic biguanide, was discontinued in the U.S. in 1976 because of its toxicity. Metformin (Glucophage) has a lower incidence of this particular toxicity.

17. Who is at increased risk for lactic acidosis from metformin use?

Because metformin is renally excreted, patients with renal insufficiency are at risk for drug accumulation and subsequent lactic acidosis. Case reports of metformin overdose are rare, but presumably accumulation of the drug after overdose will also cause lactic acidosis.

18. What is the treatment for biguanide toxicity?

Treatment of biguanide-induced lactic acidosis is primarily supportive, with attention to correction of the acid-base abnormalities. Hemodialysis has been used to enhance drug removal and treat the acidemia.

19. *Extra credit:* Insulin that has been exogenously administered can be found in patients with high insulin levels along with low levels of what quantitative marker substance?

C peptide.

BIBLIOGRAPHY

1. Bailey CJ: Metformin: An update. Gen Pharmacol 24:1299–1309, 1993.
2. Boyle PJ, Justice K, Krentz AJ, et al: Octreotide reverses hyperinsulinemia and prevents hypoglycemia induced by sulfonylurea overdoses. J Clin Endocrinol Metabol 76:752–756, 1993.
3. Ciechanowski K, Borowiak KS, Potocka BA, et al: Chlorpropamide toxicity with survival despite 27-day hypoglycemia. J Toxicol Clin Toxicol 37:869–871, 1999.
4. Cook DL: The β-cell response to oral hypoglycemic agents. Diabetes Res Clin Prac 28(Suppl):S81–S89, 1995.
5. Erickson T, Arora A, Lebby TI, et al: Acute oral hypoglycemic ingestions. Vet Hum Toxicol 33:256–258, 1991.
6. Gan SC, Barr J, Arieff AI, Pearl RG: Biguanide-associated lactic acidosis: Case report and review of the literature. Arch Intern Med 152:2333–2336, 1992.
7. Klonoff DC, Barrett BJ, Nolte MS, et al: Hypoglycemia following inadvertent and factitious sulfonylurea overdosages. Diabetes Care 18:563–566, 1995.
8. Lalau JD, Lacroix C, Compagnon P, et al: Role of metformin accumulation in metformin-associated lactic acidosis. Diabetes Care 18:779–784, 1995.
9. Moore DF, Wood DF, Volans GN: Features, prevention and management of acute overdose due to antidiabetic drugs. Drug Safety 9:218–229, 1993.
10. Murray L: Oral hypoglycemic agents. In Haddad LM, Shannon MW, Winchester JF (eds): Clinical Management of Poisoning and Drug Overdose, 3rd ed. Philadelphia, W.B. Saunders, 1998, pp 650–655.
11. Quadrani DA, Spiller HA, Widder P: Five-year retrospective evaluation of sulfonylurea ingestion in children. J Toxicol Clin Toxicol 34:267–272, 1996.
12. Spiller HA, Villalobos D, Krenzelok EF, et al: Prospective multicenter study of sulfonylurea ingestion in children. J Pediatr 131:141–146, 1997.
13. Szlatenyi CS, Capes KF, Wang RY: Delayed hypoglycemia in a child after ingestion of a single glipizide tablet. Ann Emerg Med 31:773–776, 1998.

12. ANTICONVULSANTS

Robert J. Hoffman, M.D.

1. How do anticonvulsants prevent seizures?

Generally speaking, anticonvulsants prevent seizures by raising the seizure threshold, decreasing activity of epileptogenic foci, or both. They all work in the central nervous system (CNS) to either increase inhibitory tone or decrease excitatory tone. The CNS is perpetually balanced somewhere between coma (sedation) and seizure (excitation). Fortunately, most people maintain the appropriate balance between the two.

2. *Extra credit:* What inorganic substance was the earliest of the more commonly used anticonvulsants?

Bromide.

3. What are the mechanisms of action of the anticonvulsants?

The excitatory system involves glutamate as a neurotransmitter, and excitation is transduced through the N-methyl-d-aspartate (NMDA) receptors and sodium channels in CNS neurons. Sedation results predominantly from gamma-aminobutyric acid (GABA) as a neurotransmitter, which is transduced through GABA receptors.

Mechanism of Action of Anticonvulsants

DRUG	MECHANISM OF ACTION	CLINICAL RESULT
Barbiturate	↑ Cl⁻ influx at GABA receptor	↑ sedation
Benzodiazepine	↑ Cl⁻ influx at GABA receptor	↑ sedation
Carbamazepine	Prolonged Na⁺ channel inactivation	↓ excitation
	Adenosine agonism	↑ sedation
Ethosuximide	Unknown	Unknown
Felbamate	Blocks NMDA receptors	↓ excitation
	Prolonged Na⁺ channel inactivation	↓ excitation
	↑ GABA activity	↑ sedation
Gabapentin	↑ GABA activity	↑ sedation
Lamotrigine	Inhibition of glutamate and aspartate	↓ excitation
	Prolonged Na⁺ channel inactivation	↓ excitation
	↑ GABA activity	↑ sedation
Phenytoin	Prolonged Na⁺ channel inactivation	↓ excitation
	↑ adenosine agonism	↑ sedation
Topiramate	Prolonged Na⁺ channel inactivation	↓ excitation
	↑ GABA activity	↑ sedation
Valproic acid	Prolonged Na⁺ channel inactivation	↓ excitation
	↑ GABA activity	↑ sedation
Vigabatrin	↑ GABA activity	↑ sedation

4. Are there any common presentations of anticonvulsant toxicity?

Typically, CNS symptomatology manifests. Sedation or confusion, dizziness, nystagmus, and ataxia are all suggestive of anticonvulsant toxicity, and any of these problems in a patient being treated with anticonvulsants should immediately suggest toxicity. Additionally, seizure may result from carbamazepine overdose in any patient; seizure also may result from phenytoin overdose but only in epileptic patients.

5. What are the therapeutic serum concentrations for anticonvulsants?

ANTICONVULSANT	THERAPEUTIC SERUM CONCENTRATIONS	
	mg/L	μmol/L
Carbamazepine	4–12	17–51
Ethosuximide	40–100	283–708
Phenobarbital	15–40	65–172
Phenytoin	10–20	40–79
Valproic acid	50–120	347–833

6. How does chronic anticonvulsant toxicity occur and manifest?

Chronic toxicity typically is caused by a change in drug dosing or drug metabolism, which may result from illness or drug-drug interaction after the patient starts or stops taking medications in addition to their anticonvulsants. Chronic toxicity typically results in the insidious onset of symptoms such as confusion, sedation, dizziness, nystagmus, and ataxia.

7. How do drug-drug interactions affect anticonvulsant pharmacokinetics?

Patients who take multiple medications experience several possible effects. Always keep this in mind in symptomatic patients who recently have changed medications.

Drug Interactions of Anticonvulsants

DRUG	INCREASES LEVEL OF	DECREASES LEVEL OF	ANTICONVULSANT EFFECT DECREASED
Carbamazepine	None known	Doxycycline Felbamate Haloperidol Lamotrigine Phenytoin Primidone Valproic acid Warfarin	Benzodiazepines Felbamate Phenobarbital Phenytoin Primidone Valproic acid
Felbamate	Carbamazepine Phenytoin Valproic acid	Carbamazepine	Carbamazepine Phenytoin
Gabapentin	None known	None known	None known
Lamotrigine	None known	None known	Carbamazepine Pehnobarbital Phenytoin
Phenobarbital	Valproic acid	Carbamazepine Contraceptives Corticosteroids Doxycycline Griseofulvin Lamotrigine Phenytoin Propranolol Quinidine Theophylline Valproic acid Warfarin	Ammonium chloride Antacids Folic acid Pyridoxine Warfarin

(Table continued on next page.)

Drug Interactions of Anticonvulsants (cont.)

DRUG	INCREASES LEVEL OF	DECREASES LEVEL OF	ANTICONVULSANT EFFECT DECREASED
Phenytoin	Primidone Warfarin	Amiodarone Carbamazepine Contraceptives Corticosteroids Cyclosporine Disopyramide Doxycycline Furosemide Levodopa Theophylline Tolbutamide Valproic acid	Calcium Diazepam Diazoxide Ethanol Folic acid Phenobarbital Rifampin Sulcrafate Theophylline Vigabatrin
Valproic acid	Felbamate Lamotrigine Phenobarbital Primidone	Carbamazepine	Carbamazepine Phenobarbital Phenytoin Primidone
Vigabatrin	None known	Phenytoin	None known

8. Which anticonvulsants are cardiotoxic?

Phenytoin is a class IB antidysrhythmic. Interestingly, most cardiac dysrhythmias and cardiac arrests resulting from phenytoin are the result of both its antidysrhythmic activity and adverse reaction to the propylene glycol diluent in parenteral phenytoin preparations. This cardiotoxicity is related to the rate of infusion of intravenous phenytoin and is the reason intravenous phenytoin loading typically is performed over a 20–40-minute period of time. Cardiotoxicity has never been reported as a result of oral phenytoin overdose.

Carbamazepine is particularly cardiotoxic, a function of its structural similarity to tricyclic antidepressants (TCAs) and its ability to block sodium channels. Carbamazepine toxicity can result in QRS complex widening, atrioventricular (AV) block, and ventricular arrhythmias, similar to TCA overdose, and they are treated in the same manner—with sodium bicarbonate bolus and infusion.

Valproic acid is known to cause cardiac arrest in overdose, but the mechanism is unclear.

9. *Extra credit:* Hirsutism is common in patients who have taken what anticonvulsant for long periods of time?

Diphenylhydantoin or phenytoin.

10. What are the clinical manifestations of phenytoin toxicity?

Phenytoin toxicity typically results in progressively more severe symptoms as the serum phenytoin concentration increases. Dizziness and nystagmus (> 15 µg/ml), ataxia (> 30 µg/ml), lethargy and confusion (> 40 µg/ml), dysarthria, vomiting, choreoathetoid movements, hyperactive deep tendon reflexes, and ophthalmoplegia are seen. Hypotension, bradycardia, and cardiac arrest may be seen with intravenous infusion. Oral suspension administered intravenously may cause anaphylaxis or cardiac arrest.

11. How is phenytoin toxicity treated?

- Supportive care and observation
- Cardiac monitoring to detect cardiac conduction abnormality or dysrhythmia in the event that the phenytoin was administered intravenously
- Possibly, enhanced elimination of phenytoin with multiple-dose activated charcoal

12. What are the clinical manifestations of carbamazepine toxicity?

Symptoms of carbamazepine toxicity do not readily correlate with serum carbamazepine concentrations. Levels above 40 mg/L, however, do tend to be associated with increased incidence of coma, seizures, and cardiotoxicity.

Nystagmus, ataxia, dysarthria, stupor, encephalopathy, myoclonus, dystonia, choreoathetosis, and seizures may result from acute or chronic toxicity. Acute carbamazepine toxicity may cause nausea, vomiting, hypothermia, hypotension, tachycardia, and cardiac conduction abnormalities. Children tend to manifest a higher incidence of dystonia, choreoathetosis, and seizures and a lower incidence of cardiotoxicity.

Less common adverse effects of chronic administration include the syndrome of inappropriate antidiuretic hormone release (SIADH), Stevens-Johnson syndrome, lupus-like syndrome, aplastic anemia, and fatal eosinophilic myocarditis.

13. What is the treatment for carbamazepine toxicity?

- Supportive care and observation
- Cardiac monitoring to detect cardiac conduction abnormality or dysrhythmia
- Possibly, enhanced elimination of carbamazepine with multiple-dose activated charcoal

14. What are the clinical manifestations of valproic acid toxicity?

Acute toxicity from valproic acid may result in gastrointestinal and neurologic disturbances. Nausea, vomiting, mild to moderate elevation of liver enzymes, and rarely pancreatitis may occur. CNS toxicity may cause mild sedation, coma, toxic encephalopathy, or fatal cerebral edema. Ataxia, hypertonia, and tremor may also occur. Respiratory failure is common in patients with severe valproic acid overdose, and cardiac arrest may occur independently of this.

15. How is valproic acid toxicity treated?

- As usual, treatment begins with supportive care and observation.
- If an enteric-coated preparation of valproic acid is ingested, whole-bowel irrigation may be necessary.
- Reports indicate that CNS depression may respond to naloxone, which may be given to patients who are not tolerant of opioids.
- Carnitine supplementation should be given to hyperammonemic patients receiving valproic acid.
- Treatment also may include enhanced elimination of valproic acid with multiple-dose activated charcoal.

16. What metabolic disturbances are associated with valproic acid toxicity?

Valproic acid combines with carnitine to form a metabolite that is excreted in the urine, and hypocarnitinemia may result from acute or chronic valproic acid overdose. Hyperammonemia and hypocarnitinemia are both associated with valproic acid exposure. Hypocarnitinemia may be associated with hyperammonemia. This hyperammonemia is not a result of hepatotoxicity and does not correlate with encephalopathy as it does in other medical states.

Chronic toxicity and adverse effects of chronic valproic acid use may result in hepatic steatosis similar to Reye's syndrome or fatal hepatitis. Leukopenia and thrombocytopenia are also results of chronic valproic acid use, although they technically are not metabolic effects.

17. How are toxic levels of anticonvulsants reduced by enhanced elimination?

Typically, the treatment consists of discontinuation of the anticonvulsant, supportive care and observation, serial assessment of serum anticonvulsant concentration, and resumption of anticonvulsant use when the patient has a therapeutic anticonvulsant level.

Patients who do not have a seizure disorder are not harmed by decreasing the serum anticonvulsant concentration, and multiple-dose activated charcoal may be used to lower serum levels of phenytoin, carbamazepine, valproic acid, and phenobarbital. Charcoal hemoperfusion and hemodialysis are of little or no benefit and are not indicated.

In patients who do have a seizure disorder, the serum anticonvulsant concentration should be actively lowered with extreme caution because decreasing the serum anticonvulsant concentration to a subtherapeutic level may precipitate seizures.

18. What are the adverse reactions and clinical manifestations of toxicity from newer anticonvulsants?

Toxic Effects of Newer Anticonvulsants

ETHOSUXIMIDE	GABAPENTIN	LAMOTRIGINE	TOPIRAMATE	VIGABATRIN
Sedation	Ataxia	Ataxia	Ataxia	Sedation
Vomiting/diarrhea	Slurred speech	Nystagmus	Dizziness	Psychosis
Psychosis	Dizziness	Stevens-Johnson	Diplopia	
Stevens-Johnson	Sedation	syndrome*	Sedation	
syndrome*		Life-threatening	Confusion	
Aplastic anemia*		rash*	Weight loss*	
Lupus-like				
syndrome*				

* Effects are either idiosyncratic or result from chronic exposure; they are *not* expected from acute overdose.

19. Other than preventing and treating seizures, what are anticonvulsants used for?

Other medical and psychiatric purposes include:
- Chronic pain
- Hyperactivity
- Addictive behaviors (e.g., cocaine abuse)
- Other psychiatric and behavioral disorders (e.g., bipolar disorder, pervasive developmental disorder)

20. How do seizures from drug overdose differ from epileptic seizures?

Seizures that result from a drug overdose are radically different from seizures with an epileptogenic focus. Toxic exposure or drug overdose causes a global effect in the CNS that leads to seizure, whereas in epileptogenic seizures, one particular area of the brain has aberrant activity that predisposes it to seizures. In cases of epilepsy, the appropriate strategy of seizure control is to decrease the electrical activity in that particular area. In the case of overdose, the patient needs a global increase in CNS inhibitory tone.

21. How are seizures that result from drug overdose managed?

Practically speaking, the difference between treatment for epileptogenic seizures and treatment for toxic exposure seizures is the drugs used to treat the seizures. In overdose, the first line of therapy is administration of parenteral benzodiazepines such as lorazepam, midazolam, or diazepam; barbiturates follow as the second line of therapy. Classically, phenobarbital has been used, but it has a delayed onset of action and peak action, and clinical effects may not become evident for 45–60 minutes. Pentobarbital and secobarbital are also appropriate choices because they are quicker acting. Other treatment options include sedative-hypnotics such as propofol, and, ultimately, general anesthetics may be considered as treatment for status epilepticus.

22. What is the role of phenytoin in treating toxin-induced seizures?

There isn't one. Although phenytoin and fosphenytoin are routinely used for epilepsy and status epilepticus, these agents are not effective in treating toxin-induced seizures. In fact, phenytoin may worsen clinical outcome and, in some cases, may make death from overdose more likely.

23. Which poisons cause toxic seizures that require unique treatments?

Special Cases of Seizures from Overdose

SEIZURE CAUSE	TREATMENT
Isoniazid and certain mushrooms (e.g., *Gyromitra* species)	Pyridoxine (vitamin B_6)
Anticholinergic agents	Physostigmine
Carbamates and organophosphages (e.g., nerve gases)	Atropine and pralidoxime
Hypoglycemia	Dextrose

BIBLIOGRAPHY

1. Alberto G, Erickson T, Popiel R, et al: Central nervous system manifestations of a valproic acid overdose responsive to naloxone. Ann Emerg Med 18:889–891, 1989.
2. Farrar HC, Harold DA, Reed MD: Acute valproic acid intoxication: Enhanced drug clearance with oral-activated charcoal. Crit Care Med 21:299–301, 1993.
3. Fischer JH, Barr AN, Rogers SL, et al: Lack of serious toxicity following gabapentin overdose. Neurology 44:982–983, 1994.
4. Ishikura H, Matsuo N, Matsubara I, et al: Valproic acid overdose and L-carnitine therapy. J Anal Toxicol 20:55–58, 1996.
5. Karsarkis EJ, Kuo CS, Berger R, et al: Carbamazepine-induced cardiac dysfunction. Characterization of two distinct clinical syndromes. Arch Intern Med 152:186–191, 1992.
6. Mauro LS, Mauro V, Brown D, et al: Enhancement of phenytoin elimination by multiple dose activated charcoal. Ann Emerg Med 16:1132–1135, 1987.
7. McQuay H, Carroll D, Jadad AR, et al: Anticonvulsant drugs for management of pain: A systematic review. Br Med J 311:1047–1052, 1995.
8. Mellick LB, Morgan JM, Austen WG: Presentations of acute phenytoin overdose. Ann Emerg Med 7:61–67, 1989.
9. Spiller HA, Krenzelok EP, Cookson E: Carbamazepine overdose: A prospective study of serum levels and toxicity. J Toxicol Clin Toxicol 28:445–458, 1990.
10. Wyte CD, Berk WA: Severe oral phenytoin overdose does not cause cardiovascular morbidity. Ann Emerg Med 20:508–512, 1991.

13. ANTICOAGULANTS

Carson R. Harris, M.D.

1. What are the categories of anticoagulants?

Hydroxycourmarin anticoagulants:	*Indanedione anticoagulants:*
Fumarin	Valone
Warfarin	Pindone
Coumachlor	Diphacinone
Bromadiolone	Chlorphacinone
Brodifacoum	

2. What does sweet clover have to do with anticoagulants?

In the early 1920s, livestock was inadvertently fed moldy sweet clover hay and developed hemorrhagic bleeding disorders. It was later discovered that the coumarin in sweet clover is oxidized to the anticoagulant 4-bishydroxycoumarin by fungi in moldy sweet clover, which caused the bleeding.

3. What are the usual circumstances of anticoagulant ingestion or overdose?

Accidental and suicidal intent are the usual circumstance of anticoagulant poisoning.

4. Name some uncommon circumstances of poisoning.

Herbal tea preparations, especially tonka beans, melilot, and woodruff, may lead to hemorrhagic diathesis. Coumarin contamination of herbal tea purchased outside the United States has been reported. Contaminated talcum powder was responsible for the death of 177 infants in Ho Chi Minh City (Saigon) in 1981 through transdermal absorption. In addition, homicidal anticoagulant poisoning has been attempted.

5. How does warfarin anticoagulant overdose cause toxicity?

Oral anticoagulants inhibit the synthesis of vitamin K1-dependent clotting factors (factors II, VII, IX, and X) by the liver. (Remember the clotting cascade?) The existing clotting factors are not affected, but, once they are degraded, no new factors are produced. The rate of degradation occurs at different rates with factor VII (proconvertin) being the first to decrease in the plasma, followed by factors IX (Christmas factor), X (Stuart factor), and II (prothrombin). Once these factors are significantly reduced, clinical effects become apparent (usually 2–3 days).

6. *Extra credit:* The name *warfarin* is actually an acronym of the name of the patent holder plus the suffix from the word *coumarin*. Who is the patent holder of this anticoagulant?

Wisconsin Alumni Research Foundation.

7. Where does bleeding occur with an anticoagulant overdose?

Overdose with anticoagulants typically leads to bleeding in multiple organ sites. The more common sites seen are the genitourinary and gastrointestinal (GI) tracts. Central nervous system and respiratory system bleeding may manifest as stroke, epistaxis, or hemoptysis.

8. Are there any abnormal laboratory tests with an anticoagulant overdose?

Abnormal laboratory tests include leukocytosis, anemia, prolonged bleeding time, elevated prothrombin time (PT), and activated partial thromboplastin time (PTT). Platelets are usually normal as are liver function tests. Rarely do coumarin anticoagulants cause elevation of liver enzymes.

9. What are superwarfarins? How do they differ from warfarin?

The superwarfarins are long-acting anticoagulants primarily used in rodenticides and are 4-hydroxycoumarin derivatives with a 4-bromo (1,1-biphenyl) side chain. Superwarfarins have far longer action on vitamin K–dependent clotting factors than warfarin, and vitamin K therapy may be required for 2–3 months instead of days. They diminish vitamin K–dependent gamma-carboxylation of glutamic acid residues in prothrombin factor precursors that are 100 times greater on a molar basis than that of warfarin. In addition, they may have a half-life up to 120 days (warfarin, 42 hours). Animal studies suggest that one-time ingestions of brodifacoum rat bait can cause clinical bleeding as well as severe coagulation abnormalities that require large doses of vitamin K_1 and that can last months; in contrast, a single ingestion of warfarin-containing bait does not usually induce abnormalities in coagulation.

10. Name some nonmedicinal agents that contain anticoagulants.

	ANTICOAGULANT	PRODUCT
Hydroxycourmarin Anticoagulants	Fumarin	Coumarfuryl, Rat-A-Way, Tomarin, Lurat, Kill-Ko Rat, Mouse Blues, Ratafin, Fumasol, Krumkil
	Warfarin	d-Con, Warf, Dethmor, Warfarat, Dethnel, Rosex, Solfarin, Rattunal, Marfrin, Ratorex, Coumafene, Zoocoumarin, Kypfarin, Warficide, Ratox, Rax, Rodex, Tox-Hid, Liqua-Tox, Eraze, Final, Banaret, Sorexa-Plus, Biotro
	Coumachlor	Tomorin, Ratilan, Coumachlore, G-2G-23133
	Bromadiolone	Maki, Deadline, Bromone, Super-Cais, Contrac, Temus, Candien 1500, Ratimus, Sup'operates
	Brodifacoum	Talon, Havoc, PP-581, Volid, Volak, Klerat, Matikus, WBA 8119
Indanedione Anticoagulants	Valone	P.M.P., Isoval, Isotrac, Incco, Motomco, Tracking Powder
	Pindone	Pival, Pivalyn, Tri-Ban, Pivacin, Chemrat, Pivaldione, Paracakes, Contrax-P
	Diphacinone	Diphacin, PID, Diphenadione, Ramik, Promar, PCQ, Contrax-D, Rodent Cake, Kill-Ko, Rat Bait
	Chlorphacinone	Rozol, Liphdione, Caid, Delta, Drat, Quick, Microzul, Muriol, Ramucide, Afnor, LM-91, Topitox, Raviac, Ratomet, Rozol Tracking Powder

11. Which drug interactions cause excess anticoagulation?

Common drugs leading to excess anticoagulation include those that inhibit warfarin metabolism: cimetidine, ciprofloxacin, trimethoprim-sulfamethoxazole, erythromycin, and metronidazole. Other drug interactions resulting in increased anticoagulation include propranolol, piroxicam, and omeprazole.

12. How do I treat a patient with an accidental warfarin or superwarfarin ingestion?

Because most accidental or one-time ingestions of plain warfarin-related or superwarfarin-related rodenticides are pretty limited, they will not require GI decontamination and will not need emergency department management or admission to the hospital. A PT is unnecessary if the patient is clinically asymptomatic. The patient or parents should be advised to watch for signs of bleeding or bruising.

13. What is the initial management of a person with an intentional ingestion of an anticoagulant?

Patients who intentionally overdose generally ingest quite a bit and should be monitored in an intensive care setting, especially if they present with acute bleeding. Remember that airway obstruction can occur from severe epistaxis or oropharyngeal bleeding. The PT, complete blood count, and activated PTT should be checked. The PT may be obtained every 12 hours for 48 hours even if the baseline PT is minimally prolonged.

14. What about GI decontamination in these patients?

Gut decontamination must be approached with caution. Emesis induced by syrup of ipecac could raise intracranial pressure and lead to CNS bleeding. Emesis also may cause significant GI hemorrhage. Insertion of a gastric lavage tube could cause oropharyngeal, esophageal, and gastric bleeding; therefore, it should be done with care and caution. Activated charcoal (50–100 gm for adults; 15–50 gm for children) in an aqueous slurry may be administered through the lavage tube.

15. Are there any methods to enhance elimination?

Cholestyramine, 12–16 gm daily in divided doses, may reduce the half-life by interrupting the enterohepatic recirculation of warfarin and increasing the total clearance of oral anticoagulants. Forced diuresis, hemodialysis, hemoperfusion, and peritoneal dialysis have not been effective. Exchange transfusions may be effective in a life-threatening overdose.

16. How do I manage a patient who is actively bleeding after overdosing on a warfarin anticoagulant?

For severe hemorrhage, the deficient clotting factors (II, VII, IX, and X) must be replaced. This can be achieved by giving whole blood or plasma (fresh frozen plasma). Vitamin K_1 (phytonadione) is useful in reversing deficiencies in vitamin K-dependent coagulation factors II, VII, IX, and X, restoring the PT to normal levels, and decreasing or stopping the bleeding episodes.

17. How do you administer vitamin K_1 for superwarfarin ingestion?

Vitamin K_1 (phytonadione, Mephyton) can be administered orally, subcutaneously, intramuscularly, and intravenously. The oral route is best because a maximal subcutaneous or IM dose is 5 ml per injection site. If there is uncertainty about the amount ingested, vitamin K_1 may be given orally (15–25 mg for adults; for children under 12, give 5–10 mg) 3–4 times daily. If a parenteral dose is necessary, colloidal solution of phytonadione, Aquamephyton, may be given subcutaneously, intramuscularly (5–10 mg for adults; 1–5 mg for children under 12), or diluted and given intravenously at a slow rate not to exceed 1 mg/min in adults. Doses up to 100–125 mg/day for many weeks or months may be required in a severe rodenticide overdose.

18. How often should I check the PT?

The PT or international normalized ration (INR) should be monitored every 6–12 hours initially to gauge treatment effect. In most cases, bleeding is usually controlled in 3–6 hours but may take longer. PTs often will not begin to return to normal for at least 3–4 days.

19. What happens if vitamin K_1 is given too rapidly by intravenous route?

The IV route has been noted to cause anaphylactoid reactions. The patient may experience flushing, cyanosis, dizziness, hypotension, and bronchoconstriction. Anaphylactoid reactions may occur during or a few minutes after direct intravenous infusion of undiluted vitamin K_1. Cerebral thrombosis and death have been associated with intravenous and intramuscular administration of vitamin K.

20. What other treatment may be used to reverse a coumarin overdose?

Factor II-IX-X concentrate may be used in conjunction with intravenous vitamin K_1 (2.5 mg). Maximal effect is typically noted at 30 minutes with improvement of the PT and PTT.

Factor II-IX-X concentrate is more easily controlled but carries a risk of serious blood-borne diseases such as hepatitis and AIDS. It is, therefore, reserved for patients with life-threatening hemorrhage.

21. What rashes or skin conditions are associated with warfarins?

Other than ecchymosis and purpura from overanticoagulation, macular, papular, vesicular, urticarial, and purpuric skin lesions can occur. Skin necrosis is an idiosyncratic reaction that tends to occur in obese women on anticoagulant therapy for thromboembolism. Necrosis typically appears about 3–6 days after initiation of therapy and predominantly in the adipose tissue of the thighs, breasts, and buttocks. Therapy is primarily supportive.

22. What is the "purple toe" syndrome?

Systemic cholesterol microembolization may be seen in patients on anticoagulant therapy.

23. Describe the anticoagulant side effects of heparin.

Heparin neutralizes thrombin by an interaction with antithrombin III heparin cofactor prolonging the PTT. Heparin also inhibits platelet function, increases vascular wall permeability, inhibits the proliferation of vascular smooth muscle cells, and inhibits delayed hypersensitivity reactions. Heparin-induced thrombosis-thrombocytopenia syndrome has a 30% mortality rate and is associated with thrombotic and hemorrhagic complications.

24. Does heparin have nonbleeding side effects?

Hyperkalemia may occur when patients have been given 3 or more days of heparin therapy through inhibition of aldosterone production. Decreases in aldosterone levels may result in decreased excretion of potassium. Elevation of serum potassium levels occurs in about 7% of patients. It is reversible once heparin is discontinued.

25. What are LMWHs?

Low–molecular-weight heparins (LMWHs) have been separated with an average molecular weight of 4000–6500. They have an attenuated effect on coagulation and prolongation of the activated PTT compared with unfractionated heparin. Enoxaparin (Lovenox), dalteparin (Fragmin), and ardeparin (Normiflo) are approved LMWH products in the U.S.

26. Define the heparin flush syndrome.

The heparin flush syndrome is seen when the heparin solution used to "flush" arterial and venous catheters to maintain patency and vascular access is unmonitored, leading to an iatrogenic hemorrhage.

27. What is the treatment for heparin overdose?

Discontinuation of heparin. Because heparin has a short half-life, cases of minor bleeding are of no consequence.

28. *Extra credit:* Protamine sulfate is an approved antidote for the hemorrhagic effects of heparin overdose. What is the natural source of this antidotal substance?

It is derived from the sperm of salmon and other related species of fish.

29. What is the role of protamine?

If bleeding is severe or a significant heparin overdose has been administered, protamine sulfate should be considered. The neutralization of heparin by intravenous injection of protamine sulfate is rapid and takes less than 1 minute. The dose of protamine sulfate is about 1 mg for each 100 U of heparin administered. If 1 hour has elapsed since the heparin injection, 0.5–0.75 mg of protamine sulfate can be given for every 100 U of heparin; if more than 2 hours have elapsed, 0.25–0.375 mg of protamine sulfate can be given for each 100 U of heparin.

BIBLIOGRAPHY

1. Akle CA, Joiner CL: Purple toe syndrome. J R Soc Med 74:219, 1981.
2. Ellenhorn MJ, Schonwald S, Ordog G, et al (eds): Ellenhorn's Medical Toxicology: Diagnosis and Treatment of Human Poisoning, 2nd ed. Baltimore, Williams & Wilkins, 1997.
3. Hoffman RS: Anticoagulants. In Goldfrank LR, Flomenbaum NE, Lewin NA, et al (eds): Goldfrank's Toxicologic Emergencies, 6th ed. Stamford, CT, Appleton & Lange, 1998, pp 703–726.
4. Hui CH, Lie A, Lam CK, Bourke C: "Superwarfarin" poisoning leading to prolonged coagulopathy. Forensic Sci Int 78:13–18, 1996.
5. Jähnchen E, Meinertz T, Gilfrich HJ, et al: Enhanced elimination of warfarin during treatment with cholestyramine. Br J Clin Pharmacol 5:437–440, 1978.
6. Norcross WA, Ganiats TG, Ralph LP, et al: Accidental poisoning by warfarin-contaminated herbal tea. West J Med 159:80–82, 1993.
7. Puschner B, Galey FD, Holstege DM, Palazoglu M: Sweet clover poisoning in dairy cattle in California. J Am Vet Med Assoc 212:857–859, 1998.
8. Renowden S, Westmoreland D, White JP, Routledge PA: Oral cholestyramine increases elimination of warfarin after overdose. Br Med J (Clin Res Ed) 291:513–514, 1985.
9. Ridker PM: Toxic effects of herbal teas. Arch Environ Health 42:133–136, 1987.

14. ANTIHYPERTENSIVE MEDICATIONS

Andrew Topliff, M.D.

1. What types agents are used as antihypertensives?
- Beta blockers
- Calcium channel blockers
- Angiotensin-converting enzyme (ACE) inhibitors
- Alpha$_2$ agonists
- Sympatholytic antihypertensives (ganglionic blockers, peripheral adrenergic neuron blockers, peripheral alpha$_1$-adrenergic antagonists)
- Vasodilators
- Diuretics

2. What types of antihypertensives are considered the most dangerous?
Beta blockers and calcium channel blockers have been associated with the most deaths (see Chapter 18, Beta Blockers, and Chapter 19, Calcium Channel Blockers).

3. *Extra credit:* Which antihypertensive agent has a side effect desired by some individuals suffering from alopecia?
Minoxidil.

4. Describe the general therapeutic measures for antihypertensive overdose.
Typical symptoms of antihypertensives involve hypotension sometimes accompanied by bradycardia and altered mental status. The patient is assessed in terms of total clinical presentation; for example, is there a need for intubation? Hypotension is best addressed by the administration of intravenous fluid unless there are signs of fluid overload. Catecholamines also may be used to support blood pressure. Bradycardia may not be the main cause of underlying hypotension (contractility and vasodilation may be more important mechanisms), but sometimes it can be improved by the administration of atropine or catecholamines with significant beta$_1$ effects. In the setting of certain drug overdoses, other special modalities may be considered such as calcium, glucagon, or high-dosage insulin and glucose administration.

5. What symptoms are seen in beta blocker or calcium channel blocker overdose?
The most common symptoms include hypotension, bradycardia, and conduction delays and other arrhythmias. In beta blocker overdose, mental status changes are fairly common, and occasionally seizures are seen.

6. How do ACE inhibitors work?
These widely prescribed drugs inhibit the conversion of angiotensin I to angiotensin II in the lung. Angiotensin II is a potent vasoconstrictor and is responsible for the stimulation of aldosterone release. Thus, ACE inhibitors cause some direct vasodilation and also inhibit sodium and water retention secondary to aldosterone effects.

7. How does ACE inhibitor overdose present?
Severe toxicity in the setting of an ACE inhibitor is rare but occurs occasionally, most commonly in the setting of coingestants. Hypotension may occur, but death caused solely by ACE inhibitor overdose is rare.

8. How is ACE inhibitor overdose treated?

Charcoal administration for decontamination and fluids as needed. Occasionally, naloxone is helpful in reversing hypotension. Pressors are required rarely in pure ACE inhibitor overdose.

9. Are there any other special considerations about ACE inhibitors?

ACE inhibitors can cause life-threatening angioedema, likely by bradykinin-mediated mechanisms. These symptoms frequently involve the tongue and oropharynx but can occur in any part of the body even after the individual has been on the medication for months. Patients typically do not respond to the standard therapies of antihistamines, steroids, and epinephrine and may require emergent early intubation (and obviously the discontinuation of the medication).

10. How do clonidine and other alpha$_2$ agonists decrease blood pressure?

Alpha$_2$ agonists such as clonidine, guanabenz, and guanfacine work by stimulating postsynaptic alpha$_2$ receptors, primarily in the central nervous system (CNS). This enhances inhibitory neuronal activity and leads to decreased sympathetic outflow. Peripheral alpha$_2$ receptors are also affected but to a lesser degree.

11. What symptoms are seen in clonidine overdose?

The most common signs include bradycardia, hypotension (transient hypertension may be seen first), and CNS depression. These symptoms tend to develop quickly after ingestion (< 90 minutes). Miosis and decreased respiratory drive may be seen, similar to opiate overdose. Occasionally, cardiac conduction delays may occur.

12. What is the therapy for alpha$_2$-agonist overdose?

As with any overdose, the general clinical status of the patient (ABCs) and general decontamination issues must be addressed first. Transient hypertension (unless severe) should not be treated. If treatment is needed, a short-lived, titratable antihypertensive (e.g., nitroprusside) should be used because the transient hypertension is likely to be rapidly replaced by significant hypotension. Pressors may be used as indicated for hypotension.

13. Are there any other specific therapies for alpha$_2$-agonist overdose?

Because the toxidrome of alpha$_2$-agonist overdose is similar to the opiate toxidrome, patients sometimes respond to the administration of naloxone for poorly understood reasons. Given the short half-life of naloxone (approximately 30 minutes), repeat dosing may be required for a continued response.

14. Are there other antihypertensives that also work by CNS-mediated mechanisms?

Methyldopa is a prodrug of metabolites with alpha$_2$-agonist activity. Toxicity is similar but may be delayed in acute overdose secondary to the time needed for metabolic conversion to active agents.

15. What other kinds of sympatholytic antihypertensive agents exist?

Other types of sympatholytic agents may have an effect at the ganglia or may decrease norepinephrine release from distal nerve terminals. Trimethaphan is a ganglion-blocking agent that inhibits sympathetic and parasympathetic activity. Similar agents exist that are not used in this country. Guanethidine, guanadrel, and reserpine are peripheral adrenergic blocking agents that interfere with catecholamine release from nerve end terminals. Reserpine crosses the blood-brain barrier easily and may result in significant CNS depression.

16. How do alpha$_1$ antagonists work?

Alpha$_1$ antagonists such as prazosin, terazosin, and doxazosin are also sympatholytic antihypertensive agents. They work by blocking the postsynaptic alpha$_1$-adrenergic receptor, thereby affecting the tone of smooth muscle on vascular beds (and other sites).

17. Describe the symptoms seen in alpha$_1$-antagonist overdose?

Common symptoms include postural hypotension and near syncope. Occasionally, in large overdoses, significant hypotension and CNS depression may be seen.

18. What is the therapy for an alpha$_1$-antagonist overdose?

Address the ABCs. Most individuals have self-limiting symptoms or symptoms that respond to the administration of fluids and pressors.

19. Which diuretics are used as antihypertensives?

1. **Potassium-sparing diuretics**. There are two types of potassium-sparing diuretics: aldosterone antagonists such as spironolactone (Aldactone) and those that function in the distal tubule and collecting duct as Na channel antagonists (triamterene).

2. **Thiazide diuretics**. This class, which includes hydrochlorothiazide, chlorthalidone, and metozalone, affects the distal convoluted tubule, inhibiting chloride and sodium reabsorption.

3. **Loop diuretics**. Loop diuretics such as bumetanide (Bumex) and furosemide inhibit sodium, chloride, and potassium transport in the ascending loop of Henle.

20. What toxicity is seen in diuretic overdose?

Most of the toxicity seen with diuretics is related to metabolic disturbances that develop with chronic use including hyponatremia, hypokalemia, hypomagnesemia, and hyperkalemia (in the setting of potassium-sparing diuretics). Acute overdose often leads to diuresis, hypovolemia, electrolyte disturbances, and occasionally decreased mental status. Significant hypotension is unusual, but cardiac dysrhythmias may be precipitated by metabolic disturbances.

21. What is the therapy for diuretic overdose?

Therapy should of course address the overall needs of the patient especially the general concerns (sedation, hypotension). Attention should also be given to the careful correction of hypovolemia and electrolyte disturbances with the administration of IV fluids and electrolytes as needed.

22. Which vasodilators are used to treat hypertension?

Agents that act as direct vasodilators: sodium nitroprusside, hydralazine, diazoxide, and minoxidil.

23. How do vasodilators exert their effect?

These substances cause direct relaxation of smooth muscle in vascular beds possibly by affecting the use of calcium by myocytes. This results in vasodilation without ablation of sympathetic outflow. In fact, sympathetic outflow often increases with increased heart rate and contractility.

24. What effects are seen in the acute overdose of vasodilators?

- Light-headedness
- Syncope, often with a compensatory tachycardia
- Altered mental status (occasionally)

25. How is vasodilator overdose treated?

Intravenous fluids. Occasionally, the initiation of a catecholamine vasopressor may be needed (choose one with less beta effect) because heart rate often is elevated.

26. *Extra credit:* What antihypertensive compound's molecule contains five cyanide groups and, when used for hypertensive crisis, has an active metabolite that can reach toxic concentrations?

Sodium nitroprusside.

27. What special considerations are there for nitroprusside toxicity?

Sodium nitroprusside releases cyanide as it degrades, which can cause significant toxicity especially if the nitroprusside is used for more than 24 hours, if the infusion is too fast, or if the patient is malnourished or has renal failure. Therapy involves use of the cyanide treatment kit (sodium nitrite and sodium thiosulfate). In some institutions, thiosulfate is routinely given to patients receiving nitroprusside.

BIBLIOGRAPHY

1. Ajayi AA, Campbell BC, Rubin PC, et al: Effect of naloxone on the actions of captopril. Clin Pharmacol Ther 38:560–565, 1985.
2. Curry SC, Arnold-Capell P: Nitroprusside, nitroglycerin, and angiotensin-converting enzyme inhibitors. Crit Care Clin 7:555–581, 1991.
3. DeRoos F: Miscellaneous antihypertensive agents. In Goldfrank LR, Flomenbaum NE, Lewin NA, et al (eds): Goldfrank's Toxicologic Emergencies, 6th ed. Stamford, CT, Appleton & Lange, 1998, pp 845–858.
4. Ellenhorn MJ (ed): Ellenhorn's Medical Toxicology, Diagnosis and Treatment of Human Poisoning, 2nd ed. Baltimore, Williams & Wilkins, 1997.
5. Finley CJ, Silverman MA, Nunez AE: Angiotensin-converting enzyme inhibitor induces angioedema if unrecognized. Am J Emerg Med 10:550–552, 1992.
6. Henretig F, Wiley J, Brown L: Clonidine patch toxicity: The proof's in the poop! Clin Toxicol 33:475–485, 1995.

IV. Antibiotics

15. ANTITUBERCULOUS AGENTS

Shu Shum, M.B., B.S., and Jason Chu, M.D.

1. What antituberculous agents are in use today?

First line agents	*Second line agents*
Ethambutol	Amikacin
Isoniazid	Capreomycin
Rifampin	Ciprofloxacin
Pyrazinamide	Clofazine
Streptomycin	Cycloserine
	Dapson
	Ethionamide
	Kanamycin
	Ofloxacin
	Para-aminosalicylic acid
	Rifabutin

2. How much isoniazid is toxic?

Isoniazid (INH) toxicity is based on the chronicity and acetylation phenotype of the patient. In an acute setting, a serum level higher than 30 mg/L is toxic. This translates to a toxic ingestion of greater than 18 mg/kg of body weight (using a volume of distribution of INH of 0.6–0.7 L/kg). Thus, as little as 1.5 gm can produce toxicity in an adult.

3. How is INH metabolized?

INH is metabolized in the liver by *N*-acetylation, hydrolysis, and hydrazone formation. Some people ("fast acetylators") metabolize INH faster than others (obviously, the "slow acetylators"), who are homozygous for a recessive gene. Metabolites and parent compound are excreted in the urine. *N*-acetylation is governed by genetic polymorphism, i.e., fast or slow acetylators.

4. Why are slow acetylators at greater risk for acute toxicity?

Oral absorption of INH is rapid and complete in both fast and slow acetylators. In fast acetylators, the elimination half-life of INH is 0.5–1.5 hours, and in slow acetylators, the same half-life is 2–6 hours. Thus, with a given dose, the slow acetylator has a higher serum level at a given time and may exhibit more acute toxicity.

5. Why is INH toxic?

INH competes with pyridoxal 5-phosphate for the enzyme glutamic acid decarboxylase during the conversion of glutamic acid to gamma aminobutyric acid (GABA) in the brain. Thus, less GABA is formed when INH is present. GABA is an important inhibitory neurotransmitter that regulates neuronal activity. A decreased level of GABA results in uncontrolled neuronal transmission, which causes seizures. INH also inhibits the conversion of lactic acid to pyruvate, producing lactic acidosis.

6. How can I predict the acetylation phenotype?

A patient's ethnic group may furnish a clue to his or her acetylation phenotype.

Ethnicity and Acetylation Phenotype

ETHNICITY	SLOW ACETYLATOR (%)	FAST ACETYLATOR (%)
Alaskan Eskimos	20	80
Canadian Eskimos	5	95
Egyptians	80	20
Moroccans	90	10
Chinese	15	85
Japanese	10	90
African Americans	50	50
American Indians	20	80
Jews	60	40
Caucasian American	60	40
European	40	60

7. What are the presentations of acute INH overdose?

1. Refractory seizures
2. Metabolic acidosis
3. Coma

Other signs and symptoms include blurred vision with photophobia, nausea and vomiting, hyperthermia, hyperglycemia, and a shock-like state.

8. What are the common drug-drug interactions with INH?

INH has the ability to inhibit the enzyme monoamine oxidase, giving rise to a typical tyramine syndrome with palpitation, flushing, headache, dyspnea, and sweating. Serotonin syndrome may result from interaction with serotonin reuptake inhibitors such as fluoxetine. Slow acetylators, when given INH and phenytoin (Dilantin) at therapeutic doses, may develop phenytoin toxicity due to the inhibition of phenytoin hydroxylation.

9. How is acute INH overdose managed?

Acute INH overdose should be managed aggressively and anticipatorily. With a positive history, one should prepare for the abrupt onset of seizures at any time. Intravenous access, with more than one line, should be secured immediately. The hospital pharmacist should be notified to prepare the available pyridoxine (vitamin B_6) to be given intravenously. Dosing is usually gram-for-gram replacement; that is, with each gram of INH ingested (as determined from the patient's history), one needs to give a gram of intravenous pyridoxine. This may deplete the pharmacy's store of pyridoxine; oral pyridoxine may be useful if no further parenteral pyridoxine is available.

INH is absorbed rapidly from the gastrointestinal tract. Thus, it may already be too late for gastrointestinal decontamination by the time the patient presents in the emergency department. One may still proceed with lavage, charcoal, and cathartics; however, this should be done only when the acute emergency of seizures, coma, and acidosis has been managed based on advanced cardiac life support (ACLS) principles.

10. Is there special treatment for seizures?

Seizures should be managed with high doses of ultrafast-acting benzodiazepines, such as midazolam or lorazepam, with a loading dose to control the seizures activities followed by an intravenous infusion. Pyridoxine may be crucial in controlling refractory seizures. An empiric dose of 1 gm of pyridoxine for every gram of INH ingested or, alternatively, an empiric 5-gm dose over 15–30 minutes may be given. Thiopental infusion with continuous electroencephalogram (EEG) monitoring may be required to control the continuous seizure.

11. How safe is pyridoxine therapy?

Pyridoxine is safe if given in the recommended dosages. Higher doses given acutely or lower doses given chronically can cause a sensory peripheral neuropathy. Other effects include tachypnea, postural reflex abnormalities, paralysis, and convulsions.

12. Do I have to admit all patients with INH overdose?

After absorption, symptoms decline rapidly after an overdose, so patients can be discharged if they remain asymptomatic for several hours.

13. What are the symptoms of chronic INH toxicity?

Anorexia, nausea, and vomiting are common complaints. Jaundice is an important warning sign of impending hepatic failure and should be taken seriously. Peripheral neuropathy, optic neuritis, and psychosocial complaints are common. Pellagra (dermatitis, diarrhea and dementia) may be induced by the chronic INH therapy. Allergic reactions such as fever, rash, and a lupus-like syndrome may develop, but they dissipate with withdrawal of the drug. Agranulocytosis, thrombocytopenia, and anemia may occur. Patients with glucose 6-phosphate-dehydrogenase (G-6-PD) deficiency may develop hemolytic anemia during therapy.

14. Is there a way to predict the neurologic side effects?

Neurologic effects include encephalopathy, optic neuritis, optic atrophy, and peripheral neuropathy. The peripheral neuropathy is dose related and is seen more often in patients who take INH without pyridoxine, slow acetylators and malnourished, alcoholic, uremic, and diabetic patients. Treatment is vitamin B_6 supplementation.

15. Why is INH hepatitis important to know about?

A dreaded, sometimes lethal complication of chronic INH therapy is hepatitis. Ten percent of patients taking INH will have liver enzyme elevation; 10% of this subgroup will develop an overt hepatitis; and 10% of those who developed hepatitis will die, giving an overall mortality of 0.1%. Patients who are on chronic INH therapy should be monitored closely, with monthly clinical evaluation and liver function tests. The decision to continue therapy with INH should be thoroughly analyzed if any abnormalities arise.

16. What are the risk factors for INH-induced hepatitis?

Age is the most important factor; the risk of INH-induced hepatic injury increases in patients older than 35 years. Slow acetylators who are on combination therapy with INH and rifampin are at increased risk to develop hepatitis.

17. Why do I have to worry about pellagra?

Pellagra (diarrhea, dementia, and dermatitis) is caused by niacin deficiency. INH decreases tryptophan conversion to niacin, resulting in niacin deficiency.

18. *Extra credit:* What was the first biologically derived chemotherapeutic agent for the treatment of tuberculosis?

Streptomycin

19. *Extra credit:* What antitubercular drug has an adverse reaction that causes red-orange discolorations of secretions, urine, and contact lenses?

"Red man syndrome" occurs from the discoloration of the body secretions by excessive rifampin that stains the cutaneous tissue.

20. What are the common acute toxic effects of rifampin?

In acute overdose, rifampin may produce flu-like symptoms, including anorexia, nausea, and vomiting. Altered mental status, periorbital edema, dyspnea, and pulmonary edema may occur. Death from acute rifampin overdose is rare but has been reported.

21. Describe the common drug-drug interactions with rifampin.

Rifampin induces the microsomal cytochrome P450 mono-oxygenase system, specifically the enzymes CYPIIB, CYPIIC8, CYPIIC9, CYPIIIA3, and CYPIIIA4. With the induction of these oxidative enzymes in the liver, the rate of metabolism for the substrate increases, leading to a lower steady-state level of a drug. Thus, it is impossible to list all the drugs that rifampin interacts with. When the clinical situation arises, one should consult with a drug information center or the regional poison center.

Drugs that Interact with Rifampin

Acetaminophen	Clarithromycin	Indinavir	Sulfonylureas
Alprazolam	Codeine	Ivermectin	Tamoxifen
Amiodarone	Corticosteroids	Lidocaine	Testosterone
Amitriptyline	Cyclobenzaprine	Lovastatin	THC
Anticoagulants	Cyclosporines	Methadone	Theophylline
Barbiturates	Dapsone	Oral contraceptives	Tocainides
Benzodiazepines	Digitoxin	Paclitaxel (Taxol)	Troleandomycin
Beta-blockers	Diltiazem	Quinidine	Verapamil
Calcium antagonists	Estrogens	Ritonavir	Warfarin
Carbamazepine	Hydantoin	Salmeterol	Zonisamide

22. How should one approach a patient with acute rifampin overdose?

Apply ACLS protocol with particular attention to the airway. After stabilization, gastrointestinal decontamination should be considered, particularly with multiple doses of activated charcoal to break the enterohepatic recirculation. Hemodialysis does not reduce serum rifampin levels significantly. The red discoloration (see question 16) requires no treatment because the color fades away gradually.

23. What are the toxic effects of ethambutol?

Adverse effects at therapeutic doses include gastrointestinal symptoms, pruritus, joint pain, dizziness, confusion, disorientation, peripheral neuritis, and optic neuritis. The optic neuritis is dose related and causes blurred vision and loss of color vision. In overdose, nausea, abdominal pain, confusion, hallucinations, fever, and optic neuritis can occur (especially with doses > 10 gm).

24. What are the toxic effects of pyrazinamide?

Pyrazinamide can cause hepatic dysfunction with therapeutic use. About 15% of patients on 3 gm/day develop hepatitis. Hepatic function should be monitored regularly. If the liver functions tests are elevated, pyrazinamide should be discontinued.

25. What are the toxic effects of streptomycin?

Streptomycin is an aminoglycoside antibiotic and has the same toxicities as other aminoglycosides. It can cause a dose-related neuromuscular blockade. Nephrotoxicity and ototoxicity can occur. In pregnancy, streptomycin can cause hearing impairment and cranial nerve VIII damage to the fetus. It is listed as pregnancy category D.

26. Name the toxicities associated with the second-line medications.

Amikacin is an aminoglycoside and has all the toxicities of aminoglycosides. It can cause nephrotoxicity and ototoxicity.

Capreomycin can cause renal tubular damage, Bartter's syndrome, and ototoxicity.

Clofazime has gastrointestinal effects, CNS effects and red-brown discoloration of the skin and eyes.

Cycloserine mainly causes neurotoxicity such as confusion, coma, tremors, vertigo, seizures and a pellagra-like syndrome. Toxicity is increased with concomitant INH usage.

Dapsone usually causes anorexia, nausea, and vomiting. Neurotoxicity can manifest as headache, dizziness, agitation, confusion, paresthesias, psychosis, peripheral neuropathy, or coma. In overdose, dapsone causes methemoglobinemia. Patients with G-6-PD deficiency are at high risk for hemolysis.

Ethionamide can cause gastrointestinal upset, hepatitis, hypoglycemia, alopecia, rashes, and neurologic symptoms such as sensory neuropathies, depression, psychosis, tremors, and seizures.

Fluoroquinolones cause gastrointestinal symptoms (e.g., nausea, vomiting, diarrhea, and elevation of liver enzymes) and neurologic symptoms (e.g., headache, dizziness, drowsiness, seizures, and hallucinations). They are associated with joint and cartilage tenderness and hypersensitivity.

Rifabutin use is associated with elevation of liver enzymes, thrombocytopenia, neutropenia, uveitis, and loss of taste. It is related to rifampin and discolors body fluids orange and is an inducer of the P450 enzyme system.

BIBLIOGRAPHY

1. Ellenhorn MJ, Schonwald S, Ordog G, et al (eds): Ellenhorn's Medical Toxicology: Diagnosis and Treatment of Human Poisoning, 2nd ed. Baltimore, Williams & Wilkins, 1996.
2. Goldfrank LR, Flomenbaum NE, Lewin NA, et al (eds): Goldfrank's Toxicologic Emergencies, 6th ed. Stamford, CT, Appleton & Lange, 1998.
3. Hardman JG, Limbird LE, Molinoff PB, et al (eds): Goodman and Gilman's The Pharmacological Basis of Therapeutics, 9th ed. New York, McGraw-Hill, 1996.
4. Jeffery EH: Human Drug Metabolism: From Molecular Biology to Man. Boca Raton, FL, CRC Press, 1993.
5. Leikin JB, Paloucek FP: Poisoning and Toxicology Compendium. Hudson, OH, Lexi-Comp, 1998.
6. Nolan CM, Goldberg SV, Buskin SE: Hepatotoxicity associated with isoniazid preventive therapy: A 7-year survey from a public health tuberculosis clinic. JAMA 281:1014–1018, 1999.
7. Price Evans DA: Genetic Factors in Drug Therapy: Clinical and Molecular Pharmacogenetics. New York, Cambridge University Press, 1993.

16. ANTIMALARIAL DRUGS

G. Randall Bond, M.D.

1. Is there really a potential for exposure to antimalarial drugs?

Antimalarials are in many medicine cabinets. More than 50 million Westerners travel to the developing world each year. Most travelers take medication to prevent infection from malaria and may experience side effects. Some patients begin treatment for malaria while abroad and bring unused medications home, where the patient or family members ingest them intentionally or unintentionally.

2. What agents are available for prevention of malaria?

The most commonly used medication for prevention of malaria is **mefloquine**. In areas without resistance, **chloroquine** may be used. Alternatives include **doxycycline**, **primaquine**, and **proguanil** with or without atovaquone or chloroquine.

3. *Extra credit:* What antimalarial substance was worth many times its weight in gold in 17th century Europe?

The bark of *Cinchona* tree, which contains quinine.

4. *Extra credit:* In 1658, this staunch Protestant and Puritan leader refused the cinchona remedy offered to him on his deathbed because it was commonly known as "Jesuit bark"; he subsequently died. Who was this Englishman?

Oliver Cromwell.

5. Are side effects common with prophylactic antimalarial agents?

Yes. These agents often cause nausea, abdominal cramping, and headache. Almost all can produce hypersensitivity reactions including asthma, angioedema, and rash, although these are uncommon. Hypersensitivity-induced agranulocytosis, thrombocytopenia, or hepatitis may occur. Red blood cell (RBC) oxidant stress from primaquine can produce hemolysis in glucose-6-phosphate dehydrogenase (G6PD)–deficient individuals. Mefloquine can cause sleep disturbance with vivid dreams and, rarely (1/13,000), an acute psychosis. Doxycycline may cause photodermatitis.

6. What agents are used for treatment of malaria?

For treatment, chloroquine (if acquired in a sensitive area), mefloquine, or a combination of pyrimethamine with sulfadoxine (Fansidar) may be used. Because of parasite resistance to the drugs, a combination of quinine and doxycycline is often required. Travelers sometimes bring home medications that are not available in the United States including halofantrine and artemisinin derivatives (from the Chinese herb *qinghaosu*).

7. Do antimalarials have common symptoms after overdose?

No. The pattern of toxicity varies significantly even with the two most toxic agents, quinine and chloroquine.

8. Describe the symptoms of quinine overdose.

Patients often experience a well-known syndrome known as **cinchonism**. Characteristics include nausea, vomiting, decreased hearing acuity, tinnitus, and headache. With quinine toxicity, visual disturbances, including blindness, are classic. Cardiac effects include a prolonged PR interval, QRS complex, QT interval, and ST depression with or without T wave inversion. Torsades de pointes, ventricular tachycardia, and fibrillation can occur but do so rarely. Hypotension caused by vasodilation and myocardial depression may occur.

9. What causes the cardiac effects?

Quinine blocks the cardiac sodium and potassium ion channels. Sodium channel blockade produces a negative inotropic effect, slowed rate of depolarization, slowed conduction, and increased action potential duration. Inhibition of the potassium channels results in an increase in the effective refractory period. This repolarization delay predisposes to the unique ventricular tachycardia, torsades de pointes.

10. How are these cardiac effects treated?

The sodium channel manifestations should be treated with sodium bicarbonate alkalization to achieve a serum pH of 7.45–7.50, the same treatment as for patients with a serious cyclic antidepressant overdose. Because hypertonic sodium bicarbonate may result in hypokalemia, potentially exacerbating potassium channel blockade, patients should be monitored carefully for further QTc prolongation. Intervention for torsades de pointes, including magnesium administration, potassium supplementation, and overdrive pacing, may be necessary. Obviously, no class IA, IC, or III antidysrhythmic agents (those with sodium channel and potassium channel blocking activity) should be used, but type IB agents may be useful. In one case, extracorporeal membrane oxygenation (ECMO) was used to support a patient until drug metabolism occurred.

11. Is there a specific treatment for the blindness?

No. The injury is from a direct retinal toxin, not vasospasm. Attempts to reverse vasospasm, including nitrites and stellate ganglion block, have been unsuccessful. The toxicity is related to serum level so efforts to enhance elimination may be helpful.

12. Is the blindness permanent?

Usually not. Improvement in vision may occur rapidly but is usually slow, occurring over a period of months. This happens centrally at first followed by improvement in peripheral vision. The pupils may remain dilated even after normal vision has returned. Those with the greatest exposure may develop optic atrophy.

13. Is there a way to enhance elimination of quinine?

Multiple-dose activated charcoal decreases quinine half-life from approximately 8 hours to about 4.5 hours and increases clearance by over 50%. Reduction of the half-life has not been proven to improve clinical outcome. Nonetheless, because ophthalmic, central nervous system (CNS), and cardiovascular toxicity are related to serum concentration, reducing levels as quickly as possible is prudent. Activated charcoal should be administered every 2–4 hours. Other measures, such as peritoneal dialysis, hemodialysis, charcoal hemoperfusion, and exchange transfusion, are not helpful.

14. What are the signs and symptoms of chloroquine overdose?

Nausea, vomiting, diarrhea, and abdominal pain can occur, although they are less common than with quinine overdose. Chloroquine is rapidly absorbed, and apnea, coma, hypotension, and cardiovascular compromise can occur suddenly. Electrocardiographic abnormalities include QRS prolongation, atrioventricular block, ST-T depression, increased U waves, and QT interval prolongation; however, these, too, occur less often than with quinine. Significant hypokalemia invariably is associated with cardiac manifestations.

15. What is the treatment for chloroquine intoxication?

As always, establish an airway; make sure adequate FiO_2, tidal volume, and ventilatory rates are established. After intubation, 2 mg/kg of IV diazepam should be given over 30 minutes, followed by 1–2 mg/kg per day for 2–4 days. Simultaneously, epinephrine should be administered by IV drip, starting at 0.25 µg/kg/min and increased until a systolic blood pressure > 100 mmHg is achieved.

16. Does this treatment really work?

Yes. Chloroquine used to be "recommended" as a suicidal agent in France, prompting a Parisian study of the treatment protocol in question 16. Only 1 of 11 patients in the control group improved, whereas 10 of 11 patients in the treated group improved. The success of the treatment has been reported in several additional case studies.

17. Can elimination of chloroquine be enhanced by dialysis or other measures?

No. Chloroquine has a large volume of distribution and is highly protein bound, so methods to enhance elimination have not proven successful.

18. Are people who take chloroquine or hydroxychloroquine for arthritis at risk for visual changes?

Yes. These patients should have periodic visual field exams to make sure they do not develop insidious visual toxicity.

19. Do patients experience any side effects from taking mefloquine?

Occasionally, therapeutic use of mefloquine results in significant CNS effects such as dysphoria, clouded consciousness, toxic encephalopathy, anxiety, depression, giddiness, and seizures. These side effects can occur 2–3 weeks after treatment but are self limited. Two overdose patients who took very high doses experienced agitated delirium with psychosis, ataxia, dizziness, and speech difficulties. Residual damage persisted at 1 year.

20. Because halofantrine is related to mefloquine, does it have similar toxicity?

No. Halofantrine has few CNS effects but has significant impact on the potassium channel. The prolongation of the QT interval is proportional to the dose and the serum halofantrine concentration. Fifty percent of children receiving a therapeutic course of halofantrine have a QTc > 440 msec. Prolonged QTc and associated dysrhythmias (especially torsades de pointes) are expected in overdose. If halofantrine is used with other drugs that cause QTc prolongation, particularly mefloquine, arrhythmias are more likely.

21. What problems are caused by the folate metabolism–inhibitors proguanil, pyrimethamine, dapsone, and sulfadoxine?

These agents commonly cause hypersensitivity reactions in prophylactic use. In case of overdose, folate supplementation should be considered.

22. Describe the dapsone overdose syndrome.

Dapsone overdose results in nausea, vomiting, and abdominal pain. More significantly, it produces RBC oxidant stress, which leads to methemoglobinemia and, to a lesser extent, sulfhemoglobinemia. The onset may be rapid. Hemolysis, including delayed hemolysis, may cause cardiac and neurologic symptoms from end-organ hypoxia. Significant methemoglobinemia should be treated with methylene blue. Sulfhemoglobinemia is permanent but quantitatively insignificant.

23. What about pyrimethamine?

Currently, pyrimethamine is available only as a preparation with sulfadoxine (Fansidar). In children, ingestion can cause nausea, vomiting, rapid onset of seizures, fever, tachycardia with consequent blindness, deafness, and mental retardation.

24. What are the side effects of the newer agents such as the artemisinin derivatives?

Low-frequency side effects include nausea, vomiting, abdominal pain, diarrhea, and dizziness. Animal studies and rare reports of CNS side effects during therapeutic use in humans (higher incidence of seizures, transient cerebellar symptoms, and delayed awakening from cerebral malaria) suggest that these effects could occur following intentional self-poisoning. When symptoms occurred during treatment, no neurologic difference was noted in long-term follow-up.

BIBLIOGRAPHY

1. Davis TME: Adverse effects of antimalarial prophylactic drugs: An important consideration in the risk-benefit equation. Ann Pharmacother 22:1104–1106, 1998.
2. Goldfrank LR, Osborn HH: Antimalarial agents. In Goldfrank LR, Flomenbaum NA, Lewin NE, et al (eds): Goldfrank's Toxicological Emergencies, 6th ed. Stamford, CT, Appleton & Lange, 1998, pp 741–747.
3. Ingram RJH, Ellis-Pegler RB: Malaria, mefloquine and the mind. N Z Med J 110:137–138, 1997.
4. Luzzi GA, Peto TWA: Adverse effects of antimalarials. Drug Safety 8:295–311, 1993.
5. MacDonald RD, McGuigan MA: Acute dapsone intoxication: A pediatric case report. Pediatr Emerg Care 13:127–129, 1997.
6. Mai N, Day N, Van Chuong L, et al: Post-malaria neurological syndrome. Lancet 348:917–921, 1996.
7. Miller LG, Panosian CB: Ataxia and slurred speech after artesunate treatment for falciparum malaria. N Engl J Med 336:1328, 1997.
8. Nosten F, Price RN: New antimalarials: A risk-benefit analysis. Drug Safety 12:264–273, 1995.
9. Riou B, Barriot P, Rimailho A, Baud FJ: Treatment of severe chloroquine poisoning. N Engl J Med 318:1–7, 1988.
10. Rouviex B, Bricaire F, Michon C, et al: Mefloquine and an acute brain syndrome. Ann Intern Med 110:577–578, 1989.
11. Sowunmi A, Fehintola FA, Ogundahansi AT, et al: Comparative cardiac effects of halofantrine and chloroquine plus chlorpheniramine in children with acute uncomplicated falciparum malaria. Trans Royal Soc Trop Med 93:78–83, 1999.
12. Wolf LR, Otten EJ, Spadafora MP: Cinchonism: Two case reports and review of acute quinine toxicity and treatment. J Emerg Med 10:295–301, 1992.

V. Cardiac Drugs

17. DIGITALIS AND THE CARDIAC GLYCOSIDES

Louis J. Ling, M.D.

1. *Extra credit:* **What drug has been described as having the smallest therapeutic-to-toxic dose ratio of any commonly used medication?**

Digitalis.

2. *Extra credit:* **What physician is credited with discovering the use of Digitalis in treating the condition then known as dropsy?**

William Withering, in 1785.

3. What is a cardiac glycoside and where do you find them?

Cardiac glycosides are chemicals with a steroid ring, an unsaturated lactone ring, and one to four sugars (or glycosides) attached. The most common cardiac glycoside medication is digoxin, but other preparations still include digitoxin and ouabain (which older doctors still remember). They are found in plants such as foxglove, oleander, and lily of the valley and in toads.

4. What kind of toads?

Toads in the *Bufonidae* family, such as the Colorado River toad, the cane toad, and American tropical toad, secrete a toxin from special glands in their skin. It is used as an aphrodisiac and is found in some natural medications from the Far East. Some patients lick these *Bufo* toads to "get high."

5. What are the beneficial cardiac effects of digoxin?

Digoxin increases contractility by freeing cytoplasmic calcium to actin and myosin during contractions. It blocks the sodium-potassium (Na-K) pump, increases Na and calcium (Ca) in the cell, and keeps K out of the cell. It causes vasodilatation and decreases afterload.

6. Describe the electrocardiographic (ECG) findings of digoxin.

In therapeutic doses, common manifestations are prolonged P-R interval, short Q-T, ST scooping and depression, especially laterally, and decreased T waves. At higher doses, digoxin suppresses the sinoatrial node, increases automaticity, and decreases conduction at the atrioventricular node. This can result in tachycardia or heart block.

7. How do patients with digoxin toxicity typically present?

1. In **acute** overdose, the patient takes a large amount of digoxin (or licks too many toads), which causes sudden acute symptoms.

2. Some patients on **chronic** therapy have a gradual build-up of the drug and develop insidious symptoms.

8. What is the course of an acute overdose?

Because it takes time for the levels to build up in the heart and other tissues, symptoms do not occur for the first 6 hours. Serious arrhythmia occurs within 24 hours after digoxin overdose and within 5 days of the long-lasting digitoxin.

9. How does an acute overdose correlate with drug levels?

When the drug is absorbed and in the serum over the first 6 hours, the serum drug levels will be high but the patient will be asymptomatic. Symptoms occur after the tissue levels increase and the serum levels start to fall. Early drug levels can confirm that overdose has occurred.

10. What happens with an acute overdose?

Most commonly this occurs in younger patients with healthy hearts. They frequently develop heart block and bradycardia. Because the Na-K pump is blocked keeping K out of the cells, life-threatening hyperkalemia ensues.

11. Should activated charcoal be administered even if a long time has elapsed since the ingestion?

Because digoxin is slowly absorbed, activated charcoal is very useful, and multiple-dose activated charcoal shortens the half-life because both digoxin and digitoxin have enterohepatic circulation.

12. What is the treatment after acute overdose?

Serum potassium should be followed closely. Hyperkalemia, especially with ECG changes, can be treated with the usual sodium bicarbonate, insulin, and glucose, but it probably is best treated with the Fab antibodies. Atropine is useful for bradycardias, but all serious arrhythmias or heart block greater than type I should be treated with the Fab antibodies.

13. What standard treatment is absolutely contraindicated?

Calcium, often used for hyperkalemia, should not be given because digoxin results in increased intracellular calcium and can increase arrhythmias.

14. What is the Fab antibody?

Digoxin-specific Fab (fragment, antigen binding) antibody fragments developed from sheep are a specific antidote for digoxin, but they also cross react with digitoxin and have been used for plant and toad poisoning as well. Fab binds free digoxin so well that it causes a concentration gradient that pulls the tissue-bound drug into the serum where it is inactive when bound. The total serum levels rise dramatically but free active digoxin is almost undetectable. Effects of the antibody occur within minutes to an hour, although maximum effect may take several hours more.

15. Which patients should receive the Fab antibody?

Indications include any severe ventricular arrhythmias, bradycardia unresponsive to atropine, rising potassium levels, especially potassium level > 5 mEq/L, and serum digoxin level > 15 ng/ml even in the early distribution period before the patient gets symptoms.

16. How much Fab fragment should be given?

The total body load of digoxin can be estimated in two ways. Since each molecule of digoxin is bound by one Fab antibody fragment, the dose of antidote is based on the estimated digoxin ingested or the total body load based on a steady state serum level taken at least 6 hours after ingestion. The formulas are in the package insert.

A typical patient will require 5–15 vials of antibody after an acute overdose and perhaps only 2–4 vials after a chronic overdose.

17. How does chronic overdose or toxicity occur?

Digoxin can build up slowly especially in older patients with poor renal function or after a change in dose or formulations. The addition of other drugs such as cimetidine and calcium channel blockers can increase digoxin effect. Hypokalemia and hypomagnesemia, common side effects of diuretics, can induce toxicity. Patients with advanced heart disease and chronic pulmonary disease are also at increased risk.

18. How is chronic overdose different from acute overdose?

Anorexia, nausea, and vomiting are common. Central nervous system (CNS) effects such as dizziness, fatigue, confusion, lethargy, and delirium can occur. The increased perceptions of yellow and green objects are classic, but perceptions of other colors can occur. Other visual disturbances include decreased light, blurring, or the perception of halos. Because many of these older patients are on diuretics, hypokalemia and total body potassium depletion is common. Magnesium is often depleted, and patients should receive supplementation. Serum drug levels are only minimally elevated or in the therapeutic range for some patients.

19. Can a patient die from a chronic overdose?

Absolutely, especially if patients are older and have underlying heart disease. It is important not to miss this diagnosis in the emergency department when older patients on digoxin present with nonspecific gastrointestinal and CNS symptoms.

20. So once I give the Fab antibody fragment, is that it?

Almost. In acute overdose, the Na-K pump suddenly works again, and there is a rapid influx of potassium back into the cells possibly resulting in hypokalemia. There is often a rebound in free digoxin 24 hours after the antibody is given. This rebound is delayed with renal failure. The drug-antibody complex is excreted through the kidneys, and the half-life is prolonged with renal failure. Patients who were digoxin dependent may decompensate, especially if they require digoxin for rate control.

21. Why are antibody fragments used in the antidote instead of intact antibody?

Because fragments are smaller, they are more rapidly excreted from the kidneys, cause less of an immune response, and have a wider volume of distribution to get to more digoxin faster.

22. Why was the antibody made for digoxin rather than another drug?

Digoxin is a drug that commonly causes toxicity but is taken in very small doses. Small doses of drug mean that only a small dose of antibody is needed. Larger doses of antibody are very difficult and expensive to make, and larger doses of sheep protein can cause more of an immune reaction. Therefore, digitalis was a very smart choice to pick as a target drug for an antibody.

23. What other ways are there to get cardiac glycoside poisoning besides digoxin overdose and licking toads?

Some Chinese medications such as *chu an wu* contain the toad venom. Many plants contain cardiac glycosides including foxglove leaves, lily of the valley buds, and seeds from oleander (*Thevetia peruviana*). Drinking tea made with these plants can be dangerous.

24. Is treatment the same with other cardiac glycosides as for digoxin?

Similar effects can be expected, and there is cross over with the digoxin assay and dioxin Fab antibody fragment. Therefore, whereas the serum levels may not correlate and the dose of antidote may need to be increased, the treatment concepts are the same.

BIBLIOGRAPHY

1. Antman EM, Wenger TL, Butler VP, et al: Treatment of 150 cases of life-threatening digitalis intoxication with digoxin-specific Fab antibody fragments. Final report of a multi-center study. Circulation 81:1744–1752, 1990.
2. Brubacher JR, Ravikumar PR, Bania T, et al: Treatment of toad venom poisoning with digoxin-specific Fab fragments. Chest 110:1282–1288, 1996.
3. Kinlay S, Buckley N: Magnesium sulfate in the treatment of ventricular arrhythmias due to digoxin toxicity. J Toxicol Clin Toxicol 33:55–59, 1995.
4. Linden CH: Digitalis glycosides. In Ford M, Delaney KA, Ling L, Erickson T (eds): Clinical Toxicology. Philadelphia, W.B. Saunders, 2000, pp 379–390.
5. Rich SA, Libera JM, Locke RJ: Treatment of foxglove extract poisoning with digoxin-specific Fab fragments. Ann Emerg Med 22:1904–1907, 1993.
6. Withering W: An account of the foxglove and some of its medical uses: With practical remarks on dropsy and other diseases. Med Classics 2:295–443, 1937.

18. BETA BLOCKERS

Andrew Topliff, M.D.

1. What are beta blockers used for?

Beta blockers are used for hypertension, angina, dysrhythmias, and occasionally cardiomyopathy. They are sometimes used for migraine headaches, panic disorder, and treatment of thyrotoxicosis. Ophthalmic products are available for the treatment of glaucoma.

2. What beta blockers are available?

More than 50 beta blockers exist. Beta blockers commonly used in the United States include:

Acebutolol	Carteolol	Levobunolol	Pindolol
Atenolol	Carvedilol	Metoprolol	Propranolol
Betaxolol	Esmolol	Nadolol	Sotalol
Bisprolol	Labetalol	Penbutolol	Timolol

3. How do beta blockers work?

Beta adrenergic receptors are coupled to G proteins, which serve to increase adenylate cyclase activity and increase intracellular levels of cyclic adenosine monophosphate (cAMP). This activates protein kinases with subsequent phosphorylation of a variety of ion channels and enzymes.

In $beta_1$ agonism this results in eventual increase in intracellular calcium. Calcium then binds troponin and causes conformational changes. Actin myosin cross-linkage and subsequent adenosine triphosphate (ATP)–dependent contraction can then occur (and thus increased cardiac contractility). $Beta_1$-receptor antagonism is the mechanistic goal of most beta blockers. However, other beta receptors and occasionally even alpha receptors may be involved, especially in the setting of overdose.

4. Describe the important differences among beta blockers.

Lipophilicity (how readily the drug dissolves in fat and how well it crosses fatty cell membranes such as the blood-brain barrier) can vary greatly. Propranolol is the most lipophilic, has more membrane-stabilizing activity, and thus causes more effects in the lipid-laden central nervous system (CNS) in overdose including seizures.

Protein binding varies from 10% to 90%.

Half-lives vary from 8 minutes to 18 hours for some of the agents.

Metabolism is primarily hepatic transformation and then renal clearance. However, some agents (i.e., atenolol, nadolol, and sotalol) are primarily renally cleared and may accumulate in renal failure, whereas others have a tendency to accumulate in the setting of hepatic failure.

Sotalol blocks the delayed rectifier **potassium channels** responsible for repolarization. Consequently, sotalol toxicity causes prolonged QT intervals with subsequent torsades de pointes and other ventricular arrhythmias.

5. Some beta blockers vary in $beta_1$ selectivity. Does this make a difference in overdose?

Receptor specificity varies greatly among beta blockers. Some agents (i.e., metoprolol, atenolol, esmolol) are active primarily against $beta_1$ receptors, whereas other agents, such as labetalol, affect $alpha_2$, $beta_1$, and $beta_2$ receptors. However, in an overdose, even the most selective agents will lose selectivity, making these differences less important.

6. What are the typical signs and symptoms of beta blocker overdose?

Bradycardia and hypotension are commonly seen, although one third of individuals remain asymptomatic. Other cardiac effects include atrioventricular block, conduction delay, ventricular arrhythmia, and cardiac arrest. Torsades de pointes is not unusual in the setting of a sotalol overdose. Pulmonary edema also may occur. Increased airway resistance (beta$_2$ blockade), respiratory depression, and hypoglycemia may occur. Neurologic effects include sedation or coma, fatigue, confusion, and occasionally seizures (especially in propranolol overdose).

7. What unusual symptoms may be seen in beta blocker overdose?

Lipophilic beta blockers may lead to increased CNS effects such as coma. A large overdose of lipophilic beta blockers that have membrane-stabilizing activity (fast sodium channel inhibitors), such as propranolol (and possibly acebutolol), may cause seizures.

Because of its effect on potassium channels, sotalol may cause QT prolongation, torsades de pointes, and a variety of ventricular arrhythmias. Some beta blockers (e.g., acebutolol, pindolol) have beta agonist-antagonist effects, giving them possible sympathomimetic activity. It is unclear whether there would be any apparent differences seen in overdose.

8. What other overdoses might cause similar toxidromes?

Other substances that commonly cause bradycardia and sometimes hypotension include calcium channel blockers (CCBs), clonidine, digoxin, sodium channel blockers, cholinergics, opiates, and sedative-hypnotics. Medical conditions that may produce a similar clinical picture include hyperkalemia, hypothermia, myocardial infarction, and conduction delays.

In many overdoses, other aspects of the toxidrome may indicate clearly what type of substance is involved. CCBs may closely mimic beta blocker overdose, although patients may be tachycardic and tend to have less obtundation. Fortunately, treatment is similar for both overdoses.

9. Can an electrocardiogram (ECG) help differentiate beta blocker overdose from other overdoses?

ECG changes may be useful with CCBs and beta blockers, which typically exhibit PR interval prolongation and occasionally widening of the QRS. Digoxin causes PR prolongation but frequently causes identifying ST segment changes and atrial and ventricular dysrhythmias. Sodium channel blockers (e.g., type 1A antidysrhythmic agents) typically cause QRS prolongation and occasionally seizures.

10. Are toxidromes that are similar but caused by different substances treated differently?

The therapy for CCB and beta blocker overdose is similar, although calcium supplementation and the administration of vasopressors probably elicits better response in CCB overdose. Nonetheless, fluids, calcium, glucagon, vasopressors, and possibly insulin and glucose may be effective in both toxidromes. Digoxin toxicity warrants the administration of digoxin antigen-binding fragments (Fab, Digibind), and overdose of any substance that produces QRS prolongation suggests that alkalization may be beneficial. Clonidine and opiate overdose may improve with the administration of naloxone.

11. Which beta blockers are considered the most dangerous in overdose?

The characteristics that make beta blockers dangerous in overdose include lipophilicity, sodium channel activity (membrane-stabilizing activity), and potassium channel activity (due to effects on repolarization). Therefore, propranolol, which is lipophilic and membrane stabilizing, causes a disproportionate number of deaths. However, it is unclear whether this is due to drug effects, the fact that it is prescribed more often than other agents, or other factors.

12. What dose of beta blockers can be ignored?

Healthy individuals with inadvertent ingestions of less than an age-appropriate dose probably can be watched at home. However, some people become significantly ill from doses of only 2–3 times therapeutic range. This is especially true for ill patients and individuals who are dependent on sympathetic tone who become symptomatic at therapeutic doses.

13. How soon after ingestion do symptoms occur?

Symptoms occur as early as 20 minutes but may take $\geq$ 1–2 hours to develop if sustained-release products were ingested.

14. How long after ingestion should individuals be observed?

Most patients become symptomatic or develop ECG changes within 6 hours of ingestion. Thus, patients who do manifest symptoms or ECG changes 6 hours after ingestion can be discharged safely.

15. Are there any exceptions to the 6-hour rule?

Two exceptions exist: timed-release beta blocker formulations and sotalol, which is known to cause ECG changes that may persist for days after ingestion.

16. How should one pursue gastrointestinal decontamination?

Always address the patient's overall condition (e.g., respiratory status) first. Charcoal is highly effective for binding beta blockers. In a recent overdose, lavage might be useful, but in bradycardic patients, atropine may be indicated prior to lavage to prevent any vagal effects. Whole bowel irrigation can be useful if sustained-release products were ingested, but again, atropine may be indicated in bradycardic individuals before placement of a nasogastric tube.

17. What is the basic therapy for mildly symptomatic beta blocker overdose?

Individuals who are mildly hypotensive and bradycardic sometimes only require atropine (adult dose: 1 mg) and fluids. Cardiac monitoring is clearly advised.

18. *Extra credit:* What is the agent of choice for treating overdoses of the beta-blocker drugs?

Glucagon.

19. Describe the therapy for moderately symptomatic patients.

Glucagon is used for patients who are moderately ill and for patients who do not respond to atropine and fluids. Typical dosing for an adult is approximately 2–5 mg IV push followed by a 2–5-mg infusion each hour. Additional atropine may also be required. Of course, airway and other issues should be addressed as the need arises.

20. How does glucagon work?

Glucagon appears to bind to specific receptors that are combined to G proteins, which lead to increased activity of adenylate cyclase and increased amounts of cAMP. Increased cAMP activates phosphokinases, leading to the phosphorylation of calcium channels and increased levels of intracellular calcium. This in turn leads to actin-myosin contraction (increased contractility and vascular tone).

21. What is the therapy for severely symptomatic individuals?

Catecholamines are usually required. Dopamine, norepinephrine, dobutamine, isoproterenol, and epinephrine all should work. Because extremely large amounts of these drugs may be required, it is useful to begin with common dosages and rapidly titrate upward as needed.

Drugs that have significant beta$_2$ effects (isoproterenol and epinephrine) may actually worsen hypotension and should be discontinued if this effect is seen. Drugs with significant alpha effect (epinephrine and norepinephrine) may cause peripheral vasoconstriction without significantly increasing cardiac contractility. Thoughtful monitoring of vital signs and intra-arterial and pulmonary artery pressure can help establish the ideal therapeutic regimen. Phosphodiesterase inhibitors such as amrinone have been used as well.

22. If these modalities fail, are there any other options?

Pacing may be of use because it frequently corrects the bradycardia. However, it may not affect the hypotension. Intra-aortic balloon pump or extracorporeal circulation may be useful temporizing strategies until the toxidrome resolves. Large amounts of insulin and glucose have significantly improved survivability in canine models with propranolol overdose.

23. How do insulin and glucose work?

The mechanisms for this are not clear but may involve "force feeding" the heart with carbohydrates instead of the usual free fatty acids that are the mainstay of cardiac metabolism. This has been shown to affect hypotension from a variety of causes including beta blockers, CCBs, and cardiac ischemia.

24. Is dialysis useful at all?

Dialysis is unlikely to be useful except in those beta blockers with low lipid solubility and low protein binding (i.e., acebutolol, atenolol, esmolol in renal failure, and nadolol) and would most likely be useful for sotalol overdoses. Some substances that have low lipid solubility and higher protein binding may respond to charcoal hemoperfusion.

BIBLIOGRAPHY

1. Cada DJ, Covington TR, et al: Diuretics and cardiovasculars. In Drug Facts and Comparisons. St. Louis, Mosby, 1995, pp 593–599.
2. Critchley JA, Ungar A: The management of acute poisoning due to beta-adrenoreceptor antagonists. Med Toxicol Adverse Drug Exp 4:32–45, 1989.
3. Kerns W, Schroeder D, Williams C, et al: Insulin improves survival in a canine model of acute beta-blocker toxicity. Ann Emerg Med 29:748–757, 1997.
4. Kline JA, Leonova E, Raymond RM: Beneficial myocardial metabolic effects of insulin during verapamil toxicity in the anesthetized canine. Crit Care Med 23:1251–1263, 1995.
5. Neuvonen PJ, Elonen E, Vuorenmaa T, Laaska M: Prolonged QT interval and severe tachydysrhythmias: Common features of sotalol intoxication. Eur J Clin Pharmacol 20:85–89, 1981.
6. Reith DM, Dawson AH, Epid D, et al: Relative toxicity of beta blockers in overdose. J Toxicol Clin Toxicol 34:273–278, 1996.

19. CALCIUM CHANNEL BLOCKERS

David C. Lee, M.D., and Kent Clark, M.D.

1. What are calcium channel blockers (CCBs)?
This group of agents targets the slow calcium channels prevalent in the myocardium and vascular smooth muscle. They inhibit the slow influx of extracellular calcium from moving intracellularly. In the myocardium, this action leads to reduced myocardial contractility, depressed sinoatrial (SA) nodal activity, and slowed atrioventricular (AV) nodal conduction. In the periphery, this action leads to vasodilation.

2. *Extra credit:* CCBs were first introduced in the 1960s to treat what medical condition?
Angina.

3. What are the different types of CCBs?
Of the four classes of CCBs, the first three are widely used in the United States:
1. **Phenylalkylamines** (verapamil). This type of agent exerts its greatest effect on the SA and AV nodal tissue of the myocardium. This leads to its profound negative inotropic effects. Verapamil has relatively modest peripheral vasodilatory effects.
2. **Dihydropyridines** (amlodipine, felodipine, isradipine, nicardipine, nifedipine, nimodipine). This is the largest class of CCBs. These CCBs have the greatest affinity for the peripheral vascular smooth muscle causing vasodilation and decreased blood pressure, but they have little effect on the myocardium.
3. **Benzothiazepines** (diltiazem). This type of agent exhibits modest myocardial activity, leading to decreased inotropy, and modest vascular smooth muscle activity, leading to decreased blood pressure.
4. **Diphenylpiperazines** (cinnarizine, flunarizine). This class is not encountered often and is of little clinical or toxicologic importance.

4. How dangerous are the CCBs?
According to data supplied by the American Association of Poison Control Centers, CCBs are one of the five most lethal classes of pharmaceutical agents in overdose settings. Verapamil is the most likely to cause death.

5. How soon do symptoms of CCB overdose appear?
Symptoms after ingestion of the standard oral preparation typically occur within the first 1–6 hours. Sustained-release formulations may not show signs of toxicity for 24 hours.

6. When should patients with CCB overdose go to the hospital?
All patients with possible CCB overdose should seek medical attention immediately. Because the clinical status can change abruptly, these patients should be kept in a monitored setting until a toxic overdose can be ruled out.

7. How does CCB overdose manifest?
1. Myocardium effects—bradydysrhythmias, sinus arrest, varying degrees of AV blockade, congestive heart failure, and cardiogenic shock
2. Vascular smooth muscle vasodilation effects—hypotension, syncope, and profound shock
3. Central nervous system depression, lethargy, and coma
4. Seizures—rarely reported; occur more commonly in the pediatric population
5. Hyperglycemia—attributed to blockage of calcium channels on the pancreatic beta cells leading to relative hypoinsulinemia

80

8. Who is most at risk from CCB overdose?

Death from CCB overdose in the **pediatric population** has been described from ingestion of as little as 10 mg of nifedipine.

9. What is the mechanism of death from CCB overdose?

Profound cardiovascular collapse that is often recalcitrant to standard pharmacologic interventions.

10. How are CCB overdoses treated?

All patients suspected of overdose must be moved quickly to a monitored setting and receive supplemental oxygen and IV access. As in all emergencies, particular attention must be paid to the patient's airway, breathing, and circulation (ABCs). Gastric decontamination may be preformed by lavage if the patient presents within 60 minutes of the ingestion. Activated charcoal should be given in all suspected individuals, and whole bowel irrigation should be considered in a patient who has overdosed on a sustained-release preparation.

Bradydysrhythmias and hypotension should be treated initially in the standard advanced cardiac life support (ACLS) fashion with the administration of atropine and fluid bolus of normal saline. However, these measures are often do little to reverse the effects of CCB overdose.

11. Are there any antidotes?

Calcium chloride (10%) and calcium gluconate (10%) are the most widely used and accepted treatments for reversing hypotension in the setting of CCB overdose. They do not always work, however, and calcium has little effect on the bradycardia.

12. What dose of IV calcium should be used?

Calcium dosages should be given as boluses, but the ideal dose is unknown. Usually, small doses are repeated until a response is elicited. In adults, 1 gm of calcium chloride or 3 gm of calcium gluconate is repeated every 10 minutes. The suggested pediatric dose is 20 mg/kg of calcium chloride or 0.2 ml/kg of 10% calcium chloride, which should be repeated until the child responds.

13. What if the calcium does not work?

Hypotension that does not respond to fluids and calcium should be treated by addition of inotropic support. The two most widely used agents are isoproterenol and dopamine, and they may need to be given in doses much larger than usual before the patient responds.

14. What are some experimental treatments for CCB overdose?

Glucagon. Although most widely used as the treatment for beta blocker overdose, glucagon's effectiveness at reversing some of the manifestations of CCB overdose has been well documented. Glucagon acts by simulating intracellular cyclic adenosine monophosphate production, leading to increased inotropy and chronotropy independent of the calcium channels.

4-Aminopyridine. Independently, 4-aminopyridine promotes calcium influx and has been show to reverse the effects of calcium channel blockade induced in experimental animals. However, it has never been shown to increase survival and exists only as an investigational drug in the U.S.

Insulin. Insulin infusion in animal studies has been shown to reverse the cardiotoxicity of verapamil. Although the mechanism is unclear, insulin may act independent of the myocardial calcium channels. Its use is under further investigation.

15. When should patients with CCB overdose be admitted to the hospital?

Patients who have taken an unknown quantity of standard-preparation CCBs should be observed in a monitored setting. If they exhibit signs of toxicity, they should be admitted to the hospital to a monitored bed. Severe signs of toxicity should be watched in the intensive care unit. Furthermore, any patient overdosing on sustained-release preparations should be admitted and monitored for at least 24 hours.

16. When can patients with CCB overdose be sent home?

If a patient has not taken a sustained-release preparation and shows no signs of clinical toxicity after being monitored for 8 hours, he or she may safely be discharged to home. If a patient has taken a sustained-release preparation and shows no sign of clinical toxicity after being monitored for 24 hours, he or she may be discharged safely.

BIBLIOGRAPHY

1. Cox J, Wang RY: Critical consequences of common drugs: Manifestations and management of calcium channel blocker and b-adrenergic antagonist overdose. Emerg Med Rep 15:83–90, 1994.
2. Howland MA: Calcium. In Goldfrank LR, Flomenbaum NE, Lewin NA, et al (eds): Goldfrank's Toxicologic Emergencies, 6th ed. Stamford, CT, Appleton & Lange, 1998, pp 1424–1427.
3. Kline JA, Tomaszewski CA, Schroeder JD, et al: Insulin is a superior antidote for cardiovascular toxicity induced by verapamil in the anesthetized canine. J Pharmacol Exp Therapeutics 267:744–750, 1993.
4. Pearigan PD, Benowitz NL: Poisoning due to calcium antagonists: Experience with verapamil, diltiazem, and nifedipine. Drug Safety 6:408–430, 1991.
5. Plewa MC, Martin GC, Menegazzi JJ, et al: Hemodynamic effects of 3,4-diaminopyridine in a swine model of verapamil toxicity. Ann Emerg Med 23:499–507, 1994.
6. Roberts DJ: Common cardiovascular drugs. In Rosen P, Barkin R (eds): Emergency Medicine, 4th ed. St. Louis, Mosby, 1998, pp 1307–1320.
7. Thomas HT, Stone CK, May WA: Exacerbation of verapamil-induced hyperglycemia with glucagon. Am J Emerg Med 13:27–29, 1995.
8. Viccellio P, Henry MC, Yvan J: Calcium channel blockers. In Viccellio P, Bania T, Brent J, et al (eds): Emergency Toxicology, 2nd ed. Philadelphia, Lippincott-Raven, 1998, pp 695–701.

20. ANTIDYSRHYTHMICS

Mark Su, M.D.

1. How are the antidysrhythmics classified?

Despite multiple attempts at revision, the Vaughan-Williams classification is still the most commonly used. It is a system based on the different electrophysiologic properties of the drugs and their subsequent antidysrhythmic effects. The Vaughan-Williams classification has short-comings because it does not take into account that most antidysrhythmic drugs have more than one action and each may have varying effects, direct and indirect, depending on the site of action.

2. What are the four major groups of antidysrhythmic agents?

Class I   Sodium-channel blockers
Class II   Beta-adrenergic antagonists
Class III   Potassium-channel blockers
Class IV   Calcium-channel blockers

3. Are there other drugs or classes of drugs that are not classically characterized as anti-dysrhythmics but that have sodium-channel blocking properties?

Yes. Cocaine, carbamazepine, diphenhydramine, phenothiazines, and tricyclic antidepressants all have antidysrhythmic effects.

4. What are the differences among the class I antidysrhythmic agents?

In addition to sodium-channel blockade, **class IA** drugs prolong the repolarization and refractoriness of myocardial tissue, which leads to prolonged QRS and QT intervals.

Class IB drugs shorten the action potential but produce less inhibition of the fast inward sodium channel. Thus, they have little effect on the QRS, QT, or PR intervals.

Class IC drugs decrease the conduction velocity but have minimal effect on repolarization, and their potent sodium-channel blockade increases the QRS interval more than any other class I agent.

5. List the class IA antidysrhythmic agents.

Disopyramide
Procainamide
Quinidine

6. Name the clinical manifestations of procainamide toxicity.

Hypotension
Fever
Systemic lupus erythematosus–like syndrome
Widening of QRS interval
Prolongation of the QTc duration
Torsades de pointes

7. What drugs are contraindicated in patients with procainamide-induced cardiac toxicity?

Other class IA antidysrhymics (i.e., quinidine, disopyramide) and beta blockers.

8. What is the toxicity of quinidine?

Quinidine, similar to procainamide, is cardiotoxic and is associated with decreased atrioventricular (AV) conduction, intraventricular conduction abnormalities, increased QTc, T-wave inversions, and ST depression. Compared to procainamide, however, quinidine is associated with increased QTc at therapeutic concentrations.

9. What is quinidine syncope?
Quinidine syncope is thought to be from a ventricular dysrhythmia, most likely torsades de pointes.

10. Name the class IB antidysrhythmic agents.

Lidocaine	Phenytoin
Mexiletine	Tocainide

11. What organ system is most commonly affected by lidocaine and how does it manifest clinically?
The **central nervous system** is most commonly affected. Toxicity typically appears as drowsiness, weakness, a sensation of drifting away, euphoria, dysphoria, diplopia, decreased hearing, paresthesias, muscle fasciculations, and seizures.

12. What cardiac toxicity does lidocaine have?
Despite the fact that lidocaine does not commonly cause any electrocardiogram (ECG) abnormalities, sinus arrest, AV block, hypotension, and cardiopulmonary arrest can all occur. Adverse reactions have also been reported at therapeutic doses. Treatment for hypotension includes IV fluids or vasopressors and intra-aortic balloon pump. If bradydysrhythmias occur, atropine, isoproterenol, or a pacemaker can be used.

13. What physiologic conditions or medications can increase the likelihood of lidocaine toxicity?
Because 95% of lidocaine is metabolized by mixed-function oxidases in the liver, toxicity may occur with therapeutic doses in patients who have congestive heart failure, shock, liver disease, or simultaneous use of cimetidine or propranolol.

14. Is phenytoin cardiotoxic?
There has been no reported cardiotoxicity resulting from an oral overdose of phenytoin. However, hypotension and asystole have occurred secondary to the propylene glycol diluent in the intravenous solution being infused too rapidly.

15. List the class IC antidysrhythmics.
Encainide
Flecainide
Propafenone

16. Describe the toxic effects of class IC antidysrhythmics.
They have significant negative inotropic effects. Potent sodium-channel blockade can result in bradycardia, ventricular fibrillation, ventricular tachycardia, and varying heart blocks. Flecainide has also been known to cause neutropenia, and propafenone can cause hypoglycemia.

17. What is the treatment for cardiotoxicity caused by class I antidysrhythmic agents?
Hypertonic sodium bicarbonate has been used to overcome sodium-channel blockade associated with the class I antidysrhythmics and is therefore used for the treatment of wide-complex dysrhythmias associated with some of these agents.

18. In what class of antidysrhythmic is adenosine?
Trick question. Adenosine does not fit into the Vaughan-Williams classification. It is a purinergic receptor agonist that is used in the treatment of reentrant supraventricular tachycardia.

It has a very short half-life. No overdoses have been reported, but its adverse effects include asystole, bronchospasm, and hypotension. Interestingly, patients taking methylxanthines such as theophyline may require larger-than-usual doses of adenosine to exert the desired antidysrhythmic effect because of the antagonistic activity of these agents at adenosine receptors.

19. What class of antidysrhythmic is amiodarone and what toxicity does it have?

Amiodarone, an iodinated compound with a structure similar to thyroxine, is used to treat life-threatening dysrhythmias that are resistant to other medications. It is a class III antidysrhythmic but has effects of all four classes in addition to an antithyroid effect. Toxicity includes negative inotropy and other noncardiac effects including pulmonary fibrosis, hypothyroidism, corneal microdeposits, and photosensitivity. Additionally, when used concomitantly with certain cardioactive drugs (e.g., digoxin, quinidine, procainamide, phenytoin, flecainide), it is known to increase their serum levels.

20. In what class of antidysrhythmic is bretylium? What toxicity does it have?

Like amiodarone, bretylium is a class III agent used to treat resistant ventricular dysrhythmias, including those following myocardial infarction. Bretylium blocks potassium channels but has no effect on sodium channels or automaticity. It also initially causes the release of norepinephrine from sympathetic ganglia with resulting hypertension. However, it later inhibits the release of norepinephrine with ensuing hypotension. IV administration is associated with nausea and vomiting.

BIBLIOGRAPHY

1. Benowitz NL: Lidocaine, mexiletine, and tocainide. In Haddad LM, et al (eds): Clinical Management of Poisoning and Drug Overdose, 2nd ed. Philadelphia, W.B. Saunders, 1990, pp 1371–1379.
2. Desai AD, Chun S, Sung RJ: The role of intravenous amiodarone in the management of cardiac arrhythmias. Ann Intern Med 127:294–303, 1997.
3. Drayer D: Basic clinical pharmacology of the antiarrhythmic drugs procainamide and quinidine. Cardiovasc Rev Rep, pp 44–52, 1990.
4. Kowey P: Pharmacologic effects of antiarrhythmic drugs. Arch Intern Med 158:325–332, 1998.
5. Leatham EW, Holt DW, McKenna WJ: Class III antiarrhythmics in overdose: Presenting features and management principles. Drug Saf 9:450–462, 1993.
6. Lewin N: Antidysrhythmic agents. In Goldfrank LR, Flomenbaum NE, Lewin NA, et al (eds): Goldfrank's Toxicologic Emergencies, 6th ed. Stamford, CT, Appleton & Lange, 1998, pp 860–871.
7. Roden DM: Antiarrhythmic drugs. In Hardman JG, et al (eds): Goodman and Gilman's The Pharmacologic Basis of Therapeutics, 9th ed. New York, McGraw-Hill, 1996, pp 839–874.

VI. Psychopharmacologic Medications

21. CYCLIC ANTIDEPRESSANTS

Paul Bolger, M.D., and Mark B. Mycyk, M.D.

1. Describe how cyclic antidepressants treat depression.

Depressive disorder is thought to be associated with a central neurotransmitter deficiency (serotonin, dopamine, norepinephrine). It is postulated that the first-generation cyclic antidepressants (or tricyclic antidepressants, as they were classically called when released in the 1960s) work by inhibiting the reuptake of these transmitters, thereby increasing their availability within the synapse.

2. How are the cyclics different from the newer antidepressant medicines?

The cyclic antidepressants (CAs) are so named because they all contain a classic ring chemical structure. Unlike the newer generation of selective serotonin reuptake inhibitors (SSRIs), which are relatively selective in their activity, each of the cyclics demonstrates activity at a number of different receptor sites. These various secondary effects are related to the much higher frequency of adverse effects associated with CA use.

3. *Extra credit:* Most cyclic antidepressants have such a low therapeutic index that serious intoxication can be caused by as little as how many times the normal therapeutic dose?

Less than 10 times the normal dose.

4. Why are the cyclic antidepressants considered to be so toxic?

Unfortunately, in addition to inhibiting the reuptake of neurotransmitters, the cyclics also exert secondary effects that are potentially catastrophic even in small overdoses. These are the major secondary actions implicated in most adverse effects:

1. **Sodium channel inhibition.** The cyclics inhibit fast sodium channels in the myocardium in the same way that the class IA antiarrhythmics do (also known as the quinidine-like effect), thus prolonging phase 0 myocardial depolarization. Impaired phase 0 depolarization slows conduction through the ventricular system and appears as a widened QRS on an electrocardiogram (ECG). Inhibited sodium channels have the further effect of inhibiting calcium entry into the myocardial cells, thus diminishing cardiac contractility.

2. **Anticholinergic activity.** Inhibited cholinergic response produces the classic anticholinergic syndrome of dry skin, mydriasis, diminished bowel sounds, hallucinations, delirium, and, most importantly, tachycardia and hyperthermia.

3. **Alpha-adrenergic inhibition.** Cyclic antagonism at the alpha receptors causes peripheral vasodilation. At toxic doses, hypotension further contributes to tachycardia.

5. Describe the clinical presentation of CA overdose.

Patients with acute CA overdose present with symptoms that range anywhere on a clinical spectrum from the mild signs of an anticholinergic syndrome to life-threatening seizures, wide-complex arrhythmias, and hypotension. It is not uncommon for someone with a very recent ingestion to present without symptoms and deteriorate rapidly (< 1 hr). Any patient with a reported cyclic overdose requires immediate attention and evaluation.

6. What is a helpful clinical indicator of severe CA overdose?

The most helpful screening tool is ECG evaluation. A single prospective study identified the QRS duration as the most sensitive indicator of serious cyclic overdose. In the setting of an acute cyclic overdose, 30% of patients with a QRS width > 100 msec developed seizures, and 50% of patients with a QRS width of > 160 msec developed cardiac arrhythmias. No patients with a QRS width < 100 msec developed seizures or cardiac arrhythmias. Although not as sensitive, a rightward axis shift in the terminal 40 msec of the QRS seen most easily in lead AVR is also an indicator of serious CA overdose. Unfortunately, no other clinical or laboratory measures have been found to be helpful in predicting serious CA toxicity.

7. Describe the initial management of a patient with a cyclic overdose.

Because these patients have a tendency to deteriorate rapidly, attention to the ABCs (airway, breathing, circulation) is the first priority. IV access and cardiac monitoring should be established immediately. A 12-lead ECG should be evaluated quickly for QRS prolongation or rightward axis shift. Serum and urine screens for other coingestants may also be indicated. After initial stabilization and screening, rapid gastrointestinal decontamination with oral activated charcoal is recommended. If the patient does not have a secured airway, intubation before charcoal administration is indicated. Gastric lavage is recommended if the patient presents within an hour after ingestion, because CAs are potentially life-threatening agents. Syrup of ipecac is contraindicated, and whole bowel irrigation is probably not useful.

8. What do we do with an ECG demonstrating a QRS width > 100 msec?

In the setting of cyclic overdose, a QRS width should be considered normal only if it is < 100 msec, even though up to 20% of the general population have normal baseline ECGs with a QRS width of 100–120 msec. If the QRS is prolonged, sodium bicarbonate should be administered. The exact mechanism of sodium bicarbonate efficacy continues to spark controversy, but the mechanism is probably a combination of the sodium load along with serum alkalization. Because cyclics poison the myocardial sodium channels in much the same way that quinidine does, it makes sense that the sodium load is an effective antidotal treatment for reducing the QRS width and other arrhythmias. However, it has also been demonstrated that alkalizing the serum increases plasma protein binding of the cyclics, thereby decreasing freely available active drug. Moreover, acidosis further exacerbates cardiac irritability.

9. How should an ECG with arrhythmias other than QRS widening be treated?

In the setting of a cyclic overdose, sodium bicarbonate is considered the antiarrhythmic of choice. QRS widening is simply an early sign of later, more fatal arrhythmias such as ventricular tachycardia, supraventricular tachycardia, and atrioventricular dissociation. A patient who presents with an acute CA overdose and a wide-complex tachycardia should receive sodium bicarbonate first. Class IA and IC antiarrhythmics are contraindicated because they potentiate sodium-channel blockade. Lidocaine has been suggested as a useful adjunct but only as second-line therapy in refractory arrhythmias.

10. How should sodium bicarbonate be administered?

Even the means of administering sodium bicarbonate optimally is controversial. It is common practice to administer sodium bicarbonate as a 1–2-mEq IV bolus push until the QRS narrows to normal limits or the arterial blood pH reaches 7.50–7.55. Traditionally, some authors have suggested that alkalization after initial bolus therapy by adding 3 ampules of 50 mEq doses of sodium bicarbonate to a liter of D5W solution and continued infusion at a rate of 150–200 cc/hour for 4–6 hours may be helpful. However, it makes more sense to push sodium bicarbonate ampules as indicated by the QRS width as long as serum pH does not exceed 7.55, because alkalemia may also cause cardiac excitability. Alkalization to increase protein binding of CAs also may be augmented by hyperventilation of the intubated patient.

11. How should seizures be treated in the setting of a cyclic overdose?

Because seizure-related hypoxia leads to acidosis, prolonged seizures further aggravate cardiac toxicity and need to be expeditiously terminated. Benzodiazepines such as diazepam or lorazepam are most effective immediately. If seizures are refractory to benzodiazepines, phenobarbital is the next useful adjunct.

12. Because cyclic overdose demonstrates so many features of classic anticholinergic poisoning, can physostigmine be used as an antidote?

Physostigmine is a reversible cholinesterase inhibitor that has almost immediate effect in reversing the hallucinations and mental status changes associated with pure anticholinergic poisoning. It was once part of the coma cocktail and administered routinely by prehospital personal and emergency department (ED) staff. However, in patients with anticholinergic symptoms from cyclic poisoning, physostigmine has been shown to precipitate seizure activity or cardiac asystole and is now contraindicated in cyclic overdoses. Physostigmine is an effective antidote when used appropriately for treatment of a noncyclic-induced anticholinergic syndrome; unless the practitioner is certain there is no cyclic coingestants, caution should be maintained.

13. *Extra credit:* What is the trade name of physostigmine?

Antilirium.

14. Should serum CA levels guide therapy?

Cyclic levels unfortunately do not correlate well with toxicity. However, because other drugs have been known to cause QRS widening in overdoses, a cyclic level may be helpful in confirming the presence of a cyclic ingestion.

15. When is it safe to discharge someone with a cyclic ingestion but an otherwise unremarkable work-up?

Serious cyclic toxicity typically presents early after ingestion. In fact, most fatalities occur within the first 2 hours after ingestion, and most signs of any toxicity related to a cyclic will manifest within 6 hours of observation. Thus, patients who have ingested a cyclic but manifest no signs of toxicity generally can be discharged from the ED as long as they have had continuous cardiac monitoring for 6 hours. Remember that these patients also need an appropriate psychiatric evaluation after they have been medically cleared. It is interesting to note that the generic "6-hour" observation rule in the field of toxicology has only been validated in cyclic poisoning but extended (without appropriate studies) to the management of other poisonings.

BIBLIOGRAPHY

1. Boehnert M, Lovejoy FM: Value of QRS duration versus serum drug level in predicting seizures and ventricular arrhythmias after an acute overdose of tricyclic antidepressants. N Engl J Med 313:474–479, 1985.
2. Crone O: Poisoning due to tricyclic antidepressant overdosage: Clinical presentation and treatment. Med Toxicol 1:261–288, 1986.
3. Ellison DW, Pentel PR: Clinical features and consequences of seizures due to cyclic antidepressant overdose. Am J Emerg Med 7:5, 1989.
4. Foulke GE: Identification of toxicity risk early after antidepressant overdose. Am J Emerg Med 13:123–126, 1995.
5. Liebelt EI, Francis PD, Woolf AD: ECG lead AVR versus QRS interval in predicting seizures and arrhythmias in acute tricyclic antidepressant toxicity. Ann Emerg Med 26:195–205, 1995.
6. McCabe JL, Cobaugh DJ, Menegazzi JJ, Fata J: Experimental tricyclic antidepressant toxicity: A randomized, controlled comparison of hypertonic saline solution, sodium bicarbonate, and hyperventilation. Ann Emerg Med 32:329–333, 1998.
7. Rosenstein DL, Nelson JC, Jacobs SC: Seizures associated with antidepressants: A review. J Clin Psychiatry 54:289–299, 1993.
8. Pimentel L, Trommer L: Cyclic antidepressant overdoses. Emerg Med Clin North Am 12:533–549, 1994.
9. Weisman RS: Cyclic antidepressants. In Goldfrank LR, Flomenbaum NE, Lewin NA, et al (eds): Goldfrank's Toxicologic Emergencies, 6th ed. Stamford, CT, Appleton & Lange, 1998, pp 925–934.

22. SELECTIVE SEROTONIN REUPTAKE INHIBITORS

Evan Kahn, M.D., and Mark B. Mycyk, M.D.

1. Selective serotonin reuptake inhibitors (SSRIs) are touted as being very safe. Why dedicate a whole chapter to SSRIs if they are so benign?

Indeed, current SSRIs are extremely safe and were designed in response to the high incidence of adverse effects attributed to tricyclic antidepressants (TCAs, also known as first-generation cyclics). In fact, the safety window of SSRIs is so much larger than that of TCAs that many authors have deemed the greatest risk associated with SSRIs is their **lack of use** in the depressed and mentally ill population. During the period 1987–1996, only 16 cases of fatal overdoses from SSRIs were reported compared with 100–150 overdoses from TCAs. However, as with all other medicines, SSRI use is not entirely benign, especially since the number of patients being prescribed SSRIs is multiplying at an incredible rate. These drugs do have potentially lethal complications alone, in overdose, or in combination with other medicines. Evaluation and disposition of these patients should not be taken lightly.

2. Describe the antidepressant mechanism of SSRIs.

All of the SSRIs do exactly what their name indicates: they inhibit presynaptic neuronal reuptake of serotonin. It is thought that depressive disorders are related to a relative deficiency of neurotransmitters, with serotonin considered one of the most relevant. Unlike TCAs, SSRIs have very selective activity and exert minimal (not negligible) activity at other neurotransmitter-receptor sites. Specifically, trazodone and nefazodone antagonize alpha-adrenergic receptors, venlafaxine inhibits reuptake of norepinephrine and dopamine, and bupropion inhibits dopaminergic receptors.

3. What are the common features of toxic overdoses of SSRIs?

In general, acute ingestions of several magnitudes greater than the daily recommended dosage are rarely associated with any symptoms. Bradycardia is one feature commonly reported to be associated with therapeutic to supratherapeutic doses of all SSRIs. Acute ingestions up to 50 times the daily recommended dose of SSRIs are often associated with nausea, vomiting, tremor, lethargy, dizziness, and central nervous system (CNS) depression. Acute ingestions greater than 150 times the usual daily dose have been reported with death. Animal studies and several human case reports suggest that seizures are more commonly associated with SSRI overdose than previously thought, although the overall incidence remains relatively low. In the majority of deaths associated with SSRI overdose, coingestants were also implicated.

4. Discuss the management of SSRI overdose.

Treatment is mainly supportive with specific attention to the ABCs (airway, breathing, circulation). A single dose of oral activated charcoal is helpful in acute ingestion. SSRI overdose is rarely fatal; however, obtaining serum levels, urinalysis, and an electrocardiogram (ECG) to screen for other potentially more toxic coingestants is indicated.

5. What is the serotonin syndrome?

Serotonin syndrome (also known as serotonin behavioral or hyperreactivity syndrome) is a reaction most commonly precipitated by the combination of different drugs that enhance serotonin levels presynaptically by different mechanisms. Serotonin syndrome precipitated by single drug overdose is extremely rare (see Table). Although it has been recognized in animals since the

1950s and was identified in humans using monoamine oxidase inhibitors (MAOIs) combined with SSRIs in the 1960s, it was not given this name until 1982. This syndrome refers to the triad of cognitive, autonomic, and neuromuscular manifestations in the setting of serotonergic-enhancing agents. The syndrome typically appears within 24 hours of an adjustment to a dosage of a chronically used medicine or the addition of another agent to a drug regimen. Clinical signs and symptoms include confusion, agitation, disorientation, tremor, nausea, vomiting, shivers, myoclonus, diaphoresis, ataxia, hyperreflexia, delirium, coma, mydriasis, hyperthermia, and unstable blood pressure. Although concrete diagnostic criteria for serotonin syndrome are still not agreed upon, most authors have concluded that someone with mental status changes, autonomic instability, and neuromuscular changes associated with serotonergic agent use fulfills the diagnosis for serotonin syndrome.

Drugs that Affect Serotonin Levels

EFFECT	DRUG
Inhibits serotonin breakdown	MAOIs, cocaine
Inhibits serotonin reuptake	SSRIs, meperidine, dextromethorphan
Promotes serotonin release	MDMA ("ecstasy")

MDMA = methylenedioxymethamphetamine

6. What is the proper management of a patient who presents with serotonin syndrome?

Supportive therapy, recognition of the syndrome, and discontinuing the offending agents are the mainstays of treatment. Activated charcoal is appropriate in the setting of an acute overdose. If hyperthermia and muscle rigidity are present, benzodiazepines should be considered as preferential treatment, because hyperthermia in the setting of serotonin syndrome is an indicator of poor prognosis. Some innovative treatments under investigation include cyproheptadine, methysergide, and propranolol. Cyproheptadine, an antihistamine with extensive serotonergic blockade activity, is the most promising in hastening clinical recovery. Nonetheless, with appropriate supportive care only, symptoms generally resolve within the first 24 hours.

7. How is serotonin syndrome different from neuroleptic malignant syndrome (NMS)?

Although the two share many of the same clinical characteristics, serotonin syndrome is secondary to serotonin excess whereas NMS is secondary to dopamine deficiency. Some authors argue that the two are part of a continuum of the same clinical pathophysiology, especially because excess serotonin has been shown to create a dopamine deficiency, and dopamine agonists have been shown to release even more serotonin presynaptically. Unlike serotonin syndrome, NMS is almost always associated with hyperthermia and usually presents over the course of several days. The important point is that treatment of both disorders relies on rapid recognition, discontinuation of the offending agents, and aggressive supportive therapy.

8. What other atypical effects have been reported with SSRI use?

Serotonin receptor sites are not limited to neurons. Platelets have been demonstrated to have serotonin receptors, and some studies have shown an increased incidence of bleeding in patients using therapeutic doses of SSRIs. Although the exact mechanism is not clear, it may be due to SSRI-inhibited platelet production of nitric oxide or simply enhanced serotonergic agonism of the platelet serotonin receptor. The syndrome of inappropriate secretion of diuretic hormone (SIADH) has also been sporadically reported in various degrees in patients who use SSRIs chronically. Also, serotonin excess has been implicated in dopamine deficiency: some case series report parkinsonism in patients previously using SSRIs.

9. *Extra credit:* What commonly used herbal medication has SSRI-type properties?

St. John's wort.

BIBLIOGRAPHY

1. Barbey JT, Roose SP: SSRI safety in overdose. J Clin Psychiatry 59:42–48, 1998.
2. DiRocco A, Brannan T, Prikhojan A, Yahr MD: Sertraline-induced parkinsonism: A case report and an in-vivo study of the effect of sertraline on dopamine metabolism. J Neurol Transm 105:247–251, 1998.
3. Friel PN, Logan BK, Fligier CL: Three fatal drug overdoses involving bupropion. J Anal Toxicol 17:436–438, 1993.
4. Graudins A, Stearman A, Chan B: Treatment of the serotonin syndrome with cyproheptadine. J Emerg Med 16:615–619, 1998.
5. Martin TG: Serotonin syndrome. Ann Emerg Med 28:520–526, 1996.
6. Pentel PR, Keyler DE, Haddad LM: Tricyclic antidepressants and selective serotonin reuptake inhibitors. In Haddad LM, Shannon MW, Winchester JF (eds): Clinical Management of Poisoning and Drug Overdose, 3rd ed. Philadelphia, W.B. Saunders, 1998, pp 447–451.
7. Settle EC: Antidepressant drugs: Disturbing and potentially dangerous adverse effects. J Clin Psychiatry 59:25–30, 1998.
8. Stoner SC, Marken PA, Watson WA, et al: Antidepressant overdoses and resultant emergency department services: The impact of SSRIs. Psychopharmacol Bull 33:667–670, 1997.
9. Stork C: Selective serotonin reuptake inhibitors and other antidepressants. In Goldfrank LR, Flomenbaum NE, Lewin NA, et al (eds): Goldfrank's Toxicologic Emergencies, 6th ed. Stamford, CT, Appleton & Lange, 1998, pp 935–942.

23. NEUROLEPTIC AGENTS

John Alexis, M.D., and Anthony Burda, R.Ph.

1. What are neuroleptic agents?

The term *neuroleptic* has replaced terms such as *major tranquilizer* and *antipsychotic drugs*, which are often used in the treatment of a variety of psychotic and anxiety states. The early usage of the term neuroleptic encompassed all agents that possessed antipsychotic properties along with extrapyramidal effects (e.g., rigidity, tremor, bradykinesia, and akathisia). Newer "atypical neuroleptics" lack these parkinsonian effects yet are still referred to as neuroleptic agents.

2. *Extra credit:* What drug was first tried in 1950 to treat motor agitation in mental illness?

Promethazine.

3. How are neuroleptic agents classified? Give some examples of each drug class.

Since the synthesis of chlorpromazine and promethazine in 1950, several dozen neuroleptic agents have been developed and marketed for both human and veterinary use. These drugs are commonly divided into groups based on chemical structures. Each chemical group differs from the others based on pharmacologic potency and spectrum of side effects (i.e., degree of sedation, anticholinergic symptoms, adverse cardiovascular reactions, and incidence of extrapyramidal symptoms).

Examples of Different Neuroleptic Agents

NEUROLEPTIC CLASS	EXAMPLE	TRADE NAME
Phenothiazines		
Aliphatics	Chlorpromazine	Thorazine
	Promethazine	Phenergan
Piperazines	Trifluoperazine	Stelazine
	Prochlorperazine	Compazine
	Perphenazine	Trilafon
	Fluphenazine	Prolixin
Piperidines	Thioridazine	Mellaril
	Mesoridazine	Serentil
Thioxanthenes	Thiothixene	Navane
Butyrophenones	Droperidol	Inapsin
	Haloperidol	Haldol
Indoles	Molindone	Moban
Dibenzoxazepines	Loxapine	Loxitane
Diphenyl-butylpiperidines	Pimozide	Orap
Dibenzodiazepines	Clozapine	Clozaril
	Olanzapine	Zyprexa
Benzisoxazoles	Risperidone	Risperdal
Dibenzothiazepines	Quetiapine	Seroquel

4. When are neuroleptic agents indicated?

Neuroleptic medications are best known for their efficacy as antipsychotics, which reduce the hallucinations, delirium, and agitation. Many have antiemetic properties (e.g., prochlorperizine) and are used in the management of nausea, vomiting, and motion sickness. Some demonstrate

93

H_1 receptor antagonism (e.g., promethazine) and have been used for their antihistaminic properties. Agents such as droperidol are used as adjuncts in the induction of anesthesia. Neuroleptics are available in a variety of oral and parenteral forms.

5. Explain the most significant toxicologic effects of neuroleptic drug.
- In overdose settings, neuroleptics can act as **central nervous system (CNS) depressants**.
- Extrapyramidal effects such as **acute dystonic reactions** may occur.
- Due to a lowering of the seizure threshold, **convulsions** are possible.
- **Antimuscarinic-antihistaminic signs and symptoms** (e.g., tachycardia, dry mucous membranes, and decreased gastrointestinal [GI] motility) may be present.
- **Mydriasis** or **miosis** may be observed.
- Peripheral alpha$_1$ receptor blockade may be responsible for **hypotension**.
- Quinidine-like effects on the heart account for various **electrocardiographic (ECG) abnormalities** and **cardiac dysrhythmias**.
- Alterations in thermoregulation may account for **hypothermia** or **hyperthermia**.

6. Discuss neuroleptic-induced hypotension.
Neuroleptic-induced hypotension occurs because of peripheral alpha-receptor blockade. Treatment with intravenous fluids and vasopressors may be necessary. Pure alpha agonists such as norepinephrine and phenylephrine may be more effective than mixed alpha-beta adrenergic agents (i.e., epinephrine or dopamine), because unopposed beta stimulation may cause vasodilation that will exacerbate the hypotension.

7. Explain the treatment of neuroleptic-induced cardiac arrhythmias.
Death from neuroleptic overdose is rare; however, arrhythmias induced by neuroleptics can be fatal. Quinidine-like effects may cause cardiac conduction defects such as atrioventricular block, widening of the QRS interval, and prolonged QT interval. Ventricular tachycardia and fibrillation with sudden cardiac arrest have been reported and are more likely to occur with piperidine phenothiazine overdoses. Arrhythmias may be life threatening and difficult to treat. Lidocaine may be used for ventricular dysrhythmias. Manage ventricular fibrillation with cardioversion. Treat torsades de pointes with IV magnesium sulfate, isoproterenol, or atrial overdrive pacing while correcting any electrolyte abnormalities. As with the tricyclic antidepressants, widening QRS may be treated with sodium bicarbonate.
Avoid all class 1A antidysrhythmics, such as quinidine, procainamide, and disopyramide, because these may exacerbate conduction disturbance. Bretylium should be avoided because its alpha blockade may worsen hypotension.

8. What factors increase the incidence of mortality in acute neuroleptic overdose?
Acute neuroleptic overdose is rarely lethal and is usually part of a coingestion of drugs. For that reason, a patient with schizoaffective disorder who is taking both neuroleptics and antidepressants has an increased risk of death if he or she attempts suicide. Deaths are also more frequent with thioridazine and mesoridazine overdose secondary to the increased incidence of arrhythmias.

9. A patient with schizophrenia presents to your emergency department 1 hour after ingesting an unknown amount of haloperidol. Should this patient undergo gastric decontamination?
Depression of mental status, dystonic reactions, and seizures increase the patient's risk for aspiration. Uncontrolled gastric evacuation methods such as using syrup of ipecac are not recommended. Orogastric lavage is preferred if given within 1 hour of a potentially life-threatening amount of neuroleptic agent. Activated charcoal should be administered with or without a cathartic, depending on the age of the patient. After a recent ingestion, some phenothiazines may show up on KUB (kidneys-ureters-bladder) imaging.

10. What other supportive measures may you consider in neuroleptic overdose?

Airway protection and ventilatory support are mandatory in overdosed patients experiencing significant CNS and respiratory depression. Anticonvulsants such as benzodiazepines and phenobarbital can be administered to a patient experiencing seizures. For agents with significant anticholinergic symptomatology, physostigmine should be avoided. Because of large volumes of distribution and high degree of protein binding demonstrated by most neuroleptic agents, extracorporeal methods of drug removal such as hemodialysis and hemoperfusion will not remove significant amounts of drug.

11. Name some common extrapyramidal symptoms (EPSs) that can be seen with neuroleptics.

Neuroleptic agents are dopamine receptor antagonists. When antidopaminergic activities exceed anticholinergic activity, dystonia results. The fewer anticholinergic properties that are present, the greater the EPS reactions encountered. Therefore, piperazines, phenothiazines, and butyrophenones are the most likely agents to produce EPSs. The newer classes of atypical neuroleptics produce lower incidences of EPS. The following are some are some brief descriptions of EPSs:

Dystonic reactions. Dystonic reactions include oculogyric crisis (upward gaze paralysis), torticollis, retrocollis, opisthotonos (scoliosis), and tortipelvis (abdominal wall spasms). In 95% of cases, acute dystonias appear within 4 days of initiation of therapy or with an increase in drug dosage. Dystonias usually appears within 60 days of therapy. Young age, male sex, cocaine use, and a history of acute dystonia are all risk factors.

Akathisia. The restlessness, inability to sit still, and muscle discomfort of this condition often affect elderly patients and occur early in treatment (5–60 days). Lowering the dosage of the neuroleptic agent decreases its incidence.

Parkinsonism (akinesia). Parkinsonism is characterized by bradykinesia, shuffling gait, resting tremor, masked face, and rabbit syndrome (periorbital tremor). It affects 90% of susceptible patients within 72 days of therapy and occasionally responds to reduction in the dosage of the neuroleptic.

12. How are many of the extrapyramidal adverse effects best treated?

First, don't panic; the dystonias may appear dangerous but they rarely cause death. Anticholinergics or benzodiazepines are the usual treatment. Benzodiazepines are best if the patient is experiencing hyperthermia. After an acute dystonic reaction, several days of therapy may be needed to counteract the adverse effects. Intramuscular injection of either agent is usually adequate; intravenous administration is necessary only in cases of stridor. Prophylaxis with anticholinergics also can be used initially to prevent extrapyramidal symptoms.

AGENT	DOSE
Diphenhydramine (Benadryl)	50–100 mg or 1–2 mg/kg
Benztropine mesylate (Cogentin)	1–2 mg IM
Trihexyphenidyl (Artane)	1–3 mg IV or IM
Diazepam (Valium)	5–10 mg IV or IM

13. Describe tardive dyskinesia. How does it differ from other EPSs?

Tardive dyskinesia is more problematic for the patient than other EPSs. Tardive disorders (tardive dyskinesia and tardive dystonia) occur after years of neuroleptic therapy and are often irreversible. The usual symptom of tardive dyskinesia is involuntary, repetitive movements of the face, tongue, and lips. Choreoathetoid movements of the limbs are more common in tardive dystonia.

Tardive dyskinesia and tardive dystonia are often considered similar diseases; however, their epidemiology differs. Dyskinesia affects older females more commonly, whereas dystonias usually affect younger males. It has been postulated that chronic neuroleptic use causes upregulation of dopamine receptors in the striatum. Thus, the appearance of tardive dyskinesia often emerges as the neuroleptic agent is withdrawn and dopamine activity increases.

14. How is tardive dyskinesia treated?

There is no established therapy for tardive dystonia or dyskinesia. When a patient develops tardive dyskinesia, the physician should reevaluate whether the patient truly needs the neuroleptics. If not, clozapine or other atypical neuroleptics should be considered. If the dystonia continues, botulinum toxin injections may be added to the regimen. Tetrabenazine and reserpine are other alternatives if clozapine and botulinum toxin don't help. In addition, many studies show vitamin E to be of benefit. On the other hand, few studies have reported the improvement in symptoms with electroconvulsive therapy (4 case studies to date). Other drugs such as substituted benzamides sulpiride, tiapride, and remoxipride are in use internationally but have not yet been approved in the United States. The benefit of calcium channel blockers is unclear.

15. An obtunded male with a temperature of 105°F arrives in the emergency department with convulsions. He has a history of schizophrenia and is being treated with fluphenazine.

The differential diagnosis includes meningitis, CNS event, and possible anticholinergic poisoning. Neuroleptic malignant syndrome (NMS) is an uncommon yet potentially fatal complication associated with neuroleptic drug therapy. It was first described in 1960 by Delay and Lemperier and named the "syndrome malin des neuroleptiques." The syndrome is characterized by "lead pipe" rigidity, profound hyperthermia, mental status changes (e.g., lethargy and confusion), and autonomic instability characterized by profuse diaphoresis and fluctuation in heart rate and blood pressure. Akinesia, choreoathetosis, tremors, and generalized contractions may result. Creatine phosphokinase (CPK), leukocyte, and liver enzyme levels may be elevated.

NMS is an idiosyncratic reaction that affects up to 2% of patients on neuroleptics. NMS essentially is an extreme extrapyramidal reaction that likely is caused by excessive dopamine receptor blockade. It may occur with other agents that block dopamine receptors such as metoclopramide, after abrupt withdrawal of dopamine agonists such as bromocriptine or L-dopa, and during chronic lithium therapy. NMS also may occur after a rapid increase in neuroleptic dosing or following cessation of anticholinergic medication.

16. Discuss the management of NMS.

Because fever in NMS is often resistant to antipyretics, the patient should be cooled rapidly with spray mist fans and strategic ice placement. If rigidity is severe, paralytic agents and benzodiazepines may be used. Additional interventions that have shown evidence of shortening duration of the syndrome are treatment with bromocriptine or dantrolene sodium. Bromocriptine, a dopamine agonist, is given orally at a dose of 5 mg three times daily. Dantrolene sodium, which relieves muscle hyperrigidity by acting in the muscle sarcoplasmic reticulum and inhibiting the release of calcium, can be dosed at 2.5 mg/kg up to 10 mg/kg IV, followed by maintenance dosing of 2.5 mg/kg every 6 hours. Anticholinergic agents should be avoided. Symptoms may last up to 10 days, and all neuroleptics should be withheld for up to 2 weeks. In addition, evidence suggests that electroconvulsive therapy helps with NMS. If neuroleptic therapy will be reinitiated, an agent with fewer extrapyramidal effects should be selected, such as an atypical neuroleptic (e.g., clozapine).

17. What are the newer "atypical neuroleptics" and how do they differ from first-generation drugs such as the phenothiazines?

In recent years several new neuroleptic medications have become very popular, including clozapine, olanzapine, risperidone, and quetiapine. Several other agents are currently under investigation, including sertindole, ziprasidone, and remoxipride. A therapeutic advantage of this group of agents is that they are effective as antipsychotic drugs but have a lower incidence of EPSs. Reversal of tardive dyskinesia with clozapine also has been reported. The cause is probably the selective action at central serotonin $5HT_2$ and dopamine D_2 receptors in the mesolimbic system rather than the striatum such as the traditional neuroleptics.

Clozapine overdose may produce sedation or coma with marked respiratory depression, anticholinergic findings, tachycardia and arrhythmias, hypotension, seizures, and NMS. Blood dyscrasias such as neutropenia and agranulocytosis are known to occur as idiosyncratic reactions during therapeutic use and may be noted following overdose. The complete blood count (CBC) should be monitored carefully for several weeks following clozapine overdose.

Both **olanzapine** and **quetiapine** possess chemical structures similar to clozapine; however, they have not demonstrated bone marrow toxicity as with clozapine. Toxicity of these agents is characterized by CNS depression, tachycardia, hypotension, ECG changes, EPSs, seizures, and liver enzyme elevations. Anticholinergic effects may occur with olanzapine. NMS has been reported with quetiapine.

Risperidone overdose has been associated with mild CNS depression, hypotension or hypertension, tachycardia, agitation, electrolyte disturbances such as hyponatremia or hypokalemia, cardiac conduction disturbances, EPSs, and NMS.

BIBLIOGRAPHY

1. Baldessarini RJ: Drugs and treatment of psychiatric disorders. In Hardman JG, Limbird LE, Molinoff PB, et al (eds): Goodman and Gilman's The Pharmacological Basis of Therapeutics, 9th ed. New York, McGraw-Hill, 1996, pp 399–420.
2. Buckley P, Hutchinson M: Neuroleptic malignant syndrome. J Neurol Neurosurg Psychiatry 58:271–273, 1995.
3. Dawkins K, Lieberman JA, Lebowitz BD, Hsiao JK: Antipsychotics: Past and future: National Institute of Mental Health Division of Services and Intervention Research Workshop, July 14, 1998. Schizophr Bull 25:395–405, 1999.
4. Gupta S, Mosnik D, Black DW, et al: Tardive dyskinesia: Review of treatments past, present, and future. Ann Clin Psychiatry 11:257–265, 1999.
5. Lewin NA: Neuroleptic agents. In Goldfrank LR, Flomenbaum NE, Lewin NA, et al (eds): Goldfrank's Toxicological Emergencies, 6th ed. Stamford, CT, Appleton & Lange, 1998, pp 943–953.
6. Littrell KH, Johnson CG, Littrell S, Peabody CD: Marked reductoin of tardive dyskinesia with olanzapine. Arch Gen Psychiatry 55:279–280, 1998.
7. Meltzer HY, McGurk SR: The effects of clozapine, risperidone, and olanzapine on cognitive function in schizophrenia. Schizophr Bull 25:233–255, 1999.
8. Raja M: Managing antipsychotic-induced acute and tardive dystonia. Drug Safety 19:57–72, 1998.
9. Toll LL, Hulbut KM (eds): Poisondex System. Engelwood, CO, Micromedex, 2000.
10. Van Harten PN, Hoek H, Kahn RS: Acute dystonia induced by drug treatment. Br Med J 319:623–626, 1999.

24. MONOAMINE OXIDASE INHIBITORS

Paul Bolger, M.D., and Andrea G. Carlson, M.D.

1. Describe the mechanism of action of monoamine oxidase inhibitors (MAOIs).

Monoamine oxidase is an intracellular enzyme that breaks down naturally occurring and ingested monoamines. Its inhibition increases the concentration of norepinephrine, epinephrine, dopamine, and serotonin in the sympathetic nerve terminals. The increase in catecholamine concentration is what is thought to cause the antidepressant effect of the MAOIs.

Inhibition of this enzyme occurs in the central nervous system (CNS) and in the periphery. There are two commonly known subtypes of MAO: MAO-A, found in the liver and gastrointestinal tract, and MAO-B, found in the brain and platelets. Certain MAOIs preferentially inhibit one subtype, and certain substrates are exclusive to one particular subtype. MAOIs inhibit many other enzyme systems, including B_6-containing enzyme systems.

MAOIs also have amphetamine-like activity because of their structural similarity to amphetamines. Certain MAOIs are metabolized into amphetamine and methamphetamine.

2. *Extra credit:* In 1957, what MAOI was introduced into psychiatry as a "psychic energizer"?

Iproniazid was first introduced as a treatment for tuberculosis. Patients taking this medication were noted to have dramatic elevation in their moods. Media photographs from that time captured patients dancing in the hospital corridors, apparently overjoyed by their recovery from tuberculosis, when, in fact, these patients were probably experiencing euphoric side effects of iproniazid! Further studies confirmed that iproniazid inhibited monoamine oxidase and could reverse the notorious depressogenic effect of reserpine. Unfortunately, other, less-pleasant side effects of iproniazid required its replacement with the present-day medication isoniazid (INH), which does not have any significant effect on the MAO enzymes.

3. Which MAOIs are available in the United States?

MAOI	TRADE NAME	USE	MAO SUBTYPE INHIBITOR
Phenelzine sulfate	Nardil	Treatment for depression	Irreversible inhibitor of both MAO-A and MAO-B
Tranylcypromine sulfate	Parnate	Treatment for depression	Irreversible inhibitor of both MAO-A and MAO-B
Procarbazine	Matulane	Antineoplastic agent for Hodgkin's disease	Irreversible inhibitor of both MAO-A and MAO-B
Selegiline	Eldepryl	Antiparkinsonian agent	Irreversible MAO-B inhibitor

Outside of the United States, other MAOIs are in use, including reversible and irreversible inhibitors of MAO-A.

4. What is the clinical presentation of MAOI overdose?

Symptoms of MAOI overdose characteristically are related to CNS sympathetic hyperactivity from increased concentration of catecholamines at the nerve terminal. Because of the delayed onset of symptoms, patients initially may have no symptoms, even after a massive ingestion.

Toxicity symptoms include headache, agitation, hypertension, tachycardia, tachypnea, hyperthermia, flushing, sweating, agitation, muscular rigidity, myoclonus, seizures, coma, mydriasis, and nystagmus. In severe poisonings, hypotension, bradycardia, and asystole can occur, presumably because of the depletion of catecholamines available for neurotransmission. Other late effects are pulmonary edema, disseminated intravascular coagulation, rhabdomyolysis, and myoglobinuric renal failure.

5. Discuss the management of MAOI overdose.

Begin with the standard approach to any ingestion with attention to the ABCs (airway, breathing, circulation). Activated charcoal should be administered.

Initiate supportive care for cardiovascular complications. Severe hypertension is treated with a rapidly titratable agent such as nitroprusside. Hypertension can be followed quickly by profound hypotension; therefore, longer acting agents should be avoided. Beta blockers also should be avoided because they may cause unopposed alpha stimulation. Reflex bradycardia should not be treated with vagolytics such as atropine because it may worsen hypertension. Bradycardia associated with hypotension may require temporary pacing. Hypotension is treated initially with fluid resuscitation. For persistent hypotension, use a direct-acting vasopressor such as norepinephrine or epinephrine.

Advanced cardiac life support (ACLS) algorithms apply to the treatment of dysrhythmias in MAOI overdose with the exception of bretylium, which causes a release of endogenous catecholamines, possibly worsening toxicity.

Seizures, neuromuscular rigidity, and agitation are treated with benzodiazepines. Passive cooling measures (cool mist, fans) to control hyperthermia may be needed. Rhabdomyolysis is treated with aggressive hydration and diuretics.

6. What is the appropriate disposition of a patient with MAOI ingestion?

The onset of these symptoms is consistently delayed, sometimes up to 12 hours. Symptoms and death can occur for days after overdose. Thus, all patients with suspected MAOI overdose should have 24 hours of intensive care unit (ICU) observation, regardless of initial presentation. The usual "6-hour observation period" does not apply in suspected MAOI overdose.

7. Does hemodialysis have a role in the management of MAOI overdose?

Neither hemodialysis nor hemoperfusion plays a role in management of MAOI overdose. MAOIs are highly protein bound and have a large volume of distribution (V_d). Thus, only a small fraction of drug remains in the plasma after distribution. Consequently, removal of the drug from the serum will not have a great impact on total body concentration or on the concentration of the drug at the nerve terminal.

8. What clue on a routine urine drug screen can suggest MAOI ingestion?

Tranylcypromine and selegiline both have amphetamine and methamphetamine as active metabolites and may lead to a false-positive urine drug screen.

9. Is an MAOI serum level helpful in the management of overdose?

No. Although detectable levels can confirm exposure, peak plasma levels are not well characterized and rarely guide clinical management or predict outcome.

10. *Extra credit:* Which highly publicized death that significantly impacted graduate medical education may have involved an MAOI-drug interaction?

The unexplained death of 18-year-old Libby Zion in a New York hospital in 1984 became the focus of a national debate regarding resident physician training, working conditions, and supervision. Although an autopsy and review of the clinical data failed to reveal a definite cause of Miss Zion's death, one theory is that she was given meperidine during a period of agitation. Meperidine is well known to have a potential adverse reaction with MAOIs such as phenelzine, which she had been taking chronically for depression. Within an hour of meperidine administration, Miss Zion's agitation returned and her fever elevated. She suffered fatal cardiac arrest 2 hours later.

11. Name other common drugs that interact with MAOIs to produce toxicity.

Any sympathomimetic agent (see Table) can produce toxicity by causing release of catecholamines in the CNS and parasympathetic nervous system (PNS). The MAOIs cause an increased pool of catecholamines in the nerve terminals due to the inhibition of metabolism.

Common Sympathomimetic Agents

Albuterol	Epinephrine	Methylphenidate	Phenylpropanolamine
Amphetamines	Isoetharine	Norepinephrine	Pseudoephedrine
Cocaine	Isoproterenol	Pemoline	Reserpine
Dopamine	Ketamine	Phentermine	Salmeterol
Ephedrine	Methyldopa	Phenylephrine	Terbutaline

Any drug associated with increased concentration of serotonin, including codeine and dextromethorphan, can precipitate serotonin syndrome. MAOIs also can potentiate the hypoglycemic effect of insulin and sulfonylureas.

12. A young woman presents to the emergency department with a severe headache that began at a wine and cheese party. The physical examination reveals marked hypertension. Her medical history indicates only depression, for which she takes phenelzine. She denies taking more than the prescribed dosage of her medication. Can you explain her symptoms?

Yes. Foods and beverages that contain tyramine can precipitate toxicity. Tyramine acts similarly to indirect-acting sympathomimetic drugs, causing release of catecholamines in the CNS and PNS. Like MAOI overdose, patients present with hypertension, headache, tachycardia, bradycardia, hyperthermia, altered mental status, seizures, intracranial hemorrhage, or serotonin syndrome. Unlike MAOI overdose, symptoms will occur minutes to hours after ingestion of the offending agent.

Over the years, scattered case reports of the MAOI-tyramine reaction have implicated nearly seventy different food items. Such reports have resulted in over-inclusive dietary restrictions that have limited compliance of those patients taking MAOIs. Recently, both clinical investigations assessing actual food tyramine content and reviews of the literature have been performed in an attempt to clarify the necessary dietary restrictions.

Foods with Significant Tyramine Content

Aged cheeses	Improperly stored or spoiled meats
Aged or cured meats	Sauerkraut
Broad bean pods	Soybean curd, miso
Concentrated yeast extract (Marmite)	Soy sauce
Dry sausages	Tap beers

Wine and domestic bottled or canned beers, historically considered major culprits in the tyramine reaction, are considered safe when consumed in moderation.

13. How do you treat patients with MAO-drug or food interactions?

The approach to these patients is largely supportive. Care of cardiovascular complications is the same as for overdose. Any symptomatic patient should be admitted to the ICU for 24 hours of monitoring. If completely asymptomatic for 6 hours, a patient may be discharged home.

BIBLIOGRAPHY

1. Asch DA, Parker RM: The Libby Zion case: One step forward or two steps backward? N Engl J Med 318:771–775, 1988.
2. Bosse GM, Matyunas NJ: Delayed toxidromes. J Emerg Med 17:679–690, 1999.

3. Gardner DM, Shulman KI, Walker SE, Tailor SA: The making of a user friendly MAOI diet. J Clin Psychiatry 57:99–104, 1996.
4. Jacobsen E: The early history of psychotherapeutic drugs. Psychopharmacology 89:138–144, 1986.
5. Livingston MG, Livingston HM: Monoamine oxidase inhibitors. An update on drug interactions. Drug Saf 14:219–227, 1996.
6. Sauter D: Monoamine oxidase inhibitors. In Goldfrank LR, Flomenbaum NE, Lewin NA, et al (eds): Goldfrank's Toxicologic Emergencies, 6th ed. Stamford, CT, Appleton & Lange, 1998, pp 955–965.

25. LITHIUM

Helen Choi, M.D., and Frank Paloucek, PharmD

1. Lithium behaves similarly to what two ubiquitous cations in the human body and why?
Sodium and potassium. Lithium, with a valence of $^+1$, is atomic element 3 in the periodic table and belongs to the same family of metals as sodium and potassium.

2. For what condition is lithium classically indicated?
Bipolar disorder (manic-depression) and other affective disorders.

3. What other disorders is lithium used for?
During the 19th century, it was used to treat arthritis and nephrolithiasis. Currently, lithium is used for the prevention of cluster headaches and as a cell stimulator in patients with neutropenia.

4. *Extra credit:* The year 1930 saw the introduction of a lithium-containing drink called Bib-Label Lithiated Lemon-Lime Soda, which was touted to relieve the depression caused by hangovers. Still on the market, but without lithium, what is this popular drink now called?
7-Up.

5. *Extra credit:* In the 1940s and 1950s, lithium was used as a substitute for a common culinary substance that led to intoxications and its eventual withdrawal from the market. Name the substance.
Table salt.

6. What are the pharmacokinetics of lithium?
Ninety-five percent of lithium is cleared by the kidneys; its clearance is therefore dependent on the glomerular filtration rate. Five percent of lithium is secreted in sweat and salivary glands. The half-life is 20–24 hours but may be longer in patients who are chronically on lithium. It is predominantly reabsorbed after filtration in the proximal tubules; however, some lithium is reabsorbed distally at the level of the loop of Henle and the distal tubules. This reabsorption is in preference to sodium, leading to increased accumulation with intravascular volume depletion or dehydration. The steady-state volume of distribution is 0.6–0.9 L/kg with a long distribution half-life (12 hours for the central nervous system).

7. Do lithium levels correlate with toxicity?
No. Lithium levels do not predict or correlate with clinical manifestations. This may be explained by lithium's slow distribution time. The therapeutic range for lithium serum concentrations is commonly reported as 0.6–1.2 mEq/L.

8. Which organ systems does lithium affect?
Neurologic abnormalities predominate in acute and chronic lithium intoxication. A fine tremor of the hands may be appreciated initially. However, as toxicity progresses, hyperreflexia and agitation will develop followed by fasciculations, muscular irritability, choreoathetosis, clonus, seizures, and altered mental status, including confusion, lethargy, and even coma. Nystagmus, dysarthria, and ataxia also have been reported.

9. What is the mechanism of action of lithium?
The definite mechanism of action of lithium is unknown. Proposed mechanisms include:
• Competition with sodium and potassium as discussed in questions 1 and 6

- Interference with magnesium metabolism because of its similar atomic radius
- Interactions with protein kinase C and G proteins, which may ultimately decrease the brain's concentration of inositol (an important mediator of intracellular calcium release)
- Decreasing the effects of norepinephrine by interfering with the second-messenger cyclic adenosine monophosphate (cAMP)

10. List the clinical manifestations of patients with acute lithium intoxication.

In addition to neurologic manifestations, gastrointestinal (GI) symptoms of nausea, vomiting, and diarrhea predominate. Fluid loss leads to dizziness, light-headedness, and orthostatic hypotension. Nonspecific T-wave changes may develop on electrocardiogram (ECG). Because there is no direct cardiotoxic effect, malignant dysrhythmias and cardiac dysfunction are rare.

11. What are the clinical manifestations of patients with chronic lithium intoxication?

Patients on chronic lithium therapy who acutely overdose may show manifestations of both acute and chronic poisoning—a diagnostic and therapeutic challenge. The GI symptoms seen in acute toxicity are usually lacking or missed; changes in mental status prompt patient evaluation and care.

Acute Versus Chronic Lithium Intoxication

INTOXICATION	PRECEPITATING EVENTS	INITIAL SYMPTOMS	PROGRESSION
Acute	None	GI (nausea, vomiting, diarrhea)	Initial mild neurologic findings or tremor, hyperreflexia, and agitation can progress to seizures, encephalopathy, and coma
Chronic	Incorrect dosing, dehydration, drug interactions (NSAIDs or ACE-inhibitors), renal or cardiac disease	Neurologic, similar to later stages of acute intoxication; nystagmus often present.	Milder neurologic findings progress to more severe manifestations, e.g., tremors become fasciculations, seizures, coma, and death

NSAID = nonsteroidal anti-inflammatory drug; ACE = angiotensin-converting enzyme

Long-term neurologic sequelae of prolonged lithium therapy include memory deficits, Parkinson's disease, and personality changes. Other long-term complications are nephrogenic diabetes insipidus and hypothyroidism.

12. Describe the general approach to the poisoned patient.

Start with ABCs (airway, breathing, and circulation) as always, although lithium toxicity is not known to cause problems with airway or breathing. IV access should be established, and the patient should be placed on a monitor because, rarely, a prolonged QT interval may occur. Cardiogenic shock and dysrhythmias also may occur secondary to excessive GI and urinary losses and accompanying electrolyte imbalances. In addition to basic laboratory tests, a lithium concentration should be drawn at presentation. Serial concentrations should be drawn, initially at 2-hour intervals, to assess if absorption is continuing. In an acute overdose, once concentrations begin declining, expect an initial apparent half-life of less than 12 hours. This reflects tissue distribution.

13. What should GI decontamination entail?

Unless there are coingestants, activated charcoal (AC) has no role in lithium overdoses. Lithium, like iron, does not adsorb to AC. A cathartic such as sorbitol may be given if the patient does not have diarrhea. Whole bowel irrigation with polyethylene glycol-electrolyte solution should be considered, particularly if a sustained release preparation such as Lithobid was ingested.

14. How should renal elimination be enhanced?

Correcting dehydration and electrolyte imbalance is most important in maximizing lithium excretion. Loop diuretics or the less-potent thiazides are not recommended. Initially they may increase excretion, but if the patient becomes water- or salt-depleted, lithium reabsorption will increase and toxicity will worsen. Similarly, mannitol, carbonic anhydrase inhibitors, and phosphodiesterase inhibitors initially may produce a small increase in elimination but will be overcome by lithium retention and are therefore not recommended.

15. What other therapeutic modalities are there for lithium toxicity?

Because lithium is a small ion, is not protein bound, and has a small apparent volume of distribution (V_d), it is dialyzable. Hemodialysis removes 70–170 ml/min, which is 10–15 times more than the clearance of lithium by peritoneal dialysis. Indications include severe neurologic dysfunction or toxicity in the face of renal failure. Patients with hyponatremic, edematous states (congestive heart failure, anasarca, pulmonary edema) who cannot tolerate sodium repletion also should be considered for hemodialysis. The slow distribution half-life provides significant potential for the benefit of these procedures in acute overdoses and possibly acute on chronic overdose. However, in the absence of other indications, hemodialysis offers minimal benefit in chronic intoxication.

16. At what lithium levels is hemodialysis indicated?

The goal of hemodialysis is to decrease the possibility of long-term neurologic complications. A patient with two or more lithium levels of > 4.0 mEq/L and no previous acute lithium overdose should be considered for dialysis because the rate of excretion will not be fast enough to prevent a significant lithium load from entering the central nervous system.

17. A lithium level should be checked 6 hours after dialysis. Why?

Dialysis removes lithium from plasma. Once lithium from the intracellular space equilibrates with the plasma, a "rebound" level may develop. If the level is high or if neurologic symptoms persist, the patient should be dialyzed again.

18. What is the role of sodium polystyrene sulfonate (SPS)?

SPS (Kayexalate), a cation-exchange ion, is commonly used to treat hyperkalemia dispensed as a suspension in 70% sorbitol. In theory, it has the potential to bind lithium; however, animal studies have shown that large doses of SPS (up to 10 gm/kg) are required. These doses are large enough that hypokalemia is a concern. Human studies of SPS-induced hypokalemia are equivocal. Additionally, the potential for sorbitol-induced diarrhea and volume depletion resulting in increased lithium reabsorption must be considered.

BIBLIOGRAPHY

1. Bosinski T, Bailie GR, Eisele G: Massive and extended rebound of serum lithium concentrations following hemodialysis in two chronic overdose cases. Am J Emerg Med 16:98–100, 1998.
2. Dupuis RE, Cooper AA, Rosamond LJ, et al: Multiple delayed peak lithium concentrations following acute intoxication with an extended-release product. Ann Pharmacother 30:356–360, 1996.
3. Leblanc M, Raymond M, Bonnardeaux A, et al: Lithium poisoning treated by high-performance continuous arteriovenous and venovenous hemodiafiltration. Am J Kidney Dis 27:365–372, 1996.
4. Scharman EJ: Methods used to decrease lithium absorption or enhance elimination. J Toxicol Clin Toxicol 35:601–608, 1997.
5. Timmer RT, Sands JM: Lithium intoxication. J Am Soc Nephrol 10:666–674, 1999.

26. OPIOIDS

David D. Gummin, M.D., Bryan Finke, M.D., and Joseph B. Reuben, M.D.

1. What are the major opioid receptors?

Mu, kappa, and delta are the major classes of opioid receptors. Epsilon and zeta receptors as well as other minor types have also been described, although their role in humans remains to be determined. The primary receptor type responsible for respiratory depression is the mu receptor. Kappa agonism appears to cause much less respiratory depression. The sigma receptor was once thought to be an opioid receptor because it is stimulated by pentazocine and other mixed agonist-antagonists. Agonism can induce dysphoria and an acute psychotic state.

2. What differentiates an opioid from an opiate?

Opioids are the class of compounds that exert pharmacologic activity at opioid receptors. These include the opioid agonists, antagonists, and the mixed agonist-antagonists. Additionally included are endogenous morphines (endorphins). Opiates, on the other hand, are alkaloid extracts of the opium poppy, *Papaver somniferum* (e.g., morphine, codeine, thebaine). Opiates are opioids, but the reverse is not always true.

3. *Extra credit:* Ipecac used to be mixed with 10% opium to produce a drug used to induce sweating to treat fever. What was this preparation called?

Dover's Powders.

4. Describe the ocular findings of opioid intoxication.

The most classic finding is miosis, thought to occur from mu-receptor agonism at the Edinger-Westphal nucleus of the third cranial nerve. Kappa agonism also may contribute to miosis. Mydriasis is rarely reported in opioid overdose, most frequently in the setting of hypoxemia, hypotension, acidosis, or profound bradycardia. Mydriasis has also been reported with combination preparations, such as meperidine, propoxyphene, or Lomotil (diphenoxylate-atropine), and with adulterants, such as scopolamine in heroin. Nystagmus has been reported in opioid toxicity, with successful reversal by naloxone, but this is not an anticipated finding.

5. What is the differential diagnosis of miosis in toxic presentations?

COPS is a simple mnemonic to help remember the differential diagnosis of miosis:

C	**C**lonidine, **c**holinergics
O	**O**pioids, **o**rganophosphorous compounds
P	**P**henothiazines, **p**hencyclidine, **p**ontine hemorrhage
S	**S**edative hypnotics, **s**ubarachnoid hemorrhage

6. What is the life threat in opioid overdose?

All opioids induce respiratory depression. In particular, strong mu-receptor agonists depress respirations in a dose-dependent fashion. Noncardiogenic pulmonary edema can be seen with essentially all of the opioids in overdose as well, but this appears to be a complication of respiratory depression and subsequent hypoxia. A few opioid agents are implicated in cardiotoxicity, namely propoxyphene and pentazocine. Propoxyphene and its metabolite, norpropoxyphene, cause dose-dependent widening of the QRS complex in a fashion similar to that of the tricyclic antidepressants. This results from inhibition of the fast sodium channels in the cardiac conduction system and is also known as the **quinidine-like effect**. Tachydysrhythmias may result, which can be treated with either sodium bicarbonate or lidocaine.

Many opioids can induce seizures, often associated with hypoxemia, although specifically the fentanyls, meperidine, and propoxyphene are epileptogenic. Cardiac compromise or seizures from opioids are rarely, if ever, sufficient to be a life threat—the overwhelming concern in overdose is respiratory. Management of ventilation and oxygenation is the single most important aspect of treating opioid overdose.

7. What is the mechanism of opioid-induced pulmonary edema?

Noncardiogenic pulmonary edema (NCPE) is common in opioid overdose, involving up to 50% of acute overdoses and the majority of fatalities. Both hemodynamic data and fluid analysis confirm the edema to be noncardiogenic in nature. Most cases involve loss of consciousness, with presumptive hypoventilation preceding NCPE. The mechanism appears related to hypoxic stress-inducing pulmonary capillary fluid leak. No data conclusively support a receptor-mediated mechanism in NCPE, and naloxone has not been demonstrated to be of benefit. In fact, animal data suggest that naloxone may be deleterious in the setting of hypercarbia. Treatment priorities are ventilation and oxygenation. There is little benefit of diuretic administration.

8. What is MPTP?

1-Methyl-4-phenyl-1,2,3,6-tetrahydropyridine. In the early 1980s, opioid addicts in California developed a syndrome indistinguishable from idiopathic parkinsonism. These cases provided the origin of the term *frozen addicts*. It was later found that this resulted from an illicit drug laboratory's attempt to synthesize MPPP, a designer derivative of meperidine. Through poor technique, MPTP was formed, which is selectively oxidized to neurotoxic MPP+ by monoamine oxidase in cells of the substantia nigra. MPP+ selectively exterminates niagral cells and resulted in the (irreversible) syndrome.

9. *Extra credit:* In the 1980s, a new form of Mexican heroin began to appear in North America. Because its color and consistency are similar to a roofing compound, it is commonly called what?

Black tar heroin.

10. Which opioids may give false-positive results on the urine toxicology screen?

This question actually begs two answers. Most "urine tox screens" use an immunoassay (IA) technique (e.g., EMIT, FPIA, KIMS) to measure *opiates* (not *opioids*) in the urine. These assays are typically developed from morphine antigen, so that there is significant cross-reactivity with morphine-like opioids, which contain a phenanthrene ring (e.g., morphine, codeine, heroin, hydromorphone, hydrocodone). Poppy seeds in the diet actually contain enough codeine and morphine to cause a positive test (*not* a false positive!) at a standard level of detection of 300 ng/ml. Because of this, most employee evaluations, including the military and the U.S. Department of Transportation, have raised their detection cut-off for positives to 2000 ng/ml. A few drugs will cross-react (interfere) with the assay and may cause false-positives—e.g., papaverine, rifampin, ofloxacin, and phenothiazines.

Some urine drug screens will actually offer specific IAs for synthetic opioids. Examples are methadone, propoxyphene, meperidine, and fentanyl. When these tests are part of the screen, they are usually specific for the synthetic being assayed. Nonetheless, some interference may occur, and it depends on the testing method. Some possibilities are diphenhydramine interference with the propoxyphene assay and disopyramide or verapamil interfering with the methadone assay. Antagonists such as naloxone and nalmefene do *not* cause false positives in therapeutic doses.

11. Which opioid antagonist is the agent of choice in acute overdose?

To date, no agent has demonstrated itself more useful or cost-effective than naloxone in reversing the effects of opioid overdose in the emergency setting. Naltrexone and nalmefene are opioid antagonists with longer duration of action than naloxone. Nalmefene has been tried in the acute overdose setting without showing an advantage. Both have demonstrated utility in reversing opioid effects in anesthesia. Availability may limit their use in some emergency departments. A more tangible concern with use of long-acting agents to reverse acute overdose is the long duration of action, which may provide persistent antagonism during the observation of a patient while in the emergency department. If the habituated patient then leaves the department or is discharged and continues to use opioids, the agonism will initially be blocked but may manifest with severe toxicity once the antagonist wears off.

12. How is naloxone dosed in the acute overdose setting?

Opioid withdrawal in the habituated patient is extremely unpleasant, both for the patient and for the caregiver. It is additionally very time consuming and resource intensive. As such, the lowest dose of antagonist that will satisfactorily restore consciousness should be used. Small boluses of 0.4 mg of IV naloxone may be repeated every 2–3 minutes to achieve the "wake-up" dose. If 2 mg are infused without adequate response, larger repeat boluses of 2 mg each can be administered every 2–3 minutes until consciousness is restored. Propoxyphene, meperidine, methadone, fentanyl, and Lomotil (diphenoxylate and atropine) as well as the mixed agonist-antagonists require higher dosing of antagonist in overdose. In addition, massive overdose with any of the agonist drugs may require larger-than-conventional doses of antagonist for reversal. Up to 10 mg of naloxone should be administered acutely before considering that the patient has "failed a course of naloxone."

If 10 mg have been administered without any response, it is unlikely that mental status is decreased from opioid intoxication alone, and other causes of coma should be sought. Naloxone can be administered intramuscularly, subcutaneously, or endotracheally if the intravenous route is not available. Intramuscular and subcutaneous routes provided expectedly delayed onset of action.

Serum half-life of naloxone is about 1 hour. Patients with massive overdose or those presenting with intoxication from long-acting agents may have recurrence of central nervous system (CNS) and respiratory depression when the naloxone begins to wear off. In this setting, a naloxone drip may be started by infusing two thirds of the wake-up dose as an hourly infusion. Initially, calculate two thirds of the wake-up dose. Then place 10 times this amount of naloxone into a liter of saline or D5W and infuse at 100 ml/hour.

13. What are the admission criteria for an opioid overdose?

Intravenous heroin overdose that responds to standard dosing of naloxone typically can be observed for 4 hours following the last dose of naloxone. If signs and symptoms do not recur, and there are no signs of pulmonary edema, the patient may be discharged or medically cleared for further evaluation (e.g., to psychiatric or substance abuse professionals). Oral overdose requires longer monitoring, typically involving hospital admission, particularly if a long-acting or a delayed-release preparation is responsible (e.g., methadone, Lomotil, LAAM). Patients who require naloxone drip to maintain consciousness or to whom a long-acting antagonist is administered (e.g., naltrexone, nalmaphene) should be admitted for observation. Any patient who shows evidence of NCPE (tachypnea, rales, hypoxemia, or radiographic evidence of NCPE) should be admitted to a critical care unit for observation or for positive pressure ventilation where required.

14. What is tramadol?

Tramadol is a centrally acting analgesic. It is a synthetic analog of codeine with low affinity for opioid receptors (the affinity for the mu receptor is 10 times less than that of codeine). It is used for moderate and moderate-severe pain control. Tramadol may be used safely in the setting of gastrointestinal bleeding or platelet dysfunction because it does not inhibit prostaglandin synthesis. Much of its effects appear to be through modulation of central monoamine pathways by inhibiting reuptake of 5-hydroxytryptamine and norepinephrine. In overdose, the effects are similar to those of other opioids. Convulsions may occur in susceptible individuals, so this drug should probably be avoided in epileptic patients.

15. How should heroin body packers and stuffers be managed?

"Body packers" differ from "body stuffers" in terms of the quantity of heroin and the quality of the packaging. The drug carriers, called body packers or "mules," intentionally swallow or store drug packets in orifices to avoid customs or other authorities. In contrast, body stuffers hastily conceal illicit packets in orifices just prior to detection. These represent two separate dilemmas. Packers usually ingest well-sealed, prepared packets that resist leaking. However, the quantity ingested is usually very high. Stuffers, on the other hand, ingest smaller quantities of contraband, but the packaging is not fully prepared. In both instances, packets are difficult to detect and they may leak or burst. The diagnosis is difficult and should not rely solely on abdominal radiographs or computed tomography (CT) scan, which will miss the majority of packets. The overall management should include:

- Rapid detection by *combined* body cavity searches and abdominal radiographs
- Decontamination with activated charcoal
- Critical care monitoring with anticipation of toxicity

To reduce total transit time through the gut, polyethylene glycol electrolyte lavage solution (PEG-ELS) has been added to the management of asymptomatic patients. Patients may deteriorate quickly once the packets rupture. In those exhibiting signs of toxicity, emergent surgery and enterotomy have met some clinical success. Surgery is mandated in the setting of bowel obstruction due to impaction. Very high dose continuous naloxone infusion may be necessary.

16. How can clonidine overdose be confused with opioid overdose?

Clonidine is an alpha$_2$-adrenergic agonist used in the management of hypertension and various withdrawal states. It shares some pharmacologic properties (and also clinical features) with the opioids in overdose. Both alpha$_2$ and mu receptors cause G-protein–mediated potassium efflux with subsequent hyperpolarization of neurons in the CNS. In overdose, both clonidine and the mu agonists cause miosis, coma, and respiratory depression. Interestingly, naloxone can reverse the hypoventilation and CNS depression seen in clonidine or other imidazoline overdose, but does so inconsistently.

BIBLIOGRAPHY

1. Ballard PA, Tetrud JW, Langston JW: Permanent human parkinsonism due to 1-methyl-4-phenyl-1,2,3,6-tetrahydropyridine (MPTP): Seven cases. Neurology 35:949–956, 1985.
2. Bamigbade TA, Langford RM: Tramadol hydrochloride: An overview of current use. Hosp Med 59:373–376, 1998.
3. Goldfrank L, Weisman RS, Errick JK, et al: A dosing nomogram for continuous infusion intravenous naloxone. Ann Emerg Med 15:566–570, 1986.
4. Hine CH, Wright JA, Allison DJ, et al: Analysis of fatalities from acute narcotism in a major urban area. J Forensic Sci 27:372–384, 1982.
5. Kaplan JL, Marx JA, Calabro JJ, et al: Double-blind, randomized study of nalmefene and naloxone in emergency department patients with suspected narcotic overdose. Ann Emerg Med 34:42–50, 1999.
6. Levine B: Principles of Forensic Toxicology. Washington, DC, American Association for Clinical Chemistry, 1999, pp 217–220.
7. McCarron MM, Challoner KR, Thompson GA: Diphenoxylate-atropine (Lomotil) overdose in children: An update. Pediatrics 87:694–700, 1991.
8. Perrone J, Hamilton R, Nelson L, et al: Scopolamine poisoning among heroin users. MMWR 45:457–460, 1996.
9. Nelson LS: Opioids. In Goldfrank LR, et al (eds): Goldfrank's Toxicologic Emergencies, 6th ed. Stamford, CT, Appleton & Lange, 1998, pp 975–995.
10. Reisene T, Pasternak G: Opioid analgesics and antagonists. In Hardman JG, Limbird LE, Mikubiff PB, et al (eds): Goodman and Gilman's The Pharmacologic Basis of Therapeutics, 9th ed. New York, McGraw-Hill, 1996, pp 521–556.
11. Robinson T, Birrer R, Mandava N, et al: Body smuggling of illicit drugs: Two cases requiring surgical intervention. Surgery 113:709–711, 1993.
12. Schug SA, Zech D, Grond S: Adverse effects of systemic opioid analgesics. Drug Safe 7:200–213, 1992.
13. Sporer KA: Acute heroin overdose. Ann Intern Med 130:584–590, 1999.
14. Storrow AB, Wians FH Jr, Mikkelsen SL, et al: Does naloxone cause a positive urine opiate screen? Ann Emerg Med 24:1151–1153, 1994.

27. SEDATIVE-HYPNOTICS

Leon Gussow, M.D.

1. What are sedatives-hypnotics?

Technically, a **sedative** is a drug that decreases anxiety, producing a state of calm and relaxation. Despite the name, a **hypnotic** drug has nothing to do with magicians, hocus-pocus, swinging watches, or getting someone to believe he's a chicken. It is simply a medication that induces sleep. In practice, the terms *sedative* and *hypnotic* are commonly used interchangeably. Sedative-hypnotics are used clinically to treat seizures, muscle spasm, anxiety, insomnia, agitation, and alcohol withdrawal.

2. Name some examples of sedative-hypnotics.

Barbiturates	Meprobamate (Miltown)
Benzodiazepines	Methaqualone (Quaalude)
Bromides	Buspirone
Chloral hydrate	Zolpidem (Ambien)
Ethchlorvynol (Placidyl)	

3. How do barbiturates work?

Barbiturates enhance the activity of gamma-aminobutyric acid (GABA), the major inhibitor of CNS activity. They also have peripheral effects that can be significant following overdose. These include depression of myocardial and gastrointestinal activity, decreased autonomic transmission, and skeletal muscle weakness.

4. What are the different classes of barbiturates?

Barbiturates are usually grouped according to their pharmacokinetics:

GROUP	ONSET	DURATION
Ultra-short acting	Immediate after intravenous dose	Minutes
Short-acting	10–15 minutes after oral dose	6–8 hours
Intermediate-acting	45–60 minutes	10–12 hours
Long-acting	1 hour	10–12 hours

Some pharmacologists classify barbiturates according to their intended use: anesthetic, sedative-hypnotic, or anticonvulsant.

5. My patient is comatose after taking a phenobarbital overdose. Her phenobarbital level is 80 μg/ml (therapeutic levels 15–40 μg/ml). How can I enhance clearance of the drug?

Alkalinizing the urine to a pH of 7.5–8.0 will increase clearance of long-acting barbiturates such as phenobarbital. Short- and intermediate-acting barbiturates such as secobarbital (Seconal), which are almost completely metabolized by the liver, will not be affected by changes in urine pH. Urine alkalization can be achieved by giving 1–2 mEq/kg of sodium bicarbonate ($NaHCO_3$) as an IV bolus, then starting an infusion of 1 L of D_5W to which 2 or 3 ampules of $NaHCO_3$ have been added. Patients much be watched carefully for fluid overload, hypokalemia, and systemic alkalosis (arterial pH > 7.55). Multidose activated charcoal (MDAC) will also increase the clearance and decrease the half-life of phenobarbital. The adult dose of MDAC is 25 gm every 2 hours, after the initial dose of 50–100 gm of activated charcoal.

Although most cases of phenobarbital overdose will respond to meticulous cardiopulmonary supportive care and the noninvasive measures discussed above, occasionally a severe case will require hemodialysis or charcoal hemoperfusion. Indications for hemodialysis or hemoperfusion include severe phenobarbital overdose with renal or cardiac failure, acid-base or electrolyte abnormalities, unstable cardiopulmonary status, and failure to respond to standard noninvasive care. Neither of these procedures will remove significant amounts of short- or intermediate-acting barbiturates, which are more extensively bound to protein and are more extensively distributed in the tissues (not the blood).

6. I've heard of a study that showed that while MDAC accelerated the elimination of phenobarbital in intubated ICU patients with phenobarbital overdose, it did not change the patients' clinical course. Should I still be considering it?

Yes. Although that study (by Pond et al.) is frequently cited, it involved only a very small study group (10 patients), used an inadequate dose of MDAC, and had a poorly-defined endpoint. MDAC is generally safe, and its use should be seriously considered in these patients.

7. Which are safer, barbiturates or benzodiazepines?

Benzodiazepines are generally safer than barbiturates, producing less respiratory depression and minimal cardiac effects. Death from isolated benzodiazepine overdose is extremely rare.

8. Which benzodiazepines can be given by the intramuscular route?

Lorazepam and midazolam both are reliably absorbed after IM injection. However, the IM administration of chlordiazepoxide (Librium) and diazepam (Valium) is not recommended, because absorption is unpredictable.

9. What are the signs and symptoms of benzodiazepine overdose?

Signs and symptoms of benzodiazepine overdose are nonspecific. CNS depression can range from mild drowsiness to coma. Respiratory depression is less common but can occur after large overdoses. Hypotension is unusual. In one study of pediatric patients with isolated benzodiazepine ingestions, the most common symptom seen was ataxia.

10. My patient was brought to the emergency department in a coma, and I am suspecting benzodiazepine overdose. Should I administer flumazenil?

Flumazenil is a nonspecific competitive antagonist of benzodiazepines. In pure benzodiazepine overdose, it can reverse depressed mental status and coma within minutes. However, serious complications and even fatalities have been reported following the use of flumazenil in the emergency setting. There are several situations in which the use of flumazenil can be particularly dangerous.

If a patient has ingested both a benzodiazepine and a drug that can cause seizures (e.g., cocaine or amphetamines), the effect of the benzodiazepine can actually be protective. Reversing this effect can precipitate active seizures, and if this occurs the patient will not be readily treatable with additional doses of benzodiazepine. This is especially risky when an overdose patient has taken both a benzodiazepine and a tricyclic antidepressant (TCA). In this situation, seizures can cause severe systemic acidosis, significantly increasing the toxic effect of the TCA. It is also dangerous to give flumazenil to a patient who chronically uses benzodiazepines, because this might cause acute withdrawal. In most emergency department cases, the history of ingestion is not completely clear; therefore, the routine use of flumazenil in comatose or overdose patients is not indicated.

11. Can patients develop a withdrawal syndrome after cessation of chronic benzodiazepine or barbiturate use?

They sure can. Signs and symptoms are similar to those of alcohol withdrawal and include tachycardia, hypertension, hyperthermia, diaphoresis, agitation, mental status changes, and seizures. Because some benzodiazepines and barbiturates have prolonged half-lives and long-acting metabolites, onset of the withdrawal syndrome may be delayed as long as 2 weeks after the drug is stopped. Treatment is with diazepam or phenobarbital.

12. What is flunitrazepam (Rohypnol)?

Flunitrazepam is a benzodiazepine that is not approved for use in the United States but is readily available on the illicit market. It is rapidly acting, causing significant CNS depression in 30 minutes. Because of slow elimination, coma can be prolonged. In addition, when combined with alcohol, it can produce loss of inhibition and amnesia. Flunitrazepam has been associated with cases of date rape. It is not detectable on routine urine drug screens.

13. What is buspirone?

Buspirone is a relatively new antianxiety medication that does not affect the GABA receptors but instead acts as a partial serotonin agonist. It does not have hypnotic, anticonvulsant, or muscle relaxant effects. It causes minimal CNS depression when taken together with ethanol. It does not seem to cause dependence or withdrawal. There is only limited data reported on buspirone overdose.

14. What is zolpidem (Ambien)?

Zolpidem is a sedative that lacks significant antianxiety, muscle relaxant, or anticonvulsant effects. It does not have significant interactions with other drugs and does not produce additive effects with ethanol. Overdose can produce drowsiness, but coma and respiratory failure are uncommon, even after very large ingestions.

15. Chloral hydrate is often considered a safe sedative. Is it?

Not at all. It has a low therapeutic ratio and can cause significant, even fatal, toxicity. Toxic effects include CNS depression, gastrointestinal irritation, ataxia, cardiovascular instability, hepatitis, and proteinuria. The combination of deep coma and cardiac arrhythmias should suggest chloral hydrate overdose. An active long-acting metabolite, trichloroethanol, causes most of the CNS depression seen after overdose.

16. What is the drug of choice to treat the cardiovascular manifestations of chloral hydrate toxicity?

Chloral hydrate impairs myocardial contractility, shortens the cardiac refractory period, and sensitizes myocardium to the effects of catecholamines. Resulting arrhythmias include atrial fibrillation, supraventricular tachycardia, ventricular tachycardia, multifocal premature ventricular contractions, torsades de pointes, ventricular fibrillation, and asystole. The occurrence of arrhythmias increases the risk of death. Beta-blockers are the drugs of choice in these patients.

BIBLIOGRAPHY

1. Bertino JS, Reed MD: Barbiturate and nonbarbiturate sedative hypnotic intoxication in children. Pediatr Clin North Am 33:703–722, 1986.
2. Doyon S, Roberts JR: Reappraisal of the "coma cocktail": Dextrose, flumazenil, naloxone, and thiamine. Emerg Med Clin North Am 12:301–316, 1994.
3. Frenia ML, et al: Multiple-dose activated charcoal compared to urinary alkalinization for the enhancement of phenobarbital ellimination. J Toxicol Clin Toxicol 34:169–175, 1996.
4. Hojer J, Baehrendtz S, Gustafsson L: Benzodiazepine poisoning: Experience of 702 admissions to an intensive care unit during a 14-year period. J Intern Med 226:117–122, 1989.
5. Lindberg MC, Cunningham A, Lindberg NH: Acute phenobarbital intoxication. Southern Med J 85:803–807, 1992.
6. Pond SM, et al: Randomized study of the treatment of phenobarbital overdose with repeated doses of activated charcoal. JAMA 251:3104–3108, 1984.
7. Sellers EM: Alcohol, barbiturate and benzodiazepine withdrawal syndromes: Clinical Management. CMAJ 139:113–120, 1988.
8. Shubin H, Weil MH: Shock associated with barbiturate intoxication. JAMA 215:263–268, 1971.
9. Waltzman ML: Flunitrazepam: A review of "roofies." Pediatr Emerg Care 15:59–60, 1999.
10. Weinbroum AA, et al: A risk-benefit assessment of flumazenil in the management of benzodiazepine overdose. Drug Safety 17:181–196, 1997.

VII. Drugs of Abuse

28. ETHANOL

Jennifer Owens, M.D., and Leon Gussow, M.D.

1. What is the single most important laboratory test to obtain immediately in a seemingly intoxicated patient?

All patients who appear intoxicated should have a rapid bedside serum glucose measurement, if available. Hypoglycemia can cause changes in mental status and seizures that are sometimes attributed solely to the effects of ethanol. Chronic ethanol abusers are often poorly nourished and may have decreased glycogen stores. In addition, the metabolism of ethanol increases the conversion of pyruvate to lactate, impairing gluconeogenesis. Children are especially susceptible to ethanol-associated hypoglycemia, even after ingesting only small amounts of ethanol from over-the-counter products (such as mouthwashes).

2. How should one treat an intoxicated patient who is hypoglycemic? Should thiamine be given before administering intravenous D50?

Severe, prolonged hypoglycemia (serum glucose < 40 mg/dl) can cause seizures and neurologic injury. All patients who have documented hypoglycemia, and those with altered mental status if no rapid bedside glucose test is available, should receive intravenous (IV) dextrose. The adult dose is 50 cc of D50; the pediatric dose is 2 cc/kg of D25. Remember that patients with low-normal serum glucose levels may have altered mental status from central nervous system hypoglycemia; therefore, an intoxicated patient with serum glucose < 70–100 mg/dl may benefit from a trial of IV glucose. Thiamine (100 mg IV) can prevent delayed deterioration from Wernicke's encephalopathy after carbohydrate repletion and should be given to malnourished patients who receive IV glucose. However, in the hypoglycemic patient, administration of glucose should not be delayed; the common belief that thiamine must be administered *before* intravenous hypertonic dextrose is a medical myth.

3. What do the serum electrolytes I obtain on an intoxicated patient tell me?

Ingestion of methanol or ethylene glycol can also cause a patient to appear intoxicated. Unlike ethanol, these toxic alcohols often cause an increased anion gap:

Anion gap = serum sodium – (chloride + bicarbonate)

A normal anion gap is 8–12 mEq/L. An increased anion gap indicates metabolic acidosis; usually, the serum bicarbonate level will be decreased. Other likely causes of an increased anion gap metabolic acidosis to consider in an intoxicated patient include renal failure, salicylate toxicity, alcoholic ketoacidosis, diabetic ketoacidosis, recent seizure, and carbon monoxide exposure. Increased creatinine indicates renal insufficiency, which in this setting is often caused by ethylene glycol ingestion or rhabdomyolysis. Findings on urinalysis may give a clue to the cause of renal failure: calcium oxalate crystals may be seen in ethylene glycol toxicity and myoglobin (large blood on dipstick but few cells on microscopy) in rhabdomyolysis (see also Chapter 29, Toxic Alcohols).

4. *Extra credit:* In 1951, in Atlanta, Georgia, a mass poisoning occurred from bootleg whiskey that resulted in over 300 cases of poisoning and at least 40 deaths. The 60 gallons of whiskey were contaminated with what toxic chemical?

Methanol.

5. What is the presentation, cause, and treatment of alcoholic ketoacidosis?

Alcoholic ketoacidosis (AKA) is usually seen in chronic drinkers. Typically, the patient has a history of binge drinking that stopped several days before presentation because of vomiting and abdominal distress. Because many such patients are malnourished and have a decreased supply of glycogen, the body derives energy from fat, producing acetoacetate and beta-hydroxybutyrate in the process. Laboratory tests reveal ketonuria and an increased anion gap metabolic acidosis. Serum glucose is generally not elevated. Because of the profuse vomiting that often precedes presentation, there may be a concomitant metabolic alkalosis causing the serum bicarbonate to be normal or elevated despite severe acidosis. All patients with AKA should be evaluated for methanol or ethylene glycol toxicity, which can have similar presentations. Treatment of AKA involves rehydration, glucose replacement, and thiamine.

6. My patient, who appears to be drunk, is a "frequent flyer" who often visits the emergency department in a similar state. Do I have to consider anything other than ethanol intoxication on the differential diagnosis?

You bet! Physicians who fail to evaluate seemingly intoxicated patients for other or concomitant conditions are often called "defendants." At minimum, the intoxicated patient should have a rapid bedside glucose measurement and thorough examination for evidence of head trauma or infection (pneumonia, meningitis, sepsis). Gradual improvement from the intoxicated state, as would be expected from alcohol alone, should be followed and documented. Other conditions to consider on the differential diagnosis include hypoxia, hepatic encephalopathy, barbiturate or benzodiazepine toxicity, alcohol, and Wernicke-Korsakoff syndrome.

7. What is a Mickey Finn?

Also called "knock-out drops," the Mickey Finn is a mixture of ethanol and chloral hydrate, which have additive sedative effects. Similar effects can be seen when ethanol is mixed with other central nervous system depressants such as opiates, benzodiazepines, antihistamines, phenothiazines, barbiturates, and various date rape drugs (see Chapter 37, Date Rape Drugs).

8. What is a disulfiram reaction?

A common and potentially serious ethanol interaction occurs with disulfiram (Antabuse). Disulfiram blocks the oxidation of acetaldehyde to acetic acid by inhibiting aldehyde dehydrogenase. The accumulation of acetaldehyde causes flushing, tachycardia, diaphoresis, nausea, vomiting, palpitations, headache, and chest pain. Disulfiram-like reactions can also occur with chlorpropamide, metronidazole, chloramphenicol, and *Coprinus atramentarius* (the inky cap mushroom). Disulfiram has been used to help those trying to abstain from alcohol ingestion.

9. Is there an interaction between ethanol and cocaine?

Yes! When ethanol is taken concomitantly with cocaine, the compound cocaethylene is formed in the liver. Cocaethylene has effects similar to those of cocaine but is longer lasting and more cardiotoxic and lethal.

10. What are some of the adverse effects of chronic alcohol abuse?

Chronic alcoholics have an average life span 10–15 years shorter than that of moderate or nondrinkers. Ethanol affects virtually every organ system. Increased mortality results primarily from liver and cardiac disease, cancer, and trauma. Cardiovascular effects include cardiomyopathy and hypertension. Gastrointestinal effects include increased incidence of varices, gastritis, pancreatitis, fatty liver, alcoholic hepatitis, and cirrhosis. Ethanol also causes bone marrow suppression, nutritional deficiencies, and progressive cognitive dysfunction.

11. What are the manifestations of ethanol withdrawal and how is it treated?

There are various degrees of ethanol withdrawal that can be seen in chronic alcohol abusers. Symptoms of minor abstinence can begin within 6 hours after the last drink and include tremors, agitation, hyperexcitability, weakness, and vomiting. Alcoholic hallucinations are mainly visual and occur after 24–36 hours of abstinence. Alcoholic seizures ("rum fits") occur within a day or two after cessation or reduction of ethanol intake. Most episodes are brief and self-limited, with only a single seizure. If treatment is required, benzodiazepines are the drugs of choice. Delirium tremens (DTs) begin 3–5 days after the patient stops drinking. Signs and symptoms include global confusion, delusions, vivid hallucinations, autonomic hyperactivity, agitation, and combativeness. The patient is often tachycardic, febrile, hypertensive, tremulous, and diaphoretic. Although this syndrome is characteristic, it is imperative to consider carefully concurrent conditions such as infection, metabolic illness, and traumatic injury (see also Chapter 35, Withdrawal Syndromes).

12. *Extra credit:* In 1991, testimony in a United Sates Senate hearing on Indian Affairs stated that the biggest problem on the reservations among today's Native-American youth was the consumption of alcohol from what commercial product?

Lysol Disinfectant Spray, which contains 79% volume in volume ethanol.

13. What are some potential sources of ethanol aside from alcoholic beverages?

A number of over-the-counter and commercial products contain significant amounts of ethanol, including mouthwashes, aftershave lotions, hair sprays, and cough and cold remedies. Listerine mouthwash, for example, contains 27% ethanol (54 proof), more than beer and many wines. The cold remedy Nyquil is 25% ethanol. In addition to ethanol, some products may also contain other toxins (for example, Sterno canned fuel contains ethanol and methanol). Patients sometimes ingest these products because they are readily available and inexpensive or because alcoholic beverages are not allowed in their specific setting (e.g., prison, hospital).

BIBLIOGRAPHY

1. Gentilello LM, Villaveces A, Ries RR, et al: Detection of acute alcohol intoxication and chronic alcohol dependence by trauma center staff. J Trauma 47:1311–1335, 1999.
2. Hoffman RS, Goldfrank LR: The poisoned patient with altered consciousness: Controversies in the use of a "coma cocktail." JAMA 274:562–569, 1995.
3. Khan F, Alagappan K, Cardell K: Overlooked sources of ethanol. J Emerg Med 17:985–988, 1999.
4. McMicken DB, Freedland ES: Alcohol-related seizures: Pathophysiology, differential diagnosis, evaluation, and treatment. Emerg Med Clin North Am 12:1057–1078, 1994.
5. Shaw GK: Detoxification. The use of benzodiazepines. Alcohol Alcohol 30:765–770, 1995.

29. TOXIC ALCOHOLS

Shahrzad Rafiee, M.D., and Timothy Erickson, M.D.

ISOPROPYL ALCOHOL

1. What household items contain this substance?

Isopropanol is typically found in rubbing alcohol, nail-polish remover, and glues, and it has wide industrial application as a solvent. It is second to ethanol as the most commonly ingested alcohol. Isopropanol is volatile, clear, and colorless, with a bitter taste and characteristic odor.

2. What is the toxic dose?

In adults, it has been reported at 2–4 ml/kg (approximately 150–240 ml).

3. What are symptoms of clinical toxicity?

Gastrointestinal (GI) and central nervous system (CNS) complaints are the usual presenting symptoms within the first few hours after ingestion. The CNS alterations are similar to those of ethanol intoxication, but isopropanol is considered to be twice as potent in terms of CNS toxicity. Ataxia, dysarthria, confusion, stupor, and coma may develop. Pupils are typically miotic, but this may not be a reliable sign. Isopropanol and ethanol can cause brain stem depression with resulting respiratory depression, profound hypotension, or both. GI effects can result in gastritis and upper GI bleeding.

4. What is the main metabolite of isopropanol?

Isopropanol is excreted in the urine (20–50% unchanged), and the remaining 50% is metabolized in liver to acetone by alcohol dehydrogenase. The acetone is then excreted through the kidneys and lungs. Isopropanol produces no toxic acids as metabolites because acetone is a stable compound. Therefore, no metabolic acidosis occurs unless there is resulting severe hypotension or respiratory depression.

5. What is the hallmark laboratory abnormality in isopropanol ingestions?

Ketosis with little or no acidosis. The ketosis is caused by acetone (detected within 15 minutes of ingestion). Isopropyl alcohol does cause an osmolal gap. Hypoglycemia also tends to occur.

6. Is GI decontamination effective for isopropanol ingestions?

Isopropanol is rapidly absorbed from the gastric mucosa, making lavage impractical except in cases of immediate ingestion. Activated charcoal adsorbs ethanol and other alcohols poorly but may be used if coingestants are suspected.

7. Is there a role for the ethanol drip in the management of isopropanol ingestion?

No, because there is no need to block isopropanol metabolism by alcohol dehydrogenase because the resultant metabolite (acetone) is relatively nontoxic and readily excreted through the kidneys and lungs.

ETHYLENE GLYCOL

8. What common household items contain ethylene glycol?

Ethylene glycol is commonly found in antifreeze, automobile coolant systems, and hydraulic brake fluid, and it is used as a solvent in a variety of industrial processes. It is a clear, colorless, odorless, syrupy viscous fluid with a sweet taste.

116

9. What patient populations are most at risk from ethylene glycol toxicity?

Children, most commonly from accidental ingestion, although cases of child abuse have been reported that involved recurrent acidosis from forced ingestion. **Alcoholics** tend to ingest ethylene glycol deliberately as an alcohol substitute. It is also frequently used as a **suicidal agent in adults**.

10. What is the toxic dose in adults?

The lethal dose is 100 ml (1.0–1.5 ml/kg) in adults, and the lethal blood level in untreated poisoning is 200 mg/dl. It is readily absorbed after ingestion and widely distributed to tissues, and peak blood levels occur 1–4 hours after ingestion.

11. What are the clinical toxicity symptoms of ethylene glycol poisoning?

Classically, toxicity has three phases:

1. The **CNS phase** takes place 1–12 hours postingestion. Symptoms include ataxia, nystagmus, coma, myoclonic jerks, and focal or generalized seizures. Cerebral edema may also develop. In addition, GI complaints of nausea, vomiting, and abdominal can also occur.

2. The **cardiovascular toxicity phase** occurs 12–72 hours postingestion and results in mild hypertension, tachycardia, tachypnea, and hypothermia. In significant poisoning, pulmonary edema, pneumonitis, and congestive heart failure or shock may develop.

3. The **renal toxicity phase** usually occurs 24–72 hours postingestion and consists of flank pain, costovertebral angle tenderness, and oliguric renal failure. Without proper intervention, renal failure may be permanent.

Note that not all cases of ethylene glycol poisoning will manifest all three phases.

12. What are the major metabolites of ethylene glycol?

Ethylene glycol's first metabolite is **glycoaldehyde** (osmotically active, but does not cause acidosis). The conversion occurs by alcohol dehydrogenase. The subsequent metabolite, **glycolic acid**, does cause acidosis but is not significantly osmotically active. During this conversion, lactate is also produced. Another clinically significant byproduct is **oxalate**, which causes widespread tissue injury in the kidney, where it combines with calcium to form calcium oxalate crystals that causes renal tubular damage. Oxalate crystals also causes damage to organs such as the brain, liver, vessels, and pericardium, and it may cause hypocalcemia.

13. What are possible electrocardiographic (ECG) findings in a patient with significant ethylene glycol poisoning?

One third of patients may become hypocalcemic secondary to calcium oxalate crystals and exhibit the classic ECG symptoms of prolonged QT and muscle tetany. These changes may occur as early as the CNS depression phase. Also, they may present with classic findings of hyperkalemia, particularly if they are manifesting acute renal failure.

14. What are laboratory clues to the diagnosis of ethylene glycol poisoning?

Laboratory findings suggestive of ethylene glycol poisoning are an elevated anion gap acidosis and an elevated osmolal gap. Although numerous substances can elevate either the anion or the osmolal gap besides ethylene glycol and methanol, only alcoholic or diabetic ketoacidosis (DKA) elevates both. The mnemonic METAL ACID GAP can help in the differential diagnosis:

M	**M**ethanol, **m**etformin
E	**E**thylene glycol
T	**T**oluene
A	**A**lcoholic ketoacidosis
L	**L**actic acidosis
A	**A**spirin
C	**C**arbon monoxide, **c**yanide
I	**I**soniazid, **i**ron
D	**D**iabetic ketoacidosis

G   Generalized seizures (toxic)
A   Aminoglycosides (uremic causing agents)
P   Paraldehyde, phenformin

15. How is anion gap calculated?

$$\text{Anion gap} = Na - (Cl + CO_2)$$

A normal anion gap is < 12–16.

16. What is osmolality, and how is it different from osmolarity?

Osmolality is the measurement of the number of particles (in osmoles) dissolved in a kilogram of solvent. **Osmolarity** is the number of particles (in osmoles) per liter of solution.

The **osmolal gap** is the difference between the serum osmolality measured in the laboratory and the osmolarity, which is calculated from the major osmotically active molecules in the serum (sodium chloride, glucose, and urea). In the clinical setting, the solute concentrations of the body fluids are so dilute that osmolarity and osmolality are essentially equal and can be directly compared. The two terms are usually used interchangeable in the medical literature.

17. What is the osmolal gap and how is it determined?

$$\text{Calculated osmolality} = (1.86 \times Na) + (\text{blood glucose}/18) +$$
$$(BUN/2.8) + (\text{blood ethanol}/4.6)$$

This formula can be rounded off to:

$$\text{Calculated osmolality} = (2 \times Na) + (\text{blood glucose}/18) + (BUN/3) + (\text{blood ethanol}/5)$$

$$\text{Osmolal gap} = \text{measured osmolality (from lab)} - \text{calculated osmolality}$$
(from formula above)

The presence of an osmolal gap > 10 mOsm usually indicates the presence of an unknown low-molecular-weight, osmotically active substance in the serum (such as alcohols).

18. What substances cause elevations in the osmolal gap?

The mnemonic ME DIE can be used to remember the clinically important substances:
M   Methanol
E   Ethanol

D   Diuretics
I   Isopropanol
E   Ethylene glycol

19. How can you estimate the blood level of ethylene glycol based on the osmolal gap?

$$\text{Estimated blood level in milligrams/deciliter} = \text{Osmolal gap} \times 6.2$$

This is not necessarily reliable, particularly if ethanol is a coingestant of ethylene glycol. The osmolal gap may be delayed based on the competitive inhibition of ethylene glycol by ethanol. When ethanol is ingested along with ethylene glycol, the enzymatic conversion to toxic metabolites responsible for producing the metabolic acidosis may be inhibited early in the clinical course, resulting in an elevated osmolal gap without an elevated anion gap. Thus, the presence of either one of these gaps should alert you to the possibility of ethylene glycol or methanol poisoning.

20. Are there any unique urinary findings in ethylene glycol poisonings?

Crystalluria is a diagnostic finding. They are not universally present, but their presence strongly suggests the diagnosis. They may be birefringent, octahedral, envelope-shaped, needle-shaped, or dumbbell calcium oxalate crystals. Additional findings include hematuria, epithelial cells, and proteinuria.

21. What is a rapid bedside test of a patient's urine that may reveal the diagnosis of ethylene glycol poisoning?

Most ethylene glycol-containing antifreeze compounds have fluorescein as an additive. Therefore, examining the urine with a Wood's lamp may reveal fluorescence and thereby suggest the diagnosis.

22. Is there a direct way to measure serum ethylene glycol levels?

Yes, ethylene glycol levels may be determined by the laboratory. However, the results usually have a long turnaround time and often are sent to a reference laboratory. The assays are difficult to perform and may yield false positives. In chronic alcoholics, 2,3-butanediol has been mistakenly identified as ethylene glycol. When interpreting lab results, watch the units used. Levels reported in milligrams per liter (mg/L) have been mistakenly interpreted as milligrams per deciliter (mg/dl), and inappropriate therapy has been instituted as a result.

23. Is there a role for gastric decontamination of patients with ethylene glycol poisoning?

The early onset of CNS depression and seizures are relative contraindications to the use of ipecac. Gastric aspiration may be of benefit if performed within the first hour of ingestion. Ethylene glycol is poorly absorbed by activated charcoal and should be avoided unless there are coingestants that it may absorb. There is no evidence that cathartics are of benefit.

24. What are goals of care for a patient with significant poisoning?

1. **Supportive care**. Ensure airway patency and protection as needed. Treat seizures with standard anticonvulsants. For patients with significant hypocalcemia, administer either calcium gluconate or calcium chloride intravenously as replacement therapy (chloride ion delivers three times as much calcium ion in the same volume). Correct the metabolic acidosis with bicarbonate, especially with a pH < 7.20. Provide intravenous fluids to maintain brisk urine output, and carefully monitor fluid intake and output. Loop diuretics may be used to maintain urine output once adequate volume replacement has been accomplished.

2. **Antidotes**. Ethanol has been recognized as an effective antidote for ethylene glycol poisoning. Because alcohol dehydrogenase has a 100-fold greater affinity for ethanol than ethylene glycol, the administration of ethanol inhibits the conversion of ethylene glycol to its more toxic metabolites, and it allows slower renal excretion of the unchanged parent compound. The half-life is typically 2.5–5.0 hours but is increased to 17–18 hours when ethanol is given to block metabolic conversion. Most of the ethylene glycol is converted to metabolically toxic substances, of which some have a half-life of 12 hours.

25. How is the IV ethanol solution prepared?

A 5% ethanol solution is commercially available, but the volume of fluid that must be administered with this preparation is often excessive. Methods of preparing 10% ethanol infusions are as follows:

Loading dose: 600–800 mg/kg
Maintenance dose:
    Average person: 110 mg/kg/hr
    Chronic drinker: 154 mg/kg/hr
    Nondrinker: 66 mg/kg/hr

To prepare infusion, remove 100 ml of fluid from 1 L of D_5W. Replace with 100 ml of absolute alcohol (makes 10% solution of ethanol)

Goal of therapy: Most studies advocate maintaining serum ethanol levels between 100 and 150 mg/dl, but levels as low as 70 mg/dl have resulted in near complete inhibition of ethylene glycol metabolism. Blood ethanol and blood glucose levels should be closely monitored hourly after initiation of loading dose, particularly in children, who are more prone to hypoglycemia owing to lower glycogen stores.

26. What alternatives exist if IV ethanol is not available?

When there is a delay before hospital treatment, initial therapy with three to four 1- ounce shots of an 86-proof alcoholic whiskey suffices.

27. When is IV ethanol infusion indicated?

- History of ingestion when a blood level cannot be obtained in a reasonable time period
- Elevated anion gap metabolic acidosis
- Blood level > 20 mg/dl

28. Are there any other antidotes?

4-Methylpyrazole (4-MP) recently has been approved by the U.S. Food and Drug Administration for the treatment of ethylene glycol poisoning. 4-MP is a simply administered, efficacious agent that can be given orally and intravenously with minimum side effect. This agent, also known as antizol or fomepizole, is a potent inhibitor of alcohol dehydrogenase.

29. Which is more advantageous: ethanol infusion or administration of 4-MP?

According to the American Academy of Clinical Toxicology Practice Guidelines fomepizole (4-MP) has clear advantages over ethanol in terms of validated efficacy, predictable pharmacokinetics, ease of administration, and lack of adverse effects. However, ethanol has clear advantages over fomepizole in terms of long-term clinical experience and acquisition cost. The overall comparative cost of medical treatment using each antidote requires further study.

30. What are indications for hemodialysis of patients?

Hemodialysis provides definitive treatment; it removes not only ethylene glycol, but also all toxic metabolites. Indications include significant metabolic acidosis, renal dysfunction, and levels > 25–50 mg/dl. When possible ethylene glycol poisoning in children should be managed in centers capable of performing pediatric dialysis. It is continued until levels decrease below 10 mg/dl.

METHANOL

31. What household items contain methanol?

Methanol is a clear, colorless, flammable liquid with a slightly alcoholic odor. It is used most commonly in windshield washer fluid, automotive radiators, airbrakes, antifreeze additives for fuels (gasoline, diesel), octane booster, fuel for picnic stoves, and soldering torches. It is also used as a denaturing agent for ethyl alcohol, an industrial solvent, and a substitute for petroleum-derived automobile fuel.

32. What is the toxic dose in adults and pediatric populations?

Although ingestion accounts for most methanol poisonings, percutaneous absorption, especially through damaged skin, has resulted in severe toxicity. The lethal blood level of methanol left untreated is 80 mg/dl. Reported "lethal doses" vary considerably. As little as 40 ml of 15% methanol has resulted in death, whereas ingestion of 500 ml has been survived. When ethanol is not coingested, the potentially fatal methanol dose has ranged from 30–240 ml, or approximately 1 gm/kg. The minimum dose causing permanent visual deficits has not been identified. Methanol is rapidly absorbed, with peak blood levels occurring 30–90 minutes postingestion.

33. What are the clinical toxicity symptoms?

Intoxication is a common effect, starting approximately 1 hour after ingestion. Occasionally, a relatively asymptomatic period follows that may last up to 30 hours. Initial absence of symptoms does not preclude later development of significant toxicity. GI symptoms include nausea, vomiting, abdominal pain, and diarrhea. Hemorrhagic gastritis also occurs. Early visual abnormalities include blurred or decreased vision, "snowfield" blindness, and photophobia. Funduscopic examination may reveal retinal edema and hyperemia of the optic disc. Dizziness and headache are common features and precede the development of metabolic acidosis. Other findings include coma, seizures, blindness, oliguric renal failure, hyperthermia or hypothermia, cardiac failure, pulmonary edema, hypotension, and respiratory arrest.

34. What unique lab findings are consistent with methanol toxicity?

As with ethylene glycol poisoning, anion and osmolal gaps are key to diagnosis. When coingested with methanol, ethanol may inhibit the enzymatic conversion to toxic metabolites responsible for producing metabolic acidosis, resulting in an elevated osmolal gap without an elevated anion gap.

Methanol levels may be determined. Peak levels < 20 mg/dl usually are asymptomatic. Patients with levels > 50 mg/dl are acidotic. Patients with levels > 100 mg/dl have visual symptoms. Fatalities are generally associated with levels > 150 mg/dl.

35. What is the major metabolite of methanol?

The toxic ocular manifestations of methanol intoxication results from formate. Formate inhibits cytochrome oxidase in the optic nerve. The ocular lesion consists of initial hyperemia of the optic disc and peripapillary edema. This is followed by swelling of the optic nerve head and retinal vasculature. In severe cases, atrophy of the optic nerve and blindness develop.

Methanol's toxicity results from its hepatic conversion to the toxic metabolites formaldehyde and formate. These cause profound metabolic acidosis. Lactate may appear in the late phase of methanol poisoning and results from hypotension and tissue hypoxia resulting from anaerobic glucose metabolism.

36. How should methanol poisoning be managed?

Treatment should be supportive (airway patency, adequacy of respirations, seizures treated with anticonvulsants) and is similar to ethylene glycol poisoning. Ethanol is effective. It is important to initiate ethanol therapy and dialysis before visual disturbances become apparent. Indications for hemodialysis include presence of symptoms following methanol ingestion, history of ingesting 30 ml (0.4 mg/kg), methanol level of ≥ 20 mg/dl, ocular findings, and severe electrolyte abnormalities.

37. What is the morbidity and mortality of methanol toxicity?

Despite aggressive treatment, the mortality is 20%, and among survivors, 20–25% are left with permanent visual defects (decreased acuity or total blindness). Recent evidence suggests the clinical course, outcome, and development of permanent ocular deficits correlate with several key factors: severity of acidosis, delays in the therapy, and blood formate levels.

Neurologic sequelae are common following acute methanol intoxication. Cerebral edema occurs in 10% of cases. Pseudobulbar palsy, seizures, development of primitive reflexes, intellectual deficits, transverse myelitis, and persistent vegetative states also occur.

38. How can you estimate the serum methanol level from the osmolal gap?

Estimated blood level in milligrams per deciliter = osmolal gap × 2.6

BIBLIOGRAPHY

1. American Academy of Clinical Toxicology Ad Hoc Committee: Guidelines on the treatment of ethylene glycol poisoning. J Toxicol Clin Toxicol 37:537–560, 1999.
2. Brent J, McMartin K, Phillips S, et al: Fomepizole for the treatment of ethylene glycol poisoning. Methylpyrazole for Toxic Alcohols Study Group. N Engl J Med 340:832–838, 1999.
3. Trummel J, Ford M, Austin P: Ingestion of an unknown alcohol. Ann Emerg Med 27:368–374, 1996.

30. COCAINE

Leon Gussow, M.D.

1. Describe the biologic effects of cocaine.

Cocaine is a sympathomimetic. It inhibits the reuptake of epinephrine and norepinephrine in peripheral ganglia. Centrally, it increases release of norepinephrine and inhibits reuptake of dopamine and serotonin. In addition, cocaine blocks fast sodium channels (similar to the action of type IA antiarrhythmics and tricyclic antidepressants), stabilizing nerve membranes and producing local anesthesia.

2. *Extra credit:* What two potentially toxic substances were discovered during a recent drug analysis of ancient Egyptian ruins?

Cocaine and nicotine.

3. Is it true that the soft drink Coca-Cola once contained cocaine?

Yes. In the early 1900s, cocaine was an important ingredient in Coca-Cola. The drink was originally sold medicinally as a "brain tonic."

4. *Extra credit:* In the 1800s, a popular drink containing cocaine was endorsed by many famous people and even given an official seal of approval by Pope Leo XIII. What was the product's name?

Vin Mariani.

5. What does cocaine do to the cardiovascular system?

Because it induces increased sympathetic activity, cocaine produces coronary artery vasospasm and increased platelet adhesion, decreasing the supply of blood and oxygen to myocardial tissue. Concurrently, it elevates blood pressure and heart rate, increasing myocardial work and demand for oxygen. This "double whammy" can result in myocardial ischemia or myocardial infarction. Cocaine also can cause left ventricular dysfunction, ventricular and supraventricular arrhythmias, and aortic dissection. Chronic cocaine use accelerates the development of atherosclerosis and can cause myocarditis or cardiomyopathy.

6. How does cocaine affect the central nervous system?

Cocaine causes release of catecholamines in the central nervous system. Manifestations of this central hyperstimulation include tachycardia, hypertension, hyperthermia, anxiety, agitation, and seizures. Cocaine can cause ischemic or hemorrhagic stroke, which may present with headache or mental status changes and be mistaken for psychiatric illness. Cerebral vasculitis also has been associated with cocaine use. Clinically, it is important not to attribute symptoms such as headache or altered mental status to the direct effects of the drug without considering the possibility of treatable complications.

7. Does cocaine affect the lungs?

Yes, in major ways. Smoking crack cocaine can precipitate attacks of asthma or chronic obstructive pulmonary disease. Cardiogenic or noncardiogenic pulmonary edema has occurred after cocaine use. The aggressive breath-holding that crack smokers often perform can cause barotrauma injury (pneumothorax, pneumomediastinum). Severe upper airway burn injury can occur when a crack smoker inhales the heated screen from his or her pipe. These patients present with mouth and pharyngeal pain, drooling, hoarseness, and stridor that begins during an episode of pipe smoking. These symptoms are often mistakenly attributed to caustic ingestion or laryngitis.

8. What is the chance that a patient with chest pain that started during or shortly after cocaine use has sustained a myocardial infarction?

Low but real. Various studies have reported that approximately 6–31% of patients who present with cocaine-associated chest pain will be diagnosed with myocardial infarction, but even the lowest of these figures may overestimate the true incidence. Other causes of chest pain to consider in the cocaine user include pneumothorax, aortic dissection, pulmonary infarction, and musculoskeletal pain.

9. What is "crack dancing"?

Episodes of acute dyskinesia have been associated with cocaine use. This presents with choreoathetoid movements of the extremities, lip-smacking, and repetitive eye blinking. Symptoms begin minutes to hours after cocaine use and may last for several days. It has been suggested that this movement disorder is caused by supersensitivity to the effects of dopamine. Symptoms are benign and self-limiting and resolve spontaneously. Another street term for this syndrome is *boca torcida*, or "twisted mouth."

10. How does cocaine affect the kidney?

Acute renal failure can be caused by rhabdomyolysis, which presents with muscle pain, elevated creatine phosphokinase (CPK) levels, and myoglobinuria. Often, but not always, rhabdomyolysis will be preceded by episodes of seizures, hypotension, or profound hyperthermia. Renal infarcts secondary to cocaine use have also been reported.

11. Does cocaine pose a risk in pregnancy?

Absolutely. It has been associated with increased risk of spontaneous abortion, abruptio placentae, intrauterine growth retardation, and prematurity. Cocaine causes maternal hypertension, decreased uterine blood flow, and placental vasoconstriction.

12. If you had to choose one class of drugs to treat the major manifestations of cocaine toxicity, what would it be?

Agitation, cardiovascular instability, and neuropsychiatric complications of cocaine toxicity are all caused or exacerbated by increased central sympathetic activity. A **benzodiazepine** will provide sedation and also interrupt central sympathetic outflow. Many of the cardiac manifestations of cocaine toxicity (hypertension, tachycardia, chest pain, myocardial ischemia) will resolve or improve after treatment with liberal doses of benzodiazepines.

13. How should a seizing cocaine-toxic patient be managed?

Airway, breathing, and circulation (ABCs) are priorities. Ensure an open airway and maintain adequate ventilation and oxygenation. Intravenous diazepam or lorazepam may halt the seizure activity if given in adequate doses. If benzodiazepines are ineffective, intravenous phenobarbital can be used. Phenytoin is not an effective or safe antiepileptic in most toxin-induced seizures. Intractable seizures may require neuromuscular paralysis and ventilatory support or general anesthesia. Remember that the paralyzed patient may still have cerebral seizure activity, which can cause permanent neurologic damage even in the absence of motor seizures. Therefore, paralyzed patients should be monitored with bedside electroencephalography. The paralytic drug succinylcholine initially may increase muscle contractions and exacerbate hyperkalemia and hyperthermia and therefore should be avoided. Use a nondepolarizing agent instead. A computed tomography (CT) scan of the head should be obtained to determine any intracranial pathology.

14. What is the syndrome of "cocaine run amok"?

Occasionally, a syndrome of excited delirium associated with hyperthermia, rhabdomyolysis, and acute renal failure can be precipitated by cocaine toxicity. These cases often end in fatality, especially if hyperthermia is not controlled immediately. In any delirious cocaine patient, it is important to obtain a rectal temperature, CPK level, and urine myoglobin while instituting rapid cooling measures.

15. How can one control the body temperature of a hyperthermic cocaine patient?

Body temperature above 104–105°F following cocaine use is life-threatening and should be lowered immediately. Completely undress the patient, spray him or her with a cool mist, and use fans to create a constant air current. Ice packs applied to the groin and axillae can be used as adjunctive measures. In addition, cooled gastric lavage and Foley catheter administration of chilled fluids can rapidly lower hyperthermic body temperatures. If seizures or muscular hyperactivity are contributing to the elevated temperature, paralysis with a nondepolarizing agent may be indicated. Rectal temperature should be monitored frequently.

16. How should ischemic chest pain that occurs during or immediately after cocaine use be managed? Is there any difference from standard treatment of ischemic pain in the person who doesn't use cocaine?

Oxygen, nitrates, and aspirin are indicated as in any other patient with ischemic chest pain. Benzodiazepines will inhibit central sympathetic activity and help control hypertension and tachycardia. Because cocaine-induced hypertension and coronary vasoconstriction are alpha-mediated phenomena, blocking beta receptors will lead to unopposed alpha effects, increasing myocardial oxygen demand, decreasing oxygen supply, and increasing lethality. Therefore, beta-blockers are contraindicated. Phentolamine (an alpha-blocker), nitroglycerin, or nitroprusside can be used to treat hypertension. Thrombolytic agents should be used with extreme caution in the setting of apparent cocaine-associated myocardial infarction. These patients tend to do well and not have major adverse events even without thrombolytics. In addition, up to 40% of patients with cocaine-associated chest pain have baseline electrocardiograms with early repolarization changes that mimic the ST elevation of a myocardial infarction. These patients also may be at increased risk for the severe hemorrhagic complications of thrombolytic therapy. Some experts recommend thrombolytics in this setting only when the patient is having clear cardiac chest pain and the electrocardiogram clearly shows new or evolving ischemic changes.

17. Is there an interaction between cocaine and ethanol?

Yes. When cocaine and ethanol are used together, the active metabolite cocaethylene is formed in the liver. Cocaethylene has effects similar to those of cocaine itself but is longer lasting, more cardiotoxic, and more lethal.

18. What substances are sometimes added to cocaine before it is sold on the street?

Substances used to adulterate cocaine before it is sold include lactose, mannitol, sucrose, caffeine, talc, heroin, phencyclidine, lidocaine, procaine, and strychnine.

19. What are "body stuffing" and "body packing"?

Some patients swallow crack cocaine to avoid having police seize it as evidence. These patients are called "body stuffers." These patients often manifest sympathomimetic signs and symptoms that are usually mild and transient. Some body stuffers will suffer seizures, which may be delayed up to 12 hours after exposure. Treatment involves observation, activated charcoal administration, and whole-bowel irrigation with polyethylene glycol solution. The "body packer" attempts to smuggle drugs (often cocaine) by wrapping them in plastic bags, condoms, or latex gloves and swallowing large numbers (often 100 or more). Because of the massive amount of the drug a packer ingests, severe toxicity and death can result if a package leaks. Treatment is similar to that of stuffers. If a package ruptures or obstructs the gastrointestinal tract, surgical removal may be indicated.

20. *Extra credit:* Which novel by Robert Louis Stevenson was allegedly written in 3 days' time while the author was on cocaine "therapy" for tuberculosis?

Dr. Jekyll and Mr. Hyde.

BIBLIOGRAPHY

1. Daras M, Koppel BS, Atos-Radzion E: Cocaine-induced choreoathetoid movements ("crack dancing"). Neurology 44:751–752, 1994.
2. Fines RE, Brady WJ, DeBehnke DJ: Cocaine-associated dystonic reaction. Am J Emerg Med 15:513–516, 1997.
3. Goldfrank LR, Hoffman RS: The cardiovascular effects of cocaine. Ann Emerg Med 20:165–175, 1991.
4. Haim DY, Lippmann ML, Goldberg SK, Walkenstein MD: The pulmonary complications of crack cocaine: A comprehensive review. Chest 107:233–240, 1995.
5. Henning RJ, Wilson LD, Glauser JM: Cocaine plus ethanol is more cardiotoxic than cocaine or ethanol alone. Crit Care Med 22:1896–1906, 1994.
6. Hollander JE, Lozano M, Fairweather P, et al: "Abnormal" electrocardiograms in patients with cocaine-associated chest pain are due to "normal" variants. J Emerg Med 12:199–205, 1994.
7. Hollander JE, Hoffman RS, Burstein JL, et al: Cocaine-associated myocardial infarction: Mortality and complications. Arch Intern Med 155:1081, 1995.
8. Hollander JE, Wilson LD, Leo PJ, Shih RD: Complications from the use of thrombolytic agents in patients with cocaine-associated chest pain. J Emerg Med 14:731–736, 1996.
9. McCarron MM, Wood JD: The cocaine "body packer" syndrome. JAMA 250:1417–1420, 1983.
10. Merigian KS, Roberts JR: Cocaine intoxication: Hyperpyrexia, rhabdomyolysis, and acute renal failure. J Toxicol Clin Toxicol 25:135–148, 1987.
11. Mouhaffel AH, Madu EC, Satmary WA, Fraker TD Jr: Cardiovascular complications of cocaine. Chest 107:1426–1434, 1995.
12. Rose JS: Cocaethylene: A current understanding of the active metabolite of cocaine and ethanol. Am J Emerg Med 12:489–490, 1994.
13. Shannon M: Clinical toxicity of cocaine adulterants. Ann Emerg Med 17:1243-1247, 1988.
14. Sporer KA, Firestone J: Clinical course of crack cocaine body stuffers. Ann Emerg Med 29:596–601, 1997.

31. AMPHETAMINES

Joseph B. Reuben, M.D., and Timothy Erickson, M.D.

1. What are amphetamines?

They are synthetic stimulant agents with sympathomimetic properties. Similar to cocaine, amphetamines act on both the central (CNS) and peripheral nervous system. Chemically, they are structured like adrenaline (epinephrine), stimulating both alpha and beta receptors.

2. List the common effects of the sympathomimetic agents such as amphetamines (by organ system).

Amphetamines produce the "fight or flight" responses:

SYSTEM	EFFECTS
CNS	Increase in mental activity, hallucinations, seizures
Respiratory	Bronchodilation
Cardiovascular	Tachycardia, hypertension
Gastrointestinal (GI)	Increase in peristalsis
Papillary	Dilation mydriasis
Glands	Increase sweating, dry mouth
Basic metabolic	Increases hyperthermia

3. Name some amphetamines, amphetamines derivatives, and hallucinogenic amphetamines.
- Dextroamphetamine (Dexedrine)
- Methamphetamine (slang names: ice, glass, crank, meth)
- Methylphenidate (Ritalin)
- Phenylisopropylamine (Benzedrine)
- Dimethoxymethylamphetamine-sodium thiopental (DOM-STP; slang names: serenity, tranquility, peace)
- 3,4-Methylenedioxyamphetamine (MDA; slang names: harmony, love drug)
- Methylenedioxymethamphetamine (MDMA; slang names: ecstasy, XTC, Adam)
- 3,4-Methylenedioxyethamphetamine (MDEA; slang: Eve)

4. *Extra credit:* What star of the 1939 movie *The Wizard of Oz* began taking amphetamines to combat a weight problem, later turned to barbiturates as a sleep aid, and eventually died from an overdose?

Judy Garland.

5. *Extra credit:* Which country was the first to have an epidemic of amphetamine abuse after World War II?

Japan.

6. *Extra credit:* How did crank derive its name?

In the 1960s, Hell's Angels motorcycle gang members and other Harley-Davidson motorcycle riders smuggled and transported amphetamines ("speed") in the crankshaft of their motorcycles.

7. **What are the routes of administration of amphetamines?**
Oral, inhalational (smoked), intravenous, and topical (mucous membranes).

8. **Name the major cardiovascular symptoms associated with amphetamine toxicity.**
Chest pain
Palpitations/tachycardia
Cardiomyopathy
Myocarditis
Hypertension
Sudden death
Arrhythmia
Myocardial infarction

9. **How should amphetamine-induced cardiotoxicities be managed?**

Management of Amphetamine-induced Cardiotoxicities

SYMPTOM	TREATMENT	COMMENTS
Hypertension/agitation	Minimize stimulus. Administer sedation agents (benzodiazepines), calcium channel blockers, IV nitroprusside.	Beware of beta blockers; resultant unopposed alpha effects can produce intense vasospasm and paradoxical hypertension.
Chest pain (due to direct cardiac toxicity [myocarditis], vasospasm, thrombus formation)	Administer benzodiazepines, nitroglycerin, morphine, or aspirin.	Avoid use of beta blockers.
Palpitations/dysrhythmia	Benzodiazepines, calcium channel blockers, lidocaine as needed. Correct hypoxia and electrolytes.	
Cardiomyopathy	Diuretics, digoxin, and afterload reduction.	

10. **Name the major neurologic signs and symptoms associated with amphetamine toxicity.**
Anxiety/agitation
Delirium/hallucinations
Aggression/hyperactivity
Euphoria
Headache
Seizure
Stroke
Cerebral hemorrhage/edema

11. **How should amphetamine-induced neurotoxicities be managed?**

Management of Amphetamine-induced Neurotoxicities

SYMPTOM	TREATMENT
Agitation, aggression, hallucination	Benzodiazepines, antipsychotic agents (Haldol), minimize external stimuli, physical restraints (when necessary)
Seizures	Benzodiazepines, phenobarbital
Headache, cerebral hemorrhage, stroke	Correction of hypertension, neurosurgical intervention

12. List other systemic toxicities, and their treatments, secondary to amphetamine use.
- Hyperthermia—rapid cooling measures, spray mist, ice, dantrolene
- Rhabdomyolysis—control hyperthermia, alkalization, calcium replacement, fluids, diuretics, mannitol
- Renal failure—treat rhabdomyolysis, hemodialysis
- Obstetric complications (contractions, decreased fetal blood flow, intrauterine demise, abortion)—treatment per obstetric consultation
- Complications of IV drug abuse (endocarditis, HIV, cellulitis)—appropriate antibiotics and surgical debridement as needed per vascular consult
- Anorexia/weight loss—psychologic/psychiatric intervention

13. Is urinary acidification indicated for amphetamine toxicity?
No, and it may worsen renal failure by exacerbating rhabdomyolysis particularly in the setting of profound hyperthermia.

14. What are the popular hallucinogenic amphetamines?
Use of synthetic amphetamines with hallucinogen properties has become widespread among young people and college students at "raves" (marathon dance events). Some slang names for these drugs include ecstasy, Adam, and Eve. Rave parties also commonly involve use of gamma hydroxybutyrate (GHB) and ketamine.

15. What electrolyte abnormalities are commonly associated with amphetamine toxicity?
1. **Hyperkalemia** (secondary to hyperthermia and rhabdomyolysis)
2. **Hypernatremia** (secondary to dehydration)
3. **Hyponatremia** (secondary to excessive water intake). +SIADH

16. Can amphetamine use be diagnosed in the laboratory?
Yes. A qualitative urine drug screen may detect typical amphetamines for up to 72 hours after use. However, newer hallucinogenic amphetamines may not be detected. In addition, a positive test for amphetamines may be masked by adding Drano, bleach, or salt tablets to the urine sample. Suspicion should be raised if the urine is too alkaline or if the specific gravity is greater than 1.035.

17. What can cause false-positive drug screens?
False-positives can result from ephedrine, pseudoephedrine, and phenylpropanolamine, which are found in several over-the-counter medications.

18. Name the symptoms of amphetamine drug withdrawal.

Agitation	Fatigue	Mood swings
Anxiety	Increased appetite	Other drug and alcohol abuse
Craving drug	Irritability	Paranoia
Depression	Lethargy	Sleep disturbances
Exhaustion	Loss of pleasure	Suicidal ideation

BIBLIOGRAPHY

1. Aaron CK: Sympathomimetics. Emerg Med Clin North Am 8:513–526, 1990.
2. Chan P, Chen JH, Lee MH, Deng JF: Fatal and nonfatal methamphetamine intoxication in the intensive care unit. Clin Toxicol 32:147–155, 1994.
3. Dar KJ, McBrien ME: MDMA-induced hyperthermia: Report of a fatality and review of the current literature. Intensive Care Med 22:995–996, 1996.
4. Ellenhorn MJ, Schonwald S, Ordog G, et al (eds): Ellenhorn's Medical Toxicology: Diagnosis and Treatment of Human Poisoning, 2nd ed. Baltimore, Williams & Wilkins, 1996.
5. Milroy CM: Ten years of ecstasy. J R Soc Med 92:68–72, 1999.
6. Schwartz RH, Miller NS: MDMA (ecstasy) and the rave: A review. Pediatrics 100:705–708, 1997.

32. PHENCYCLIDINE

Michele Zell-Kanter, Pharm.D.

1. What is phencyclidine's abuse history?

Phencyclidine (PCP) became popular as a drug of abuse in the 1970s. It is easily manufactured from inexpensive ingredients. PCP was often mistaken for marijuana, mescaline, and psilocybin and was used as an adulterant. The term PCP is derived from "PeaCePill," a name adopted in San Francisco in the 1960s.

2. *Extra credit:* PCP was originally marketed in the late 1950s as a sedative and anesthetic agent by what major pharmaceutical company?

Parke-Davis. It was thought to be free of the cardiorespiratory depression associated with many other anesthetics. Many patients developed dysphoria and agitation after PCP-induced anesthesia, and consequently it was removed from the market. Currently, PCP is used as a veterinary anesthetic, which accounts for its street names alluding to animals (see question 5).

3. *Extra credit:* In 1988, a famous musician was arrested and charged with driving under the influence of PCP. He is often called the Godfather of Soul, but what is the real name of this personage?

James Joe Brown, Jr.

4. In what forms is PCP available?

PCP can be ingested orally, smoked, snorted, or injected. It is available as a powder, tablet, liquid, crystal, or capsule.

5. What is a Sherman?

Sherman is one of the many street names for PCP; they vary by region. Other common street names include angel dust, animal tranquilizer, crystal joint, snorts, soma, and goon. In the past, "embalming fluid" was a street name for PCP. Currently, "embalming fluid" refers to any combination of PCP, marijuana, and tea leaves soaked in formaldehyde.

6. What are the signs and symptoms of PCP-intoxication?

Presentation is highly variable and can include central nervous system (CNS) stimulation or depression, cholinergic or anticholinergic effects, and adrenergic effects. Clinical findings may wax and wane over the course of intoxication. Generally, patients present with abnormal behavior, dysphoria, and altered consciousness and thought processes. They may be confused, delusional, and disoriented and have auditory or visual hallucinations. Catatonia, myoclonia, dystonia, and choreoathetoid movements have been reported. Patients may become violent and require restraints and sedation. Generalized seizure activity can occur with large overdoses. Hypertension and nystagmus are hallmark clinical findings of PCP. Nystagmus can be horizontal, vertical, or rotatory. Patients may develop coma, usually of brief duration. Agitation and psychosis are common after coma is resolved. Patients may become hyperthermic and develop rhabdomyolysis.

7. Describe the causes of PCP-induced morbidity and mortality.

PCP fatalities result from patients taking life-threatening risks (jumping out of windows from tall buildings, running into traffic naked) or attempting suicide. Respiratory depression or arrest and intracerebral hemorrhage may also be causative.

8. Are there special pediatric considerations?

Children may become PCP intoxicated by passive inhalation or by ingestion of PCP-containing cigarette butts. Typically, children younger than 5 years present with lethargy, CNS depression, ataxia, nystagmus, and episodes of staring. Other signs of intoxication include apnea, seizures, abnormal posturing, and miosis.

9. What pharmacokinetic parameters are important?

PCP is well absorbed by all routes of administration, including through the skin from product handling. Depending on the route of administration, clinical effects can be seen within minutes (if smoked) to 1 hour (if ingested). Signs and symptoms of toxicity can last 4–6 hours after acute administration, with complete resolution within 24–48 hours. Symptomatology in chronic users or in patients who ingest packets containing PCP can last for days to weeks. PCP is a lipophilic weak base ($pK_a = 8.6$) and is ionized in acid media including the cerebrospinal fluid. Its volume of distribution is about 6.0 L/kg, and it is 80% plasma protein bound. The half-life of PCP varies from 7 hours to more than 3 days. Metabolism occurs in the liver by oxidative hydroxylation and glucuronidation. PCP's metabolites and about 10% of unchanged drug are excreted in the urine.

10. Should a PCP level be ordered to ensure the diagnosis?

Quantitative PCP levels in serum and urine are difficult to obtain and do not correlate with clinical effects. Qualitative urine samples for PCP may remain positive for up to 4 weeks in patients who are chronic abusers. Ketamine has been reported to cause a false-positive urine drug screen for PCP.

11. What other laboratory tests are pertinent?

Measure serum electrolytes, blood urea nitrogen (BUN), creatinine, glucose, and creatine phosphokinase (CPK). Monitor for development of rhabdomyolysis and renal failure.

12. Is there an antidote for PCP?

There are no antidotes. Supportive care should be given, and activated charcoal can be administered. Patients should be placed in a quiet, darkened room. Hemodialysis and hemoperfusion are not effective in removing PCP because of its large volume of distribution.

13. Is urinary acidification useful?

No, because (1) only a small percentage of PCP is eliminated unchanged in the urine and (2) urinary acidification increases the risk of myoglobinuric renal failure.

14. How should the agitated or violent patient be treated?

External stimuli should be minimized. If restraints are used, remember that these patients are at risk for developing rhabdomyolysis and hyperthermia. Benzodiazepines and haloperidol are effective.

15. What about PCP-induced seizures and hypertension?

IV benzodiazepines are the treatment of choice for seizure activity. Mild to moderate hypertension is usually self-limited. Severe hypertension has been associated with intracranial hemorrhage and should be aggressively treated.

16. What is Special K and how is it related to PCP?

Special K is a street name for ketamine. Ketamine is chemically related to PCP and is similarly abused by adolescents and young adults. It appears to be less potent and of shorter duration than PCP. Repeated usage may result in psychosis. Hallucination recurrences occur without additional drug abuse.

BIBLIOGRAPHY

1. Baldridge EB, Bessen HA: Phencyclidine. Emerg Med Clin North Am 8:541–550, 1990.
2. Holland JA, Nelson L, Ravikumar PR, et al: Embalming fluid–soaked marijuana: New high or new guise for PCP? J Psychoactive Drugs 30:215–219, 1998.
3. Shannon M: [Letter to the editor]. Pediatr Emerg Care 14:180, 1998.
4. U.S. Food and Drug Administration: Ketamine abuse. FDA Drug Bull 9:24, 1979.
5. Weiner AL, Vieira L, McKay CA, Bayer MJ: Ketamine abusers presenting to the emergency department: A case series. J Emerg Med 18:447–451, 2000.
6. Wright RO, Woolf AD: Phencyclidine. In Haddad LM, Shannon MW, Winchester JF (eds): Clinical Management of Poisoning and Drug Overdose, 3rd ed. Philadelphia, W.B. Saunders, 1998, pp 552–558.
7. Young JD, Crapo LM: Protracted phencyclidine coma from an intestinal deposit. Arch Intern Med 152:859–860, 1992.

33. LSD AND OTHER HALLUCINOGENS

Leon Gussow, M.D.

1. What is a hallucinogen?

A hallucinogen is a drug that causes hallucinations, in which the user sees or hears things that are not in fact there. Most street drugs commonly regarded as hallucinogens do not cause true hallucinations. Rather, they produce distorted perceptions and are sometimes referred to as "illusogens."

2. Okay then, what drugs are "illusogens"?

Lysergic acid diethylamide (LSD), mescaline, psilocybin, morning glory, and nutmeg will produce illusions. Phencyclidine, jimson weed, and some of the synthetic designer amphetamines have illusogenic properties.

3. *Extra credit:* Where did the acronym for the hallucinogenic chemical LSD originate?

From the German *Lyserge Saure Diethylamid*. Hofmann originally synthesized LSD from ergot alkaloids in 1943 and discovered its powerful psychotropic properties when he inadvertently ingested it.

4. What kinds of illusions are produced by LSD?

The acute effects of LSD include an intensified and altered sense of sound and color. Objects may be perceived to be surrounded by **halos** in the visual field. Apprehension of time, shape, and distance is altered. Typical perceptual distortions include **synesthesia**, which is the illusion that stimulus of one of the five senses is perceived through another sensory modality. For example, music may be "seen" as shifting patterns of color (this was the inspiration for the light shows that often accompanied rock music concerts during the "psychedelic" 1960s). In addition, objects moving across the visual field may leave behind a **trail** of individual afterimages. Thought processes can be altered, leaving the user with the mistaken impression that she or he has discovered the meaning of life or the secret soul of the universe. The user can become depressed, anxious, and paranoid, with **feelings of depersonalization** and **ego fragmentation**. This reaction can be extremely frightening and is commonly referred to as a "bad trip." Usually, however, the user is alert, oriented, and aware that the perceptual and psychological distortions being experienced are effects of the drug. These effects peak at 2–4 hours after ingestion and have a duration of 6–12 hours.

5. *Extra credit:* Where did the word *psychedelic* originate?

The Psychedelic Sounds of the 13th Floor Elevators was the 1966 debut album by the 13th Floor Elevators, the legendary Texas band led by Roky Erickson who coined the term "psychedelic."

6. *Extra credit:* This 1968 rock musical referred to the hallucinogen LSD as "STP." What was the name of this musical?

Hair.

7. *Extra credit:* Which popular Beatles song allegedly made numerous references to LSD?

"Lucy in the Sky with Diamonds."

8. My patient, a 17-year-old male just brought by ambulance from a local rock concert, seems to be hallucinating and seeing illusions. What should be included in the differential diagnosis aside from LSD intoxication?

As with any case of altered mental status, you first want to get a rapid bedside glucose measurement to check for hypoglycemia. Other toxic causes of hallucinosis include alcohol or sedative-hypnotic withdrawal, amphetamines, cocaine, phencyclidine, and anticholinergics. It is important to consider infectious processes (meningitis, encephalitis) and metabolic disorders (hyperthermia, electrolyte disturbances, hyper- or hypothyroidism). Hypoxia can cause anxiety and altered mental status. Finally, psychiatric disease (schizophrenia, psychosis) can present in this manner.

9. Aside from altered perception, what are the other effects of LSD?

Within minutes after ingestion, LSD can cause sympathomimetic manifestations including tachycardia, hypertension, marked mydriasis, tremor, nausea, flushing, and chills.

10. Does LSD produce any chronic effects?

Yes. Some LSD users will experience "flashbacks," in which LSD-induced perceptual and psychological distortions recur without reexposure to the drug. These tend to become less frequent and vivid over time. Although the neurochemical cause of these flashbacks is not known, these episodes can be triggered or exacerbated when LSD abusers are treated with selective serotonin reuptake inhibitors. In addition, LSD use can be followed by persistent personality change, psychosis, depression, and lack of motivation. It is not clear whether LSD causes these effects or simply unmasks underlying psychological disorders.

11. In what forms is LSD distributed?

LSD can be found as capsules, powder, or tablets. Blotting paper, often bearing distinctive illustrations, can be impregnated with LSD ("blotter acid"). In addition, LSD is available on squares of gelatin ("windowpanes") or as drops on small tablets ("microdots") or sugar cubes.

12. How should an acute LSD intoxication be managed?

The goal in treating patients having a "bad trip" from LSD is to reduce anxiety, reassure that the drug effects will wear off, and provide a quiet, nonthreatening environment. This is often called "talking the patient down." Benzodiazepines can be used for sedation as needed. Phenothiazines, which may reduce the seizure threshold and induce dystonic reactions, are not recommended. Severe sympathomimetic effects not responsive to benzodiazepines (e.g., hypertension) can be treated with phentolamine or nitroprusside. Because LSD is rapidly absorbed, gastric decontamination is probably not beneficial; in addition, gastric lavage or induced emesis may increase the patient's dysphoria. Physical restraints should be avoided if at all possible.

13. What are the earliest effects seen after LSD ingestion?

Sympathomimetic manifestations occur within 5–10 minutes after ingesting LSD. These include mydriasis (dilated pupils), tachycardia, and anxiety. Hallucinations and mental changes occur 30–60 minutes later.

14. Can LSD ingestion cause fatality?

Yes, but generally not from the pharmacologic effects of the drug. Deaths usually occur from delirium-induced self-injury, traumatic accidents, or subsequent depression and suicide.

15. What are the psychiatric effects of LSD?

These effects, which may not be dose related, include anxiety, paranoia, panic, dangerous behavior, hallucinations, acute psychotic reaction, and depressive reactions.

16. Another patient was just brought by ambulance from the rock concert. She is actively hallucinating and has mydriasis. What other toxins should I think of besides LSD?

Although mydriasis is often seen in LSD intoxication, it is not diagnostic. Other items in the differential diagnosis include jimson weed (*Datura stramonium*), atropine, psilocybin mushrooms, and psychedelic amphetamines (e.g., 3,4-methylenedioxyamphetamine [MDA], methylenedioxymethamphetamine [MDMA]).

17. What are the chronic effects of LSD ingestion?

LSD use can cause a variety of long-term psychiatric syndromes, including psychosis, major affective disorder, worsening of existent psychiatric problems, personality change, and recurrent flashbacks.

18. Is LSD used more often at concerts by the Rolling Stones, Pink Floyd, or the Grateful Dead?

A study performed at Soldier Field in Chicago during the summer of 1994 found that, among concert-goers treated at stadium first aid stations, LSD use was not uncommon at concerts by the Grateful Dead but not reported at all when Pink Floyd or the Stones were playing.

19. Can a person get high by licking toads?

Members of the toad genus *Bufo* have glands that produce many biologically active compounds. Despite a long-standing belief that bufotenine, found in the venom of all *Bufo* toads, is hallucinogenic, this has not been confirmed by scientific studies. However, 5-methoxy-N,N-dimethyltryptamine (5-MeODMT), found only in the venom of *Bufo alvarius*, is an active hallucinogen. Ingestion can also cause salivation, seizures, and cardiac dysrhythmias. The venom of other *Bufo* species contains digoxin-like substances and can cause a syndrome similar to digoxin toxicity.

BIBLIOGRAPHY

1. Brown RT, Braden NJ: Hallucinogens. Pediatr Clin North Am 34:341–347, 1987.
2. Erickson TB, Aks SE, Koenigsberg M, et al: Drug use patterns at major rock concert events. Ann Emerg Med 28:22–26, 1996.
3. Green RC: Nutmeg poisoning. JAMA 171:1342–1344, 1959.
4. Ingram AL: Morning glory seed reaction. JAMA 190:107–108, 1964.
5. Lyttle T, Goldstein D, Gartz J: Bufo toads and bufotenine: Fact and fiction surrounding an alleged psychedelic. J Psychoactive Drugs 28:267–290, 1996.
6. Markel H, Lee A, Homes RD, et al: LSD flashback syndrome exacerbated by selective serotonin reuptake inhibitor antidepressants in adolescents. J Pediatr 125:817–819, 1994.
7. Schwartz RH: LSD: Its rise, fall, and renewed popularity among high school students. Pediatr Clin North Am 42:403–413, 1995.

34. MARIJUANA

Maerry L. Lee, M.D., and Timothy Erickson, M.D.

1. What are hallucinogens?

Hallucinogens are agents used recreationally for their mind-altering properties. Examples include marijuana, phencyclidine (PCP), lysergic acid diethylamide (LSD), 3,4-methylenedioxyamphetamine (MDA), and 3,4-methylenedioxymethamphetamine (MDMA), which is also known as Adam, ecstasy, E, and XTC.

2. What is marijuana?

Marijuana is a psychoactive material (tetrahydrocannabinol [THC]) obtained from the leaves and flowers of the hemp plant *Cannabis sativa*. Marijuana, the most commonly used illegal substance in the United States, is the number one cash crop in the U.S., with earnings estimated at $32 billion a year. Hashish is a derivative of the cannabis plant that contains higher concentrations of THC.

3. List some of the common street names for marijuana.

Ace	Indiana hay	Pot
Brick	Jamaican	Puff the magic dragon
Bush	Joint	Reefer
Colombian gold	Kif	Rope
Dope	Mary Jane	Smoke
Ganja	MJ	Tea
Hagga	Macohna	Weed
Hashish	Panama red	Yerba

4. What are the acute effects of marijuana?

Acute effects include alteration in sensation, perception, cognition, and psychomotor functions. Patients also experience a sense of euphoria, relaxation, and various sensory alterations. Conjunctival injection, increased appetite, dry (cotton) mouth, decreased intraocular pressure, decreased testosterone levels, and urinary retention are also common. Patients have a loss of motor skills and exhibit poor judgment. Smoking a large quantity of marijuana can produce a range of effects, including mild anxiety, paranoid behavior, acute psychosis, problems dealing with reality, and obsessional thought content characterized by delusions, hallucinations, illusions, and bizarre behavior.

5. How long does the acute effect last?

The bioavailability of THC is directly related to the route of ingestion. If smoked, it takes about 15 seconds for the lungs to absorb the THC and transport it to the brain. The effects peak in 10–30 minutes and may last for 1–4 hours.

6. How long will marijuana be detected in a urine drug screen in chronic users and sporadic users?

At least 3 weeks and up to 8 weeks for chronic users and 3 days for sporadic users.

7. Will passive inhalation of marijuana (e.g., attending a rock music concert) result in a positive urine test?

No. The detection limits are set high enough to avoid this false-positive.

8. Are there any long-term effects for chronic users?

Yes. There is a sixfold increase in the incidence of schizophrenia; cancer of the mouth, jaw, tongue, and lungs in 19–30-year-olds; and nonlymphoblastic leukemia in children of marijuana-smoking mothers. There is also decreased sperm motility and number as well as an increase in abnormal morphology. T- and B-cell activity is depressed by THC.

9. What are the symptoms of marijuana withdrawal syndrome?

Sleep disturbances
Irritability
Decreased appetite
Nausea
Restlessness

10. Is marijuana intoxication life-threatening?

In children, marijuana can induce coma. In adults, the danger is more related to poor judgment and the loss of motor skills. Operating a motor vehicle or other machinery while under the influence of marijuana could lead to loss of life or limb (or lower one's in-service exam score).

In addition, marijuana is often used in combination with other illicit drugs that pose life threats. PCP is often combined with marijuana ("superweed" or "wicky stick") to obtain a more intense hallucinogenic experience.

11. Are there any special considerations to remember in the treatment of marijuana intoxication?

Be alert for the patient who develops an acute **psychotic reaction** with hallucinations, delusions, illusions, and agitation. This reaction is usually seen in inexperienced drug users or those who take too large a dose. Psychosis is usually transient and can be managed with benzodiazepines. In patients who have the genotype for schizophrenia, even a modest dose can produce a schizophrenic type of psychosis. The usual drug therapies for schizophrenia are needed. Also, **pneumomediastinum** has been described secondary to deep inhalation, leading to alveolar overdistention and rupture during marijuana smoking.

12. Does anything enhance the clearance of marijuana from the system?

No. THC accumulates in lipid tissue, is highly protein bound, and is enterohepatically recirculated. Thus, it is slowly eliminated from the body.

13. What substances result in a false-positive urine result?

Substances that can result in false-positives include ibuprofen, fenoprofen, and naproxen. However, false-positives from these substances occur only rarely because the minimum detection limit is set too high in the standard drug screen.

14. What will result in a false-negative urine test?

Dilution, detergents, diuretic use, table salt, vinegar, and other contaminants may cause false-negative results.

15. *Extra credit:* In Burma during World War II, the members of the famous Merrill's Marauders concocted an intoxicating drink with marijuana. This beverage usually made the drinker almost uncontrollable. What did the soldiers call their homemade brew?

Bullfight brandy.

16. *Extra credit:* What pesticide was once sprayed on marijuana fields by law enforcement officials to destroy the crops of its toxic effects?

Paraquat

BIBLIOGRAPHY

1. Cone EJ: In vivo adulteration: Excess fluid ingestion causes false-negative marijuana and cocaine urine test results. J Anat Toxicol 22:460–473, 1998.
2. Cone EJ, Johnson RE: Contact highs and urinary cannabis excretion after passive exposure to marijuana smoke. Clin Parmacol Ther 40:247–256, 1986.
3. Heishman SJ, Huestis MA, Henningfield JE, Cone EJ: Acute and residual effects of marijuana: Profiles of plasma THC levels, physiological, subjective and performance measures. Pharmacol Biochem Behav 37:561–565, 1990.
4. Huestis M: Pharmacology and toxicology of marijuana. Ther Drug Monit 14:131–138, 1993.
5. Liu RJH: Important considerations in the interpretation of urine drug tests. Forensic Sci Rev 4:51–65, 1992.
6. Mathers DC, Ghodse AH: Cannabis and psychotic illness. Br J Psychiatry 161:648–653, 1992.
7. Naha G, Latour C: The human toxicity of marijuana. Med J Aust 15:495–497, 1992.
8. Perez-Reyes M: Marijuan smoking: Factors that influence the bioavailability of tetrahydrocannabinol. In Chiang CN, Hawks RL (eds): Research Findings on Smoking of Abused Substances. Washington, DC, U.S. Department of Health and Human Services, 1990, pp 42–62, NIDA research monograph 99.
9. Pollan M: How pot has grown. NY Times Magazine, Feb 19, 1995, pp 31–57.
10. Pope HG, Yurgelun-Todd D: The residual cognitive effects of heavy marijuana use in college students. JAMA 275:521–527, 1996.
11. Schonberg SK: Marijuana. Pediatr Rev 18:27–29, 1997.
12. Schwartz RH, Hawks RL: Laboratory detection of marijuana use. JAMA 254:788–792, 1985.

35. WITHDRAWAL SYNDROMES

Rotem Friede, M.D., and Timothy Erickson, M.D.

1. **What are the characteristics of withdrawal syndromes?**
   - Preexisting physiologic adaptation to a drug or toxin, the continuous presence of which prevents physiologic derangements
   - Decreasing concentrations of that substance

ETHANOL

2. **Describe the different syndromes of alcohol withdrawal and when they are seen.**
   Alcoholic hallucinosis occur at 24–36 hours. Alcoholic seizures may occur at 7–48 hours and peak at 24 hours. Delirium tremens (DTs) is seen at 3–5 days but may be seen up to 14 days.

3. **What are the characteristics of alcoholic hallucinosis?**
   Characteristics are mostly visual and appear to occur in patients with insufficient thiamine stores. Another common trait is formication, the sensation of ants crawling on the skin. This often promotes itching and excoriation.

4. **When are alcohol withdrawal seizures (AS), or "rum fits," commonly seen?**
   Up to 48 hours after the cessation of alcohol ingestion in a chronic alcoholic.

5. **What are the characteristics of AS?**
   They are often brief tonic-clonic events with a short postictal period. They may recur, but status epilepticus is rare in AS. Approximately, 40% are single seizures and 3% are status epilepticus. All patients with first-time AS should have a thorough evaluation, including a complete blood count (CBC), serum electrolytes, calcium, magnesium, chest x-ray, urinalysis, computed tomography (CT) scan of the brain, and lumbar puncture. The yield on these clinical investigations is extraordinarily high. One third of all patients who develop DTs have alcoholic withdrawal seizures as the precipitating event. The seizures may occur despite the presence of an elevated serum ethanol level.

6. **What symptoms characterize DTs?**
   Florid confusion, agitation, and sympathetic storm (tachycardia, hypertension, hyperthermia, and tremulousness).

7. **What combination of DT symptoms carries a grave prognosis?**
   Hyperthermia, motor activity, and fluid depletion.

8. **What is the mortality of DTs?**
   In cases with concurrent illnesses, the rate is approximately 5% if aggressive cooling, supportive care, and fluid resuscitation are not instituted.

9. **What other drug poisonings simulate DTs?**
   Amphetamine, phencyclidine (PCP), anticholinergics, cocaine, monoamine oxidase inhibitor (MAOI)–meperidine interactions, MAOI-serotonin interactions, and MAOI overdose.

OPIOIDS

10. Describe the different stages of opioid withdrawal.

Stages of Opioid Withdrawal

STAGE	TIME FRAME	CHARACTERISTICS
Anticipatory	3–4 hours after last "fix"	Fear of withdrawal, craving, drug-seeking behavior
Early withdrawal	8–10 hours	Anxiety, restlessness, yawning, nausea, sweating, nasal stuffiness, lacrimation, rhinorrhea, dilated pupils, stomach cramps, drug-seeking behavior
	1–3 days	Severe anxiety, tremor, restlessness, piloerection, nausea, vomiting, diarrhea, muscle spasm, muscle pain, hypertension, tachycardia, fever, chills, impulse-driven drug-seeking behavior
Protracted abstinence	6 months	Hypotension, bradycardia, insomnia, loss of energy, appetite, stimulus-driven cravings

11. Where did the phrase "going cold turkey" originate?

Cold turkey is a reference to the goose-flesh appearance of the skin from piloerection that occurs during opiate withdrawal.

12. Where is opioid withdrawal mediated and what adrenergic agent is believed to lead to the symptoms seen?

Opioid withdrawal is mediated both centrally and peripherally. Levels of norepinephrine released centrally at the locus caeruleus are noted to rise.

13. What is the current treatment of the opiate withdrawal syndrome?

1. Long-acting opioid agents such as methadone
2. Centrally acting agents to block the unpleasant withdrawal symptoms
3. A simple tapering scheme if the agent is a prescribed medication

14. What is the role of clonidine in the treatment of opioid withdrawal?

Clonidine acts on central alpha$_2$ receptors and leads to decreased firing at the locus caeruleus with subsequent decrease in norepinephrine release.

SEDATIVE-HYPNOTICS

15. Which agents are considered sedative-hypnotics?

Barbiturates
Ethanol
Ethchlorvynol
Meprobamate
Methaqualone
Benzodiazepines

16. Describe gamma aminobutyric acid (GABA)–minergic withdrawal.

GABA synaptic activity is diminished such that the inhibitory control of excitatory neurotransmitters and pathways such as glutamate, *N*-methyl-D-aspartate (NMDA), norepinephrine, and dopamine is lost. This results in the clinical syndrome of withdrawal–central nervous system excitation (seizures, tremors, hallucinations) and autonomic stimulation (tachycardia, hypertension, hyperthermia, diaphoresis).

17. What are the first signs of central nervous system excitation associated with withdrawal?
A fine intention tremor that can be detected in the outstretched hand or protruding tongue.

18. What is the treatment for withdrawal?
Restoration of inhibitory control by administration of GABA agonists. Long-acting agents that can be administered in a loading dose are ideal. Diazepam is the benzodiazepine of choice. However, any benzodiazepine that can be administered intravenously will suffice. Phenobarbital has also been used successfully because of its long half-life and wide margin of safety. High-dose intravenous barbiturates are advantageous in refractory cases because they can open up GABA chloride channels directly. It is also important to correct fluid, electrolyte, and nutritional deficiencies as well as to evaluate and treat any concurrent infections. Also, place the patient in a dimly lit room with minimal external stimuli.

19. Explain the difference in the withdrawal symptoms between sedative-hypnotics (e.g., benzodiazepines, barbiturates) and alcohol.
The symptoms of sedative-hypnotic withdrawal may develop as late as 14 days after cessation of the drug, depending on the pharmacokinetic profile; alcohol withdrawal begins as quickly as 48 hours after cessation.

BENZODIAZEPINES

20. What symptoms help to differentiate benzodiazepine withdrawal from anxiety?
Presence of tinnitus
Involuntary movements
Perceptual changes

21. What are the two most common symptoms of benzodiazepine withdrawal?
Mood swings and convulsions.

22. List the different syndromes related to benzodiazepine withdrawal.
    1. **Acute sedative-hypnotic type withdrawal** is commonly seen 1–2 days after stopping a short-acting benzodiazepine or 2–4 days after a longer acting benzodiazepine. It is associated with anxiety, insomnia, nightmares, seizures, psychosis, hyperpyrexia, and death.
    2. **Subacute prolonged benzodiazepine withdrawal** occurs approximately 1 day after stopping benzodiazepine but improves with time. It is associated with anxiety, insomnia, nightmares, muscle spasm, and psychosis.
    3. **Symptom reemergence** resumes after stopping benzodiazepine use. It has the same symptoms as those that occur prior to taking benzodiazepines.

BACLOFEN

23. What is baclofen and what type of patients are prescribed baclofen?
Baclofen is an antispasmodic agent that works on muscles. Patients are prescribed baclofen for muscle relaxation and for multiple sclerosis.

24. Describe the withdrawal syndrome associated with baclofen withdrawal.
Withdrawal occurs after abrupt cessation of use of the drug for many months and may last up to 8 days. It occurs within 12–96 hours of cessation and may lead to grand mal seizures, auditory and visual hallucinations, paranoid ideas, insomnia, buccolingual dyskinesia, hyperactivity, and grandiose ideas.

25. What is the treatment?
Reinstallation of the drug with gradual tapering dose.

COCAINE

26. What are the three phases of the cocaine abstinence syndrome?

PHASE	DURATION	CHARACTERISTICS
First phase ("crash phase")	0–4 days	Dysphoria, depression, irritability, anxiety, and insomnia followed by hypersomnolence, exhaustion, and drug craving
Second phase	1–10 weeks	Anergia, anxiety, listlessness, and drug craving
Third phase ("extinction phase")	Lasts indefinitely	Normalization of mood and actions but also episodic drug craving that is often triggered by environmental cues

27. What is most notable about cocaine withdrawal?

The intense psychological depression and the drug-craving behavior.

TRICYCLIC ANTIDEPRESSANTS

28. What are the symptoms of tricyclic antidepressant withdrawal?

Cholinergic rebound is seen with anorexia, nausea, vomiting, diarrhea, diaphoresis, myalgia, malaise, headaches, chills, insomnia with vivid dreams, akathisia or parkinsonism, hypomania, or mania.

ANTIHYPERTENSIVES

29. What antihypertensive agents are associated with a withdrawal syndrome?

Clonidine
α-Methyldopa
Propranolol
Metoprolol
Oxprenolol
Guanethidine
Reserpine

30. List the usual signs and symptoms of the abrupt withdrawal of antihypertensive treatment.

- Blood pressure remains low for several days and then rises to its pretreatment level without any accompanying symptoms.
- Blood pressure remains low or rises slowly, but the patient experiences symptoms and signs of sympathetic overactivity such as anxiety, tremulousness, tachycardia, headache, and sleeplessness.
- Blood pressure rises rapidly within hours of cessation of treatment. Blood-pressure rise usually stops near the level of pretreatment blood pressure (rebound hypertension).
- Blood pressure exceeds the highest known pretreatment levels ("overshoot" hypertension).

31. What rare sequelae are associated with abrupt withdrawal of antihypertensives and in what time frame are they seen?

Malignant hypertension
Accelerating angina
Myocardial infarction
Ventricular arrhythmia
Left ventricular failure

These sequelae begin within 24–72 hours of withdrawal of the agent.

32. How is antihypertensive withdrawal managed?

Immediately reinstitute all discontinued antihypertensive medications and sedate the patient. If the blood pressure elevation is severe, administer the antihypertensives intravenously.

33. What are the characteristics of the clonidine withdrawal syndrome?

Hypertension, tachycardia, sweating, anxiety, insomnia, abdominal pain, nausea, and palpitations are seen 2–3 days after cessation. Rarely, malignant hypertension and cardiac dysrhythmias occur.

34. What drug class used for the treatment of hypertension must immediately be discontinued if used with clonidine?

Beta blockers because they may lead to unopposed alpha-adrenergic effects that may worsen hypertension in the setting of withdrawal.

CAFFEINE

35. What are the signs and symptoms of caffeine withdrawal?

Headache
Sleepiness
Drowsiness
Impaired concentration
Work difficulty
Flu-like symptoms

36. What accounts for the severity of withdrawal?

Dose of caffeine taken by the patient.

37. What is the time frame of the withdrawal syndrome?

Withdrawal occurs 12–24 hours after the last dose of caffeine and resolves within 2–4 days.

38. *Extra credit:* Which former U.S. First Lady with a long-running addiction to alcohol and drugs later underwent successful rehabilitation?

Betty Ford.

BIBLIOGRAPHY

1. Erwin WE, Williams DB, Speir WA: Delirium tremens. South Med J 91:425–432, 1998.
2. Farrell M: Opiate withdrawal. Addiction 89:1471–1475, 1994.
3. Greenberg OA: Ethanol and sedatives. Neurol Clin 11:523–534, 1993.
4. Goldfrank LR, Flomenbaum NE, Lewin NA, et al (eds): Goldfrank's Toxicologic Emergencies, 5th ed. Norwalk, CT, Appleton & Lange, 1994.
5. Miller NS, Gold MS: Management of withdrawal syndromes and relapse prevention in drug and alcohol dependence. Am Fam Physician 58:139–146, 1998.
6. Roy-Byrne PP, Sullivan MD, Cowley DS, Ries RK: Adjunctive treatment of benzodiazepine discontinuation syndrome: A review. J Psychiatric Res 27(Suppl 1):143–153, 1993.

36. TOXIC INHALANTS

Steven E. Aks, D.O.

VOLATILE SUBSTANCE ABUSE

1. What is the sudden sniffing death?

Sudden sniffing death occurs after volatile inhalant abuse. After inhaling a solvent or other volatile substance, the victim may become startled or may engage in sudden energetic activity. Shortly after initiating the activity, the patient develops a dysrhythmia and collapses. Volatile agents create light-plane anesthesia. Like certain outmoded anesthetics, these agents are dangerous because they sensitize the myocardium to endogenous catecholamines. This sensitization creates a state of irritability, and ventricular dysrhythmias and possibly asystole can develop when the patient experiences a sudden surge of catecholamines.

2. Describe the modes of inhaling volatile substances.

There are three major ways that individuals abuse these inhalants: sniffing, huffing, and bagging. **Sniffing** is the practice of inhaling the agent directly from its product container. For example, a person might sniff glue directly from the tube or sniff propellant directly from a can of spray paint. **Huffing** involves saturating a rag with the agent, placing the rag or cloth over the nose and mouth, and breathing in and out through the rag. **Bagging** is the practice of discharging a chemical into a bag, balloon, or similar vessel and inhaling in and out of the container. Because it involves breathing in and out of a closed system, bagging has the added risk of hypoxia.

3. What specific volatile substances are used as inhalants?

Products:	*Chemicals:*
Typewriter correction fluid (Wite Out, Liquid Paper)	Freons (fluorocarbons)
	Benzene
Glue	1,1,1 trichloroethane
Felt-tip marking pens	Trichlorethylene
Paint	Carbon tetrachloride (CCl_4)
Paint stripper	Methylene chloride
Gasoline	Toluene
	Miscellaneous hydrocarbons (alkanes, butane)

4. *Extra credit:* Who invented Liquid Paper?

Liquid Paper, a typewriter correction fluid, was invented by Bette Nesmith, the mother of Michael Nesmith, television star of *The Monkees* and member of the pop music group of the same name. See the Web page devoted to The Monkees: http://www.flexquarters.com/nesmith/bio.htm.

5. What are the typical signs and symptoms after acute inhalation?

Individuals who abuse volatile substances do so to experience a euphoric effect ("get high"). Adverse effects include altered mental state, slurred speech, incoherence, poor coordination, and ataxia. The patient may exhibit impaired judgment and experience hallucinations. Gastrointestinal effects include abdominal pain, nausea, and vomiting. Pulmonary effects can include cough and shortness of breath. This will be apparent if the patient has aspirated the agent. As described in question 1, if the patient is stimulated after inhaling a volatile agent, he or she may develop dysrhythmias, including supraventricular or ventricular dysrhythmias and asystole.

6. What is the toxicity of methylene chloride?

Methylene chloride is found in various paint strippers. It is metabolized slowly by the liver to its toxic metabolite carbon monoxide. Serious toxicity has been documented after inhalation in a closed space and after ingestion. In addition to the effects of carbon monoxide, the exposed patient may suffer from other solvent effects (i.e., central nervous system depression, pulmonary effects).

7. What is the specific toxicity of various inhalants?

Typical inhalants such as freons (fluorocarbons) and 1,1,1-trichloroethane will exhibit the general effects described in question 6. However, some toxic inhalants have specific effects worth special note:

Benzene is well known to cause aplastic anemia.

CCl_4 is a known hepatotoxin that can lead to centrilobular necrosis. It was once commonly used for dry cleaning and as a rug cleaner, but it has been replaced with safer products. Other agents that have been linked to hepatotoxicity include chloroform, toluene, and trichloroethylene.

Methylene chloride is metabolized to carbon monoxide.

Toluene can lead to an anion gap metabolic acidosis via the accumulation of benzoic acid. It can also lead to type I renal tubular acidosis (RTA) of the distal variety. This will manifest as a renal tubular acidification defect. The latter syndrome will appear as a metabolic acidosis, a normal anion gap, hyperchloremia, and an inappropriately high urinary pH.

8. Who is the typical user of volatile substances?

Abuse of volatile substances is common in adolescents. The majority of users are younger than 20 years old. Products containing volatile substances are readily available in hardware and other stores and are easy for young individuals to obtain. Many of these individuals come from middle-income suburban homes. One study has linked increased use to families in which there has been child abuse.

9. What will predispose a sniffer to greater cardiac toxicity?

Sudden stress
Hypercapnia
Hypokalemia
Hypoxia

10. What are poppers?

Poppers are glass ampules containing a nitrite compound that is used by adolescents and others for inhalation abuse. Poppers usually contain amyl nitrite, but another commonly used substance is isobutyl nitrite. These are popular among adolescents as a means to get high. They are also used in the homosexual population for sexual stimulation. These items are often purchased in "head shops." Some commercial names for these products include Rush, Bolt, Hardware, Heart On, Joe Aroma, Locker Room, Quick Silver, and Satan's Scent. Clinical effects include tremors, convulsions, headache, tachycardia, hypotension, and syncope. Nitrites have vasodilatory effects and provide an oxidant stress that leads to methemoglobinemia.

11. What is the treatment for toxicity from inhalants?

The treatment for volatile substance inhalation is generally supportive, because no specific treatment exists for most exposures. The patient should be removed from the source of exposure. If there is any dermal exposure, the patient should be decontaminated. An intravenous line should be started, the patient should be placed on a monitor, and oxygen should be administered to patients with respiratory difficulty or altered mental status. Treatment of dysrhythmias is somewhat controversial. In the setting of dysrhythmias there is a theoretical concern regarding the use of epinephrine because the mechanism of toxicity is sensitization of the myocardium to endogenous catecholamines. In general, advanced cardiac life support (ACLS) protocols should be followed but with judicious use of epinephrine. Patients with cyanosis should be evaluated for methemoglobinemia. Symptomatic patients with high levels of methemoglobin (> 20–25%) can be treated with methylene blue. If the patient is suffering from hepatic or neurologic effects, appropriate supportive care should be instituted.

12. What are the typical long-term sequelae of inhalant abuse?

Volatile agent abuse causes chronic neurologic, cardiac, gastrointestinal, and metabolic effects. The most important neurologic effects are impaired cognition and sensory and motor effects. Chronic cardiomyopathies have been described. Chronic users often suffer from anorexia and weight loss, and several agents have been linked to hepatotoxicity. Question 7 describes the volatile substance–induced metabolic effects (distal RTA) of toluene.

OTHER TOXIC INHALANTS

13. What are simple asphyxiants?

Simple asphyxiants cause toxicity by displacing available oxygen. If there is a high concentration of a simple asphyxiant, the patient will suffer a hypoxic insult. Examples include:
Carbon dioxide
Helium
Natural gas (methane)
Nitrogen
Propane

14. What toxic agents affect the upper airways when inhaled?

These are known as **irritant gases**. The water solubility determines where the greatest injury to the airway will be. Agents with high solubility are deposited in the upper airway and cause upper respiratory irritation. Examples include sulfur dioxide, hydrogen chloride, and ammonia.

15. What toxic agents affect the lower airways when inhaled?

Gases that have poor water solubility will affect the lower airways. Examples include oxides of nitrogen (silo filler's disease), phosgene, and ozone. Metals may also cause direct pulmonary toxicity (e.g., mercury, copper, cadmium, zinc).

16. What chemical asphyxiants are delivered through inhalation?

Carbon monoxide is odorless and colorless and is delivered via inhalation. Methylene chloride, which is metabolized to carbon monoxide, is also inhaled. **Hydrogen sulfide gas**, known for its rotten egg odor, is known as a rapid knock-down agent. **Cyanide** exposure can occur after inhalation. **Acetonitrile** can also be inhaled and is metabolized to cyanide.

17. What is metal fume fever?

Metal fume fever is an occupational disease that has been associated with inhalation of metal fumes, most commonly zinc, iron and copper. It is seen in welders who work with these metals. The symptoms often appear on Monday morning ("Monday morning fever") when a worker resumes welding after a weekend off. The symptoms include fever, shortness of breath, cough, chest pain, dry throat, and diffuse muscle aches. It is commonly misdiagnosed as a viral illness. The course of the illness is generally benign, and it resolves within several days after the patient is removed from the source of exposure. The mainstay of treatment is recognition and proper respiratory protection.

BIBLIOGRAPHY

1. Bass M: Sudden sniffing death. JAMA 212:2075–2079, 1970.
2. Brady WJ, Stremski E, Eljaiek L, Aufderheide TP: Freon inhalational abuse presenting with ventricular fibrillation. Am J Emerg Med 12:533–536, 1994.
3. Fendrich M, Mackesy-Amiti ME, Wislar JS, et al: Child abuse and the use of inhalants: Differences by degree of use. Am J Pub Health 87:765–769, 1997.

4. King GS, Smialek JE, Troutman WG: Sudden death in adolescents resulting from the inhalation of typewriter correction fluid. JAMA 253:1604–1606, 1985.

5. McLeod AA, Marjot R, Monaghan MJ, et al: Chronic cardiac toxicity after inhalation of 1,1,1-trichloroethane. Br Med J 294:727, 1987.

6. O'Brien ET, Yeoman WB, Hobby JA: Hepatorenal damage in a "glue sniffer." BMJ 2:29–30, 1971.

7. Reinhardt CF, Azar A, Maxfield ME, et al: Cardiac arrhythmias and aerosol "sniffing." Arch Environ Health 21:265–279, 1971.

8. Shesser R, Mitchell J, Edelstein S: Methemoglobinemia from isobutyl nitrite preparations. Ann Emerg Med 10:262–264, 1981.

9. Taher SM, Anderson RJ, McCartney R: Renal tubular acidosis associated with toluene "sniffing." N Engl J Med 290:765–768, 1974.

10. Wason S, Gibler WB, Hassan M: Ventricular tachycardia associated with non-freon aerosol propellants. JAMA 256:78–80, 1986.

11. White JF, Carlson GP: Epinephrine-induced cardiac arrhythmias in rabbits exposed to trichloroethylene: Potentiation by ethanol. Toxicol Appl Pharmacol 60:466–471, 1981.

37. DATE RAPE DRUGS

Kirk Cumpston, D.O., and Steven E. Aks, D.O.

1. What is date, or acquaintance, rape?

According to the Department of Justice, this can be defined as "drug-facilitated rape." An example: A man surreptitiously slips a drug into a beverage. A woman drinks the "spiked" beverage and becomes incapacitated or unconscious. While the woman is incapacitated or unconscious, she is raped.

The victim of a drug-facilitated sexual assault may exhibit signs of confusion, memory loss, dizziness, drowsiness, impaired motor skills, impaired judgment, reduced inhibition, slurred speech, or a variety of other symptoms.

2. When should acquaintance rape be suspected?

- When a patient appears intoxicated, confused, and amnestic after awakening partially clothed or naked
- If the patient wakes up in an unfamiliar location
- If the patient reports a sexual assault combined with drug or alcohol use (obviously acquaintance rape)

3. What are the acquaintance rape drugs?

1. **Flunitrazepam** (Rohypnol) is a potent benzodiazepine marketed in Mexico, South America, Asia, and Australia as a preanesthetic agent because of its hypnotic effect. It is also used for treatment of insomnia because it decreases sleep latency, prolongs deep sleep, decreases awakenings, and increases rapid-eye movement (REM) sleep. To inhibit its use as a date rape drug, Roche Pharmaceuticals has developed a new formulation that turns clear liquids a bright blue and causes dark liquids to turn murky.

2. **Gamma hydroxybutyrate (GHB)** was synthesized in 1960 and first used in the 1970s for sleep disorders because it induces REM sleep. It was also used in Europe as an anesthetic agent until it was found to induce seizure-like activity and provide poor analgesia. A study in 1977 claimed that GHB stimulated the effects of growth hormone. Although follow-up studies did not prove this, GHB is popular among bodybuilders nonetheless. GHB also has been investigated as therapy in alcohol and opiate withdrawal.

3. **Ketamine** is used as an anesthetic in emergency medicine and veterinary medicine. Abuse of ketamine produces clinical effects similar to those of phencyclidine (PCP).

4. Why are these drugs used in acquaintance rape?

Flunitrazepam can be administered intravenously, intranasally, intramuscularly, or orally. Most users buy flunitrazepam in bubble packs for $1–5 a pill. It is tasteless, odorless, and dissolves quickly in alcohol. Flunitrazepam causes euphoric, hallucinogenic, and disinhibiting effects. Heroin abusers use it to enhance the effect of low-grade heroin, and cocaine and crack abusers use it to ameliorate adverse effects of a binge.

GHB is available as a colorless, odorless liquid or gel and as a crystalline powder with a salty or soapy taste. The taste usually is masked by alcohol, marijuana, or other drugs, which increase GHB's clinical effects and possibly its aphrodisiac properties. It is quick in onset of effect, it is easily obtainable on the street or manufactured at home, and only a small quantity is needed. The victim commonly has hallucinations or amnesia, making the patient an unreliable witness.

Ketamine is used orally, intravenously, intranasally, or inhalationally. It is used in acquaintance rape because of its rapid onset and because its dissociative hallucinogenic properties make it difficult for the victim to resist the attacker or provide a reliable account of the event.

5. What is the schedule of each drug?

Flunitrazepam is a schedule IV controlled substance according to international treaty. Eight states have made it a schedule I controlled substance, with a penalty of possession similar to heroin. Importation of flunitrazepam was banned in 1996, which makes it illegal to prescribe, sell, or import in the United States.

GHB is an investigational drug for the treatment of narcolepsy. Therefore, possession of GHB is not illegal, but sale is prohibited. The Drug Enforcement Administration is considering classifying GHB as a federally controlled substance because of unauthorized manufacture of GHB for recreational use. Twenty states have controlled its use, with penalties similar to those for marijuana possession.

Ketamine is manufactured legally in the United States for medicinal use as an anesthetic in emergency medicine and veterinary medicine. Ketamine is a controlled substance in 18 states as a schedule III drug. The Department of Health and Human Services is recommending that ketamine be placed in schedule III classification.

6. What are the most common drugs actually associated with acquaintance rape?

A recent study analyzed more than 1000 urine samples from individuals claiming sexual assault where drug use was involved. Of the samples, 40% were negative and 60% were positive. Substances found included:

Alcohol (40%)
Marijuana (20%)
Benzodiazepines (6-flunitrazepam; 10%)
Cocaine (10%)
Amphetamines (5%)
GHB (5%)

Ketamine was not specifically analyzed because these cases were referred randomly by health care workers. These data suggest that a variety of drugs are involved in acquaintance rape.

7. How does one determine acquaintance rape drug use?

A high index of suspicion for acquaintance rape based on the history and presentation of the patient is critical. The usual urine toxicity screen and serum alcohol screen will detect many common drugs used in acquaintance rape, but for the newest agents, specific analysis (GHB, flunitrazepam, and ketamine) will be required.

8. What is the role of laboratory tests in the diagnosis of acquaintance rape?

Flunitrazepam. Most commercially available toxicology screens are unable to detect the small amount of flunitrazepam used in acquaintance rape. Many facilities have only class-specific detection of structurally related benzodiazepines. The most definitive detection of flunitrazepam is gas chromatography-mass spectrometry (GC-MS), the latest urine assay technique. A 2-mg dose can be detected in the urine up to 72 hours after ingestion. As with GHB, most states have or are developing programs to do the analysis along with sexual assault kits.

GHB. GHB can be difficult to detect because its half-life is 20 minutes to 1 hour and it is almost undetectable in the urine after 12 hours. The older method of detection required the conversion of GHB to gamma butyrolactone (GBL), but now GC-MS is preferred. Unfortunately, most hospitals do not have the adequate facilities to perform this test.

Ketamine. Ketamine is structurally related to PCP and is occasionally misidentified as PCP in urine toxicology screens. However, a specific test for ketamine is not widely available.

9. What is the toxicity of flunitrazepam?

Flunitrazepam is 10 times more potent than diazepam and acts on the gamma aminobutyric acid A (GABA-A) receptors. It is lipid soluble, which allows it to quickly cross the blood-brain barrier. It causes sedation in 20–30 minutes and has a duration of action of 6–12 hours. Like an intermediate benzodiazepine, its elimination half-life is on the order of 24 hours. Flunitrazepam is extensively metabolized in the kidneys. Patients present with symptoms of drowsiness, disorientation, dizziness, slurred speech, hot or cold flashes, nausea, which can progress to rapid-onset coma, amnesia, psychomotor impairment, and respiratory depression.

10. Describe the toxicity of GHB.

GHB is found naturally in the brain, and research has suggested that it acts as a neurotransmitter, affecting GHB and GABA-B receptors and causing central nervous system (CNS) depression. It increases dopamine levels and affects the opioid system. GHB takes effect in 15–30 minutes, causing drowsiness, dizziness, and disorientation. Duration of action is 3 hours, and elimination half-life ranges from 20 minutes to 1 hour, depending on the dose. GHB is metabolized to GBL and carbon dioxide in the periphery by oxidizing enzymes and the TCA cycle. The hallmark of GHB ingestion is marked agitation upon stimulation despite apnea and hypoxia. Symptoms are dose related. A dose of 10 mg/kg causes vomiting, rapid onset of coma, and amnesia. Cycles of REM and non-REM sleep occur with a 20–30-mg/kg dose. A high dose of 50 mg/kg can cause respiratory depression, bradycardia, clonic muscle contractions, anesthesia, and decreased cardiac output.

11. What is the toxicity of ketamine?

Ketamine is chemically related to PCP, and its users often claim it is superior to LSD and PCP. It takes effect in 15–20 minutes, producing analgesia. Higher doses cause dissociative anesthesia, hallucinations, delirium, respiratory depression, seizures, arrhythmias, and cardiac arrest. The effect of ketamine lasts for 20–45 minutes. It is distributed similarly to thiopental, first to highly perfused tissue, such as the heart, brain, and lungs, and then to the peripheral tissues, muscles, and fat. Finally, it is almost completely metabolized in the liver.

12. What is a Mickey Finn?

A Mickey Finn is the addition of chloral hydrate ("knock-out drops") to an alcoholic beverage. It is named for Mickey Finn, the owner of the Lone Star Saloon and Palm Garden in Chicago in the 1890s. He is purported to have put these knock-out drops in unsuspecting patrons' drinks. After drinking this cocktail, they would be rendered stuporous or unconscious, and he would rob them. His liquor license was eventually revoked.

Chloral hydrate is metabolized to trichloroethanol, which is responsible for continued hypnotic effects. Trichloroethanol has a half-life of 4–14 hours. When ethanol and trichloroethanol are both present, their respective actions are potentiated.

13. List the street names of the acquaintance rape drugs.

(See table next page.)

14. What are the general treatment and management strategies used in flunitrazepam, GHB, and ketamine ingestion?

Flunitrazepam. Supportive care of airway, blood pressure, heart rate, and respiration should be undertaken. Activated charcoal is helpful for large ingestions.

GHB. Protect airway if necessary with either rapid sequence intubation (usually needing only succinylcholine) or recovery position with bedside suction and supplemental oxygen. Atropine can be used as needed for bradycardia. Activated charcoal is not useful to decrease GHB absorption but may be helpful in the case of coingestion.

Ketamine. Supportive care of airway, blood pressure, heart rate, and respiration should be undertaken. The patient should be placed in a quiet recovery area with minimal stimulation.

15. Are there any antidotes for the acquaintance rape drugs?

There is no antidote for GHB or ketamine. For flunitrazepam, flumazenil can be used for respiratory depression. The starting dose is 0.2 mg IV. If no response, administer 0.3 mg in 1 minute, increasing to 0.5 mg per minute up to a total of 3 mg. If coingestion is suspected (e.g., tricyclic antidepressant or any drug that can cause seizures or dysrhythmias), flumazenil is not recommended.

GHB	FLUNITRAZEPAM	KETAMINE
Biosky	Circles	K
Cherry menth	Darkene	Green
Coke	The drop drug	Jet
Easy lay	Flunitrazepam	Kay
Everclear	Forget pill	Keets
Gammo-OH	La roche	Mauve
GBH	Mexican valium	Purple
Georgia home boy	Mind erasers	Special K
GHB	Pappas	Special LA
Gib	Pastas	Super acid
Goops	Peanuts	Super C
Great hormones at bedtime	Poples	
Grievous bodily harm	R05-4200	
G-riffick	R-2	
Liquid ecstasy	Reynol	
Liquid X	Rib	
Natural sleep-500	Roaches	
Nature's quaalude	Roachies	
Organic quaalude	Robinol	
Oxy-sleep	Roches	
Poor man's heroin	Rohibinol	
Salt water	Rohypnol	
Scoop	Roofenol	
Soap	Roofies	
Somatomax PM	Roopies	
Somsanit	Ropanol	
Vita-G	Rophies	
Water	Ropes	
Wolfies	Row-shay	
Zonked	Rubies	
	Ruffies	
	Trip and fall	
	Whiteys	
	Wolfies	

16. What are other forms of GHB?

GBL, when combined with NaOH, forms GHB. GBL is available for purchase over the Internet at the time of writing this chapter. One product available is called Renewtrient. 1,4-Butanediol is an industrial chemical used in the manufacture of other organic chemicals. It is converted in vivo into GHB and hence has a similar toxicologic profile.

17. What advice can be given to patients to reduce the risk of acquaintance rape?

1. Discard any beverages that have been left unattended.
2. Bring your own beverages to social gatherings, when possible.
3. Be alert to a friend's behavior that is symptomatic of a drug ingestion, and have him or her reciprocate the favor.
4. Look for signs of drowsiness, dizziness, disorientation, analgesia, and amnesia.
5. Do not leave beverages unattended in a social setting.
6. Do not accept open beverage containers from anyone other than a bartender or server.
7. Do not share or exchange beverages with anyone.
8. Do not drink beverages from a common container such as a punch bowl.
9. Do not drink anything that has an unusual appearance or taste. The new formulations of flunitrazepam cause clear liquids to turn bright blue and dark liquids to turn murky.

BIBLIOGRAPHY

1. Brandt P: Drinking in 1800s Chicago. Barfly Newspaper, March 17–31, 1999, 6:10–19.
2. Calhoun SR, Wesson DR, Galloway GP, Smith DE: Abuse of flunitrazepam (Rohypnol) and other benzo-diazepines in Austin and South Texas. J Psychoactive Subst 28:183–189, 1996.
3. Chin M-Y, Kreutzer RA, Dyer JE: Acute poisoning from gamma hydroxybutyrate in California. West J Med 156:380–384, 1992.
4. Dyer JE: Gamma hydroxybutyrate: A health-food product producing coma and seizurelike activity. Am J Emerg Med 9:321–324, 1991.
5. El Sohly MA, Salamone SJ: Prevalence of drugs used in cases of alleged sexual assault. J Anal Toxicol 23:141–146, 1999.
6. Ropero-Miller JD, Goldberger BA: Recreational drugs: Current trends of the 90s. Clin Lab Med 18:727–746, 1998.
7. Sellers EM, Lang M, Koch-Weser J, et al: Interaction of chloral hydrate and ethanol in man. Clin Pharm Ther 13:37–49, 1971.
8. Simmons MM, Cupp MJ: Use and abuse of flunitrazepam. Ann Pharmacother 32:117–119, 1998.
9. Smith KM: Drugs used in acquaintance rape. J Am Pharm Assoc 39:519–525, 1999.
10. U.S. Department of Justice: Memo to Rape Crisis Professionals, Healthcare Providers, Law Enforcement Personnel. Washington, DC, Narcotic and Dangerous Drug Section, Criminal Division, U.S. Department of Justice, 1999.

VIII. Metals

38. ARSENIC

Shahrzad Rafiee, M.D., and Timothy Erickson, M.D.

1. What is arsenic and where is it found?

Arsenic, the 33rd element on the periodic chart, occurs in organic (arsine) and inorganic (arsenites, arsenates, and elemental arsenic) forms. It is found in:

- **Rocks and soils.** Most arsenic in the terrestrial environment is found in rocks and soils. Arsenic in the surface and ground water is mostly a mixture of arsenite and arsenate.
- **Foods.** Arsenic is widely distributed in seafood (especially shellfish).
- **Human sources.** Combustion of coal, nonferrous metal smelting, and burning of agricultural wastes produce arsenic.
- **Industry.** Herbicides, fungicides, wood preservatives, desiccants, cattle and sheep dips, and dyestuffs all contain arsenic. Arsenic is also used in glass and ceramics as a metal alloy and in semiconductors and other electronic devices.

2. Extra credit: This poison, which was popular throughout Europe in the 1400s, was made by feeding arsenic to toads then distilling the juices from their dead bodies. By what name was this poison known to the people of the day?

Venin de crapaud.

3. An 80-year-old man consumes a delicious, large seafood meal the night before obtaining his yearly physical. The lab discovers a large amount of arsenic in his urine. Was his 25-year-old wife trying to murder him?

Not necessarily. Arsenic is widely distributed in food, particularly seafood. New diagnostic urine tests have been developed that distinguish the toxic inorganic forms of arsenic from the nontoxic organic arsenic found in shellfish.

4. Are there any medical uses for arsenic?

Medical uses of arsenic date back to ancient Greek and Roman times. Hippocrates prescribed a paste containing arsenic for treating ulcers. In the 1800s, a solution containing arsenite (Fowler's solution, 1% arsenite) was used to treat leukemia, psoriasis, and asthma. Fowler's solution was not withdrawn from the U.S. market until the 1950s. More than 1000 arsenic-containing compounds were produced by Erlich & Bertheim for the treatment of syphilis. Currently, the arsenic-containing drug Mel B is a treatment option for African trypanosomiasis at the meningoencephalitic stage.

5. Does arsenic have a criminal history?

Because it is tasteless and resembles sugar, arsenic has been used as an assassination tool and homicidal agent.

6. Extra credit: What 1944 movie starring Cary Grant portrayed two little old ladies who "euthanized" people with arsenic?

Arsenic and Old Lace.

7. Name the routes of exposure to arsenic.
Ingestion
Inhalation
Through the skin

8. What is the pathophysiology of arsenic toxicity?
Arsenic distributes rapidly to erythrocytes and binds to the globin portion of hemoglobin. Redistribution occurs within 24 hours to the liver, spleen, kidneys, and gastrointestinal tract. Arsenic impairs cellular respiration by inhibiting mitochondrial enzymes and uncoupling oxidative phosphorylation. Arsenic also acts on the Kreb's cycle by blocking pyruvate dehydrogenase.

9. Describe the symptoms of clinical toxicity.
Symptoms appear within 30 minutes of absorption. However, they may be delayed if the arsenic was ingested with food. Presenting symptoms are nonspecific and include headache, weakness, nausea, vomiting, and colicky abdominal pain. Hypotension and tachycardia are also common early signs. Diarrhea of arsenic poisoning is described as "rice-water" or "cholera-like" stools. Torsades de pointes has been reported in arsenic toxicity. Of the more specific physical findings, a garlic odor has been reported on the breath of individuals. Within a few hours, dark urine may be seen. Jaundice ensues in 1–2 days.
- **Central nervous system** (CNS). Symptoms include delirium, seizure, coma, and death. Arsenic also causes cortical atrophy resulting in encephalopathy.
- **Parasympathetic nervous system**. Peripheral neuropathy may appear 1–2 weeks after exposure. It mostly affects the lower extremities.
- **Cardiovascular**. A variety of electrocardiogram (ECG) changes occur, including conduction blocks, QT interval prolongation, and T wave changes. Myocarditis and pericarditis have been reported in chronic arsenic poisoning. Arsenic also causes a dilation of blood vessels and endothelial damage, resulting in hypotension and third spacing of fluids. This results in progressive hemodynamic compromise and shock.
- **Pulmonary**. Pulmonary edema, acute respiratory distress syndrome (ARDS), and respiratory failure from muscle weakness occur in conjunction with acute arsenic toxicity.
- **Gastrointestinal**. Dehydration, thirst, and corrosion of mucous membranes result in hemorrhagic gastritis. A toxic hepatitis may also occur.
- **Hematopoietic**. Hemolysis occurs after acute poisoning. Pancytopenia may result, and an absolute eosinophilia may manifest.
- **Dermatologic**. Cutaneous signs occur after systemic exposure. Erythema followed by hyperpigmentation, hyperkeratosis, brawny desquamation, and exfoliative dermatitis ensues. The hyperpigmentation is most pronounced on the eyelids, temples, neck, axilla, nipples, and groin.

10. A patient presents with abdominal pain, hematuria, and jaundice along with diminished mental status after exposure to an unknown gas. What is your diagnosis?
The triad of abdominal pain, hematuria, and jaundice are characteristics of arsine gas poisoning. Arsine toxicity occurs when arsenic-containing solutions are exposed to metals. An example is a drain-cleaning agent (containing acid and releasing hydrogen) that is placed in a container previously filled with arsenical pesticides. Arsine localizes to erythrocytes and leads to rapid, severe hemolysis, renal failure, and death. Arsine gas is a colorless, extremely toxic gas with a garlic-like odor.

11. What are Mees' lines?
These white lines on the fingernails are suggestive of nail growth arrest from chronic arsenic poisoning.

12. What studies should be obtained when considering the diagnosis of arsenic poisoning?

Blood and urine arsenic levels should be measured. Normal blood arsenic levels are < 7 μg/dl. The ideal urine test is a 24-hour urine collection. Kidney-ureter-bladder (KUB) x-ray should be obtained if radiopaque arsenic is ingested.

13. *Extra credit:* In the Reinsch test for arsenic, what common nonmetallic chemical compound can result in a false-positive test by plating out on the copper?

Sulfide.

14. Which treatment modalities are used for arsenic poisoning?

Lavage should be considered if a recent life-threatening ingestion has occurred. Activated charcoal does not significantly adsorb arsenic. Assessment and correction of intravascular volume depletion are important. Urine should be alkalinized to maintain a pH of 7 to prevent red cell breakdown products in renal tubules. If radiopaque chips are seen on KUB, whole bowel irrigation may be instituted.

Chelating agents such as British antilewisite (BAL) bind to and enhance urinary excretion of toxic metals. D-penicillamine is also used. Recent studies indicate that DMSA (succimer) is more effective than BAL, as it is for lead and mercury poisoning.

15. When are chelating agents indicated?

In symptomatic patients and those with urine arsenic levels > 200 μg/L. If renal failure occurs or exists, hemodialysis should be considered along with chelation therapy.

16. Why is BAL always given by intramuscular (IM) injection?

BAL is reconstituted in peanut oil so it cannot be given intravenously. In patients with allergies to peanuts, BAL administration is contraindicated.

17. What is lewisite?

Lewisite is an arsenic-containing vesicant gas that was used in World War I. During World War II, the continued threat of lewisite prompted researchers to develop the antidote, BAL. At the time, it was more useful topically than systemically.

18. What is blackfoot disease?

Dry gangrene of the lower extremities from atherosclerosis. This unique peripheral artery disease occurs primarily in the endemic area of chronic arsenicism on the southwest coast of Taiwan. Humic acid in well water may be the main cause of the disease.

BIBLIOGRAPHY

1. Agency for Toxic Substances and Disease Registry (ATSDR): Toxicological Profile for Arsenic (Update). Washington, DC, U.S. Public Health Service, 1998.
2. Chen CJ: Blackfoot disease. Lancet 336(8712):442, 1990.
3. DiNapoli J, Hall AH, Drake R, Rumack BH: Cyanide and arsenic poisoning by intravenous injection. Ann Emerg Med 18:308–311, 1989.
4. Ford MD: Arsenic. In Goldfrank LR, Flomenbaum NE, Lewin NA, et al (eds): Goldfrank's Toxicologic Emergencies, 6th ed. Stamford, CT, Appleton & Lange, 1998, pp 1261–1273.
5. Goyer RA: Toxic effects of metals. In Klaassen CD (ed): Toxicology: The Basic Science of Poisons, 5th ed. New York, McGraw-Hill, 1996, pp 691–736.
6. Graeme K, Pollack C: Heavy metal toxicity. Part I: Arsenic and mercury. J Emerg Med 16:45–46, 1998.
7. Lee DC, Roberts JR, Kelly JJ, et al: Whole-bowel irrigation as an adjunct in the treatment of radiopaque arsenic [letter]. Am J Emerg Med 13:244–245, 1995.
8. Mukter H, Bernhard L, Reichl FX, et al: Are we ready to replace dimercaprol (BAL) as an arsenic antidote? Hum Exp Toxicol 16:460–465, 1997.

39. LEAD

Michael Wahl, M.D., and Rotem Friede, M.D.

1. Where does the word *plumbing* come from?

It is derived from *plumbum*, the Latin word for lead, which used to line water conduits in ancient Rome. Many authors feel that the fall of the Roman empire can be traced to endemic lead poisoning. In addition to lead plumbing, the Romans used lead cooking utensils, drinking vessels, and wine vessels. The lead from the dinnerware would leach into food and drinks and be consumed by the Romans.

2. *Extra credit:* When tin and lead are mixed, a metal is formed that was widely used in colonial days to make dinnerware. What was this potentially toxic substance called?

Pewter.

3. When should lead poisoning be suspected?

Lead poisoning should be considered in any illness with gastrointestinal (GI), neuromuscular, and central nervous system manifestations, particularly in children.

4. What cognitive deficits are seen with chronic lead exposure in children?

- Decreased intelligence
- Behavioral and learning disorders
- Deficits of verbal abstraction, perceptual integration, and visuomotor function

5. What are the major routes of lead entry into the body?

- GI tract (ingestion)
- Lungs (inhalation)
- Dermal absorption—insignificant except in the case of organic lead

6. Once lead is absorbed, how is it distributed within the body?

Lead is distributed in a three-compartment model:

1. Lead is circulated initially in blood, with 95% of circulating lead attached to red blood cells.

2. It is then distributed to the soft tissues including kidneys, bone marrow, nervous tissue, and liver. Lead in the soft tissues causes the majority of symptoms and toxicities. The nervous system and the kidneys are the prime targets.

3. Lastly, lead is distributed to bone, where it is incorporated into the hydroxyapatite lattice.

7. Who is at greatest risk of lead poisoning?

1. Children. The greatest incidence of poisoning occurs in young, malnourished children who live in substandard housing with deteriorating lead paint.

2. Adults who work in occupations such as battery manufacturing, firing range clean up, radiator repair, lead smelting, construction, and demolition.

8. When is lead-based paint a possible hazard?

In any house built before 1977, because with was probably painted with lead-based paint. Usually the paint is chipping, peeling, or flaking and is readily accessible for ingestion. If it is chalking, it also can create dust, which can be inhaled. In older homes that are undergoing renovation, lead paint ingestion and inhalation can be a significant hazard in socioeconomic groups not typically associated with lead toxicity. Ingestion of lead-based pottery glaze is a recognized hazard among demented nursing home patients who are enrolled in occupational or physical therapy programs that involve pottery glazing.

9. What ethnic remedies contain high concentrations of lead?

ETHNIC GROUP	REMEDY NAME	PURPOSE
Mexican American	Arzacon (also called rueda, coral, Maria Luisa, alacaron, and liga) Greta	Both compounds are used for *empacho* (intestinal illness) and can be close to 100% lead
Southeast Asian	Pay-loo-ah (also called pelua or pejluam)	Used for rashes and fever
Indian	Ghasard	A powder used to aid digestion
	Kandu	A red powder used to aid digestion
	Bali goli	A black bean dissolved in a special solution to treat stomach aches
	Surma	A powder used as make-up but also used to treat skin infections topically
Chinese	Clamshell powder (poying tan, mai ge fen)	

10. Can gunshot wounds cause elevated lead levels?

Yes, if the bullets are retained. Lead absorption seems to occur most efficiently from pleural and synovial contact, whereas lead absorption from fat and muscle appears to be poorly absorbed. Thus, bullets in joint spaces should be removed, but bullets retained in fat or muscle can be left in place.

11. Where is lead stored in the body? How might this lead to symptoms of poisoning?

Ninety-five percent of lead in adults is stored in the bone versus 70% in children. In adults with prolonged immobilization, there is increased bone resorption where the lead is mobilized, and this may lead to significant increases in blood lead levels.

12. What are the signs, symptoms, and diagnostic evidence for acute lead poisoning?
- Signs and symptoms—anorexia, constipation, abdominal pain, behavioral changes, vomiting, hyperactivity, lethargy, fatigue, ataxia, seizures, and coma
- Laboratory results—basophilic stippling, anemia, increased urinary corporphyrins, and hemolysis
- Abdominal radiographs may show opacities
- Diagnostically, blood lead levels > 60 μg/dl correspond with acute poisoning

13. What are the signs, symptoms, and diagnostic evidence of chronic lead poisoning?

Signs and symptoms include vague aches and pains, nephritis, and peripheral neuropathy. Laboratory values may show anemia, basophilic stippling, and increased urinary aminolevulinic acid (ALA). Lead lines may be evident on radiographs. Diagnostically, blood lead levels in the range of 30–60 μg/dl along with these symptoms may indicate chronic lead poisoning.

14. Where does lead interfere in heme synthesis?

Lead blocks the action of ALA synthetase, delta-aminolevulinic dehydratase, coproporphyrinogen decarboxylase, and ferrolcheletase. Delta-ALA and coproporphyrin accumulate in the urine where they serve as markers for lead intoxication. Lead inhibits the transport of iron across mitochondrial membranes in maturing normoblasts, leading to the accumulation of protoporphyrin. Lead also causes increased fragility and decreased red cell survival because of a direct effect on the red cell membrane.

15. What classic finding on microscopic exam of hematology slides is indicative of lead poisoning?

Basophilic stippling. It is caused by the inhibition of 5'-pyrimidine nucleotidase, which impairs the cell's ability to get rid of RNA degradation products, and by the aggregation of ribosomes onto the red cell membrane.

16. What are the lead lines observed on x-rays?

In bone, lead triggers hypermineralization. The lead lines are areas of arrested bone growth, and the thickness of the lines depicts duration of lead exposure. Lead is drawn to those areas of bone that are growing rapidly, such as the femur, tibia, and radius. Lead lines are not direct lead deposits on the bone.

17. True or false: The reduction in blood lead levels seen in the United States is the result of extensive screening.

False. It has resulted from the removal of the most important sources of environmental lead such as leaded gasoline and lead abatement of contaminated homes.

18. How does the Centers for Disease Control and Prevention (CDC) define childhood lead poisoning?

A blood level of 10 μg/dl. Other laboratory tests such as erythrocyte protoporphyrin (EP) and zinc protoporphyrin (ZPP) are not necessary for the definition of childhood lead poisoning and are no longer recommended. EP and ZPP are used in the evaluation of chronic adult exposures.

19. According to the CDC, what questions should be asked to determine risk of lead poisoning in children?

1. Does the child live in or regularly visit a home built before 1950?
2. Does the child live in or regularly visit a home built before 1978 that is undergoing renovation or remodeling?
3. Specific exposure questions:
   • Does the child have a personal or family history of lead poisoning?
   • Is the child exposed to lead through occupational, industrial, or hobby sources?
   • Does the child live in close proximity to a major highway?
   • Does the child regularly consume hot tap water?
   • Does the child have a history of iron deficiency or pica (e.g., eating paint chips or dirt)?
   • Has the child been exposed to lead through cultural sources (e.g., home remedies, cosmetics, ceramic food containers)?
   • Are the child's parents migrant farm workers?
   • Do the child's parents receive poverty assistance?

20. What does screening for lead poisoning require?

1. Determine the child's risk for high-dose lead exposure. Consider the answers to the CDC's questionnaire in question 19 above and whether or not the child lives in a high-risk community. A community is considered high risk if 12% of the children who live there have elevated blood lead levels *or* if 27% of the homes in the neighborhood were built before 1950.
2. Measure blood lead levels in children who are at high risk for lead exposure.
3. Measure blood lead levels in children who are at low risk for lead poisoning (those who have a positive result on the questionnaire but who do not live in a high-risk area) in selected cases.
4. Conduct necessary follow-up lead history.

21. How can one find out if the patient lives in a high-risk area?

Lead poisoning is a reportable disease. The state department of public health collects the data and categorizes which areas are at high risk, usually by zip code.

22. What are the recommended actions for elevated lead levels in the pediatric population?

BLOOD LEAD LEVEL	RECOMMENDED ACTION
< 9	Retest in 1 year
10–14	Retest in 3–6 months; education
15–19	Retest in 2 months—if level is measured at 15–19 µg/dl twice, refer for case management; education
20–44	Clinical evaluation, education, environmental investigation, follow-up test in 1 week
45–69	Clinical evaluation, education, environmental investigation, chelation
70	Hospitalization, chelation therapy, education, environmental investigation

23. Describe the commonly used chelating agents for elevated lead levels.

1. **BAL (dimercaprol).** BAL chelates lead both intra- and extra-cellularly. Two molecules of BAL combine with one atom of lead to form a complex that is excreted in the bile and urine. In the presence of renal impairment, BAL was once the chelator of choice because its main route of excretion is in the bile. BAL is administered intramuscularly no more than once every 4 hours. It cannot be given to patients who are allergic to peanuts because it is mixed in peanut oil. Adverse reactions are mild and include painful injections, terrible sulfur odor, febrile reactions, aminotransferase elevations, nausea, vomiting, headache, conjunctivitis, lacrimation, rhinorrhea, salivation, hypertension, tachycardia, and painful sterile abscess.

2. **Calcium disodium ethylenediamine tetraacetic acid ($CaNa_2$ EDTA).** $CaNa_2$ EDTA removes lead from the extracellular compartments and increases the urinary excretion 20–50 fold. By depleting the extracellular compartment, $CaNa_2$ EDTA draws lead from the soft tissues, central nervous system (CNS), and red blood cells, reducing the lead level in these tissues. The preferred route of administration is intravenously as a continuous infusion, although it may be given intramuscularly. Infusion over 6 hours is most effective although it may be given as a slow IV push over 15–20 minutes. The course of treatment should be no longer than 5 days to allow recovery from the depletion of other metals. Repeated treatment may be given after a 2–5-day recovery period. Toxicities include acute tubular necrosis unless administered under proper conditions. Other reactions include rash, febrile reactions, fatigue, thirst, myalgia, and chills.

3. **Dimercaptosuccinic acid (DMSA or succimer).** DMSA is an orally active water-soluble chelator. DMSA may remove lead from the bone and soft tissues. It does not deplete essential metals as do BAL and $CaNa_2$ EDTA. Also, it does not increase the CNS burden of lead. Furthermore, DMSA-lead complexes can be hemodialyzed.

24. What is the role for chelating agents?

To bind inorganic lead, enhance its excretion through the GI or renal system, and, ideally, deplete soft tissues including nervous tissue of lead.

25. What are the CDC recommended guidelines for pediatric chelation therapy?

SYMPTOMS/Pb LEVELS	DOSE	REGIMEN
Encephalopathy	BAL, 450 mg/m²/day $CaNa_2$ EDTA, 1500 mg/m/day EDTA is started 4 hr after first BAL dose	75 mg/m² q 4 hr for 5 days continuous infusion *or* b.i.d.–q.i.d. for 5 days.

(Table continued on next page.)

SYMPTOMS/Pb LEVELS	DOSE	REGIMEN
Symptomatic or Pb > 70 μg/dl	BAL, 300–450 mg/m²/day CaNa₂ EDTA, 1000–1500 mg/m/day	50–75 mg/m²/day for 5 days continuous infusion *or* b.i.d./q.i.d. for 5 days EDTA is started 4 hrs after first BAL dose
Asymptomatic or Pb 45–69 μg/dl	Succimer, 700–1050 mg/m²/day, *or* EDTA, 1000 mg/m²/day	350 mg/m² t.i.d. for 5 days, then b.i.d. for 14 days continuous infusion or b.i.d.–q.i.d. for 5 days
Pb 20–44 μg/dl	Routine chelation not done Can consider succimer for 35–44 μg/dl, age < 2 yrs, rising Pb despite reduction measures	Succimer, same as above

26. What is the recommended treatment for children with acute encephalopathy from lead intoxication?

A combination of BAL at a dose of 75 mg/m² by deep intramuscular injection every 4 hours for a total daily dose of 450 mg/m². Once adequate urine output is established and 4 hours have elapsed since the first BAL dose, a continuous IV infusion of CaNa₂ EDTA is initiated at a dose of 1500 mg/m²/24 hr with maximum dose of 2000 mg/day. This combined treatment should be continued for 5 days, interrupted for 2 days, then resumed if blood lead levels are > 50 μg/dl.

27. Why is there a tendency to treat children with elevated blood lead levels more aggressively, especially those whose lead levels are in the 20–45-μg/dl range?

Evidence of the adverse effects of lead at low concentrations in children is mounting; this may be because of the child's immature blood-brain barrier. Deciding to treat or not is difficult because of the paucity of data on long-term outcome differences. There is evidence that, 1 month after chelation with DMSA, the lead level will be lower, but at 6 months, there is no difference in lead levels between placebo- and DMSA-treated children. Environmental decontamination is the most important intervention in this group.

28. What is organic lead poisoning?

It is due to exposure to tetraethyl lead (TEL), usually found in leaded gasoline. This may occur from work exposure or recreational sniffing of gasoline. Toxicity is not from TEL but from its metabolic derivatives, triethyl lead and inorganic lead. Treatment is chelation if inorganic lead levels are elevated. Otherwise, treatment entails removal from the exposure site. Inorganic lead parameters are not useful for organic lead intoxication. Symptoms are similar to the CNS manifestations of inorganic lead intoxication.

BIBLIOGRAPHY

1. Berlin CM: Lead poisoning in children. Curr Opin Pediatr 9:173–177, 1997.
2. Besunder JB, Super DM, Anderson RL: Comparison of dimercaptosuccinic acid and calcium disodium ethylenediaminetetraacetic acid versus dimercaptopropanol and ethylenediaminetetraacetic acid in children with lead poisoning. J Pediatr 130:966–971, 1997.
3. Centers for Disease Control and Prevention: Preventing Lead Poisoning in Young Children: A Statement by the Centers for Disease Control. Atlanta, CDC, 1991.
4. Committee on Drugs: Treatment guidelines for lead exposure in children. Pediatrics 96:155–160, 1995.
5. Gilfillan SC: Lead poisoning and the fall of Rome. J Occup Environ Med 7:53–60, 1965.
6. Haddad LM, Shannon MW, Winchester JF (eds): Poisoning and Drug Overdose, 3rd ed. Philadelphia, W.B. Saunders, 1997.
7. Ibels LS, Pollock CA: Lead intoxication. Med Toxicol 1:387–410, 1986.

8. Illinois Department of Public Health: Guidelines for the Detection and Management of Lead Poisoning for Physicians and Health Care Providers. Springfield, IL, Illinois Dept. of Public Health, 1996.
9. Illinois Department of Public Health: Lead Screening and Case Follow-up Guidelines for Local Health Departments. Springfield, IL, Illinois Dept. of Public Health, 1998.
10. Landrigan PJ, Todd AC: Lead poisoning. West J Med 161:153–159, 1994.
11. Lees RE, Scott GD, Miles CG: Subacute lead poisoning from retained lead shot. Can Med Assoc J 138:130–131, 1988.
12. Magos L: Lead poisoning from retained lead projectiles: A critical review of case reports. Hum Exp Toxicol 13:735–742, 1994.
13. O'Connor ME, Rich D: Children with moderately elevated lead levels: Is chelation with DMSA helpful? Clin Pediatr 38:325–331, 1999.

40. MERCURY

Michael Wahl, M.D., and Bryan Finke, M.D.

1. Where did the symbol for mercury (Hg) originate?

In A.D. 77, Pliny called mercury *hydrargyrum* ("water silver"), hence the symbol Hg. Pliny also referred to mercury intoxication as a disease of the slaves and convicts who mined it and, recognizing its respiratory hazard, advised these "workers" to cover their faces with thin bladder tissue.

2. *Extra credit:* What famous 16th century Italian sculptor and goldsmith was poisoned by fumes of mercury?

Benvenuto Cellini.

3. *Extra credit:* What great American patriot died in 1799 when, in an attempt to cure his illness, he was given a dose of mercury? (Hint: This remedy denied him his liberty and gave him death.)

Patrick Henry.

4. What are the three types of mercury exposures?

1. Elemental
2. Organic
3. Inorganic

5. Describe the main route of absorption and toxicity of elemental mercury.

Inhalation is the main route of absorption. Elemental mercury, also called quicksilver, is the only elemental metal that is a liquid at room temperature. Spilled mercury vaporizes readily and can be inhaled, where it is rapidly absorbed in the lungs. Once in the bloodstream, it distributes to all tissues and crosses the placenta and blood-brain barrier (where levels persist the longest). Acute exposure to high levels of mercury vapor can cause symptoms similar to those of metal fume fever, such as fever, chills, dyspnea, and a metallic taste in the mouth. High-level acute exposures or chronic exposure can cause a classic triad of tremor, gingivitis, and erethism. Erethism is a symptom complex that includes insomnia, pathologic shyness, memory loss, emotional lability, and depression. Elemental mercury is poorly absorbed in the gastrointestinal (GI) tract, and toxicity is rare. Nearly all ingested elemental mercury (most commonly from mercury thermometers) is excreted unchanged in the feces. Ingestion of metallic mercury is not usually a health hazard.

6. What is the main route of absorption and toxicity of organic mercury?

Ingestion is the main route of absorption of organic mercury. The largest outbreaks are linked to ingestion of organic mercurials used as fungicides and seed dressing or the consumption of shellfish and fish with high levels of organic mercury. Marine animals convert elemental mercury to organic mercury, which builds up in the tissues. The most notable example of this occurred in Minimata, Japan, in the 1940s. A vinyl chloride plant contaminated Minimata Bay with mercury for over a decade. The high number of children who were born with multiple birth defects prompted an investigation that revealed these birth defects were secondary to in utero organic mercury poisoning. In another example, over 6000 Iraqis in 1971 were exposed to methylmercury from the ingestion of bread that was made from seed treated with an organic mercurial. This seed was intended for planting only. The main toxicity consisted of neurologic symptoms, including visual field defects, hearing loss, tremor, dysarthria, mental deterioration, and death.

7. What are the main routes of absorption and toxicity of inorganic mercury?

Ingestion and dermal contamination are the main routes of absorption of inorganic mercury. Inorganic mercury is also referred to as mercury salts, which are rapidly absorbed from the GI tract. This form of mercury can be corrosive to mucosal membranes. Other than direct effects on the GI tract and mucosa, the main toxicities are neurologic and renal toxicity. Neurologic effects include tremor, nervousness, anxiety, insomnia, and personality changes. The main renal effect from ingestion of mercurial salts is acute tubular necrosis, which occurs 1 day to 2 weeks after ingestion. The lethal dose is estimated to be between 1 and 3 gm.

8. What is acrodynia?

Also known as pink disease, acrodynia is a rare, idiosyncratic reaction resulting from chronic mercury exposure. It is well described as occurring after chronic exposure to the calomel (inorganic mercury)-containing creams that were used in the pediatric population in the 1950s. Acrodynia manifests as color changes in the tips of fingers, toes, wrists, and ankles caused by mercury contamination. It has also been described with chronic inhalation exposure to elemental mercury. Acrodynia predominantly occurs in children.

9. What ophthalmologic complications are a result of mercury poisoning?

Believed to be a result of direct deposits of mercury, the anterior capsule of the eye is affected, and brown-yellow discoloration of the lens can be seen. It is an indication of exposure but not of toxicity.

10. Where does the expression "mad as a hatter" originate?

Danbury, Connecticut, was the center of the felt hat industry in the 19th century. The felting process for hats required the use of mercuric nitrate to straighten animal hair, and workers commonly absorbed toxic doses of inorganic mercury salts through the skin. People who developed the resultant psychosis were often described as "chattering away to himself like a mad hatter."

11. What laboratory testing is useful in mercury toxicity?

Screening tests, including 24-hour urine collection, electrolytes, blood urea nitrogen (BUN), creatinine, and urinalysis, are all indicated. Blood levels are useful in determining the extent of the overdose. A normal blood mercury level is < 10 gm/L.

12. List the specific antidotes for mercury poisoning.

- Elemental mercury. Oral DMSA (succimer), a chelating agent enhances renal excretion (within 2 hours).
- Inorganic salts. Immediate intramuscular administration of British anitlewisite (BAL) may prevent renal toxicity. Do not wait for confirmation blood testing!
- Organic mercury. Data suggest that oral DMSA decreases central nervous system toxicity.

Summary Table

TYPE OF MERCURY	ROUTE OF EXPOSURE	TARGET ORGAN/EFFECTS	TREATMENT
Elemental	Inhalation	CNS, lung, skin	Succimer
Organic	Oral ingestion	CNS, fetus	Succimer
Inorganic	Oral ingestion	GI, mucosa, renal, dermal	BAL, succimer

BIBLIOGRAPHY

1. Centers for Disease Control and Prevention: Mercury poisoning associated with beauty cream: Arizona, California, New Mexico, and Texas, 1996. MMWR 45:633–635, 1996.
2. Clarkson TW, Amin-Zaki L, Al-Tikriti SK: An outbreak of methylmercury poisoning due to consumption of contaminated grain. Fed Proc 35:2395–2399, 1976.
3. Gerstner HB, Huff JE: Clinical toxicology of mercury. J Toxicol Environ Health 2:491–526, 1977.

4. Goldfrank LR, Flomenbaum NE, Lewin NA, et al (eds): Toxicologic Emergencies, 6th ed. Stamford, CT, Appleton & Lange, 1998.
5. Grant K, et al: Toxicology of the Eye, 3rd ed. Springfield, IL, Charles C. Thomas, 1986.
6. Harada M: Minimata disease: Methylmercury poisoning in Japan caused by environmental pollution. Crit Rev Toxicol 25:1–24, 1995.
7. Sunderman FW: Perils of mercury. Ann Clin Lab Sci 18:89–101, 1988.
8. United States Department of Health and Human Services: Toxicologic Profile for Mercury (Update). Agency for Toxic Substances and Disease Registry. Washington, DC, USDHHS, 1994.

41. IRON

Andrea G. Carlson, M.D., and Jean L. Martinucci, M.D.

1. *Extra credit:* **Greek physicians used to give their pale, anemic patients water containing soluble iron compounds. What was their source of the iron?**

They used water in which old swords were allowed to rust.

2. How common is iron overdose?

Exposure to iron remains a common occurrence. The American Association of Poison Control Centers (AAPCC) reported 29,612 exposures to iron-containing preparations in 1998. Unintentional pediatric ingestions comprised the vast majority of reports; 80% of exposures involved children < age 6, and 94% of ingestions were considered to be unintentional. Because unintentional pediatric ingestions typically involve modest amounts, most exposures result in little or no toxicity. Thus, despite its toxic potential, death and serious morbidity from iron is uncommon.

3. What is the toxic dose of iron?

Ingestions of less than 40 mg/kg of elemental iron are generally not expected to result in serious toxicity. For this reason, many poison centers use this dose as the triage threshold for medical referral. However, adverse effects, such as nausea and diarrhea, have been reported from ingestion of supratherapeutic doses of iron as low as 10 mg/kg in adult volunteer studies.

4. Is the amount of elemental iron the same in all iron preparations?

No. Many different iron preparations are commercially available, with variable amounts of elemental iron. The three most common preparations are ferrous gluconate, sulfate, and fumarate with 12%, 20%, and 33% elemental iron by weight, respectively.

5. *Extra credit:* **What does FSG359 mean?**

This mnemonic is used to calculate the amount of elemental iron in the common salts: fumarate (33% or 1/3), sulfate (20% or 1/5), and gluconate (12% or 1/9).]

6. How many chewable vitamins would a 15-kg, 3-year-old child have to ingest to develop any symptoms of toxicity?

Minor symptoms of iron toxicity have been reported in children at doses as low as 20 mg/kg of elemental iron. Children's chewable vitamins contain up to 15 mg of elemental iron per tablet. So this child would have to ingest at least 20 tablets to reach a total dose of 300 mg, or 20 mg/kg.

7. A 17-year-old presents to the emergency department (ED) 6 hours after she took a bottle of iron tablets from her parent's bathroom cabinet. She tells you that she had abdominal pain, nausea, vomiting, and diarrhea, but she feels better now. What do you do next?

While this patient's clinical picture may suggest resolving symptoms from minor iron toxicity, she may also be on her way to real trouble. This patient may be in the "smoldering" phase (phase 2) of iron overdose, so be careful! The list below summarizes the phases of iron toxicity.

Phase 1 (0–12 hrs). Direct corrosive effects of iron result in gastrointestinal (GI) mucosal injury. Severe GI necrosis with frank hemorrhage may occur. Symptoms include vomiting, hematemesis, abdominal pain, diarrhea, hematochezia, and lethargy. Shock due to blood or fluid loss leads to hypoperfusion, which may contribute to the development of metabolic acidosis. Direct inhibition of prothrombin by iron can produce early coagulopathy in the absence of liver abnormalities.

Phase 2 (6–24 hrs). While resolution of the patient's GI symptoms may seem to indicate recovery, this phase actually represents ongoing progression of toxicity, as patients continue to

165

absorb significant amounts of iron from the intestine. Despite being known as the "quiescent" phase of iron toxicity, close evaluation during this time rarely reveals an entirely normal patient. Signs of hypovolemia and lethargy frequently remain, as does the presence of metabolic acidosis. Continued observation and treatment are indicated.

Phase 3 (6–48 hrs). Dramatic multiple organ system insult characterizes this stage of toxicity. Central nervous system effects range from coma to seizures. Cardiac depression contributes to profound shock, with worsening metabolic acidosis. Both renal and hepatic failure may occur from direct cytotoxic effects of iron. Although death may occur during any phase of iron poisoning, the potential for mortality is greatest at this time. Aggressive intervention, with hemodynamic support and antidotal therapy, is essential.

Phase 4 (2–4 days). Fulminant liver failure may occur during this stage, most likely from a direct action of iron on mitochondria as it is taken up by the reticuloendothelial system of the liver.

Phase 5 (several weeks). GI obstruction secondary to gastric or pyloric scarring may occur. This phase is rare.

8. Is a serum iron concentration helpful in the management of iron overdose?

Yes, to a degree. Serum iron concentrations are routinely drawn in an effort to determine toxicity and the need for treatment. Normal serum iron concentrations range from 50 to 150 µg/dl. Levels over 350 µg/dl are usually associated with signs of toxicity. In the past, intervention was recommended if the serum iron concentration exceeded this level. Studies since then suggest that conservative management may be appropriate for levels below 500 µg/dl. Significant toxicity frequently accompanies iron concentrations between 500 and 1000 µg/dl. Levels over 1000 µg/dl are associated with considerable morbidity.

Although an elevated serum iron concentration can support the need for intervention, a normal level does not reliably exclude the possibility of serious poisoning. Significant clinical signs of toxicity have been seen in patients with levels below 350 µg/dl. Variability in time to peak iron concentration between different preparations may also limit the usefulness of this diagnostic test, as peak levels may be missed. Interpretation of the serum iron level must always be done in the context of the patient's overall clinical picture.

9. Does the patient's serum total iron-binding capacity (TIBC) help to guide management in suspected overdose?

No. The TIBC, a measurement that quantifies the amount of iron that can be bound by transferrin in a particular volume of serum, was previously considered an essential diagnostic component of iron poisoning management. Clinicians believed that a serum iron concentration below the TIBC indicated available binding sites with negligible levels of circulating free iron, suggesting a low potential for toxicity. However, further clinical experience using this diagnostic test has revealed a host of limitations to its utility. As a result of laboratory phenomena, the TIBC is falsely elevated in the presence of high serum iron or deferoxamine. Numerous case reports demonstrate toxicity in patients whose serum iron concentrations do not exceed their TIBCs. Furthermore, reviews of acutely iron-poisoned patients have revealed that up to 40% of those with serum iron concentrations that *do* exceed the TIBC do not display any signs of toxicity. Consequently, the TIBC is neither sensitive nor specific as a marker for iron toxicity and should not be used to guide management.

10. What other laboratory findings may be seen in iron overdose?

Hyperglycemia and leukocytosis are classically observed in iron overdose. However, clinical reviews of patients with acute iron poisoning suggest that neither of these findings serve as sensitive indicators of toxicity, because both elevated iron levels and significant clinical signs of poisoning have been observed in the absence of either abnormality. An elevated anion gap metabolic acidosis, primarily due to lactic acidosis, may also be seen as may anemia from GI hemorrhage. Overall, any laboratory finding should be considered only an adjunct to the patient's clinical features of toxicity.

11. Discuss the mechanisms by which iron poisoning causes an elevated anion gap metabolic acidosis.

Four mechanisms have been proposed. First, conversion of ferrous iron (Fe^{2+}) to ferric iron (Fe^{3+}) liberates an unbuffered proton. Additionally, iron acts as a vasodilator. The hypotension that results compromises tissue perfusion, leading to lactic acidosis. The direct negative inotropic effect of iron on the heart further worsens the lactic acidosis from shock. Finally, iron acts as a cellular poison, disrupting oxidative phosphorylation. The cell becomes dependent on anaerobic metabolism, resulting in even more lactic acid production.

12. Can a negative abdominal radiograph (KUB) rule out iron poisoning?

No. Although iron is radiopaque, the absence of any opacities on an abdominal radiograph does not rule out ingestion or toxicity. Even pure iron tablets may not be visible if sufficient time has passed to allow for dissolution. The type of iron preparation is also a factor that determines its radiopacity. For example, a clinical series involving ingestion of chewable vitamins revealed that a positive KUB was obtained in 1 patient out of 30. Liquid preparations and multivitamin supplements are also not always visible on radiographs. Thus, while presence of pills on KUB may confirm a suspected ingestion and guide decontamination, their absence does not reliably exclude iron poisoning.

13. What methods of decontamination are effective?

Neither ipecac-induced emesis nor gastric lavage has been shown to remove significant amounts of iron from the stomach in overdose. Use of ipecac can also cloud the patient's clinical picture, because it will be difficult to determine whether the patient is vomiting from ipecac or from toxic effects of iron. Specialized lavage solutions, including sodium bicarbonate or phosphate, have been tried in an attempt to decrease iron's solubility and absorption. Their effectiveness has not been demonstrated, and their use may lead to significant electrolyte disturbances. The use of magnesium hydroxide to bind iron to insoluble ferric hydroxide may be effective, but large doses may result in hypermagnesemia. Activated charcoal does not adsorb iron. The use of whole bowel irrigation (WBI) has been reported with successful decontamination in a number of cases. Its use should especially be considered when visible opacities are present on KUB. Surgical removal of tablets via gastrotomy has been reported.

14. What is the antidote for iron poisoning? How does it work?

Deferoxamine (DFO) is a natural byproduct of the bacteria *Streptomyces pilosus*. DFO chelates iron, facilitating this nutrient's uptake into the bacterial cell. Clinically, DFO is used to chelate the iron that is present in toxic amounts. DFO potently binds free iron to form ferrioxamine. DFO can also remove iron bound to transferrin and in transit between transferrin and ferritin. DFO readily crosses cell membranes, removing iron from the cytoplasm and mitochondria.

15. What are indications for DFO therapy?

Because iron poisoning is a clinical diagnosis, the presence of symptoms suggestive of significant toxicity is the strongest indication for DFO administration. Additionally, support exists for treating patients with serum iron concentrations greater than 500 mg/dl with DFO.

16. What is the correct dose of DFO?

At this time, no one really knows. The manufacturer of DFO recommends an initial infusion of 15 mg/kg/hr, with a maximum daily dose of 6 gm, regardless of patient weight. Interestingly, this daily limit appears to have been established somewhat arbitrarily, with little clinical evidence to support it. In practice, actual daily doses often exceed the 6-gm limit without ill effect.

17. If the goal of DFO therapy is to chelate all of the iron, why isn't the dose of DFO determined by the amount of iron ingested?

DFO doesn't chelate all of the iron. In fact, the amount of elemental iron chelated by DFO is quite modest, only 9.35 mg of iron for every 100 mg of DFO. Administration of the manufacturer's

6-gm maximum daily dose results in chelation of only 56 mg of elemental iron, just over the amount present in one ferrous gluconate tablet. The discrepancy between the amount of iron ingested and the amount effectively chelated raises questions regarding the mechanism of DFO's effect, as well as its true clinical utility.

Several theories have been offered to account for this disparity. The bioavailability of iron is relatively low, so that much of the ingested dose is never absorbed. Furthermore, the majority of the iron that is absorbed becomes incorporated into various storage depots, including transferrin and ferritin, and does not exert any toxic effect. Most likely, very little free iron is ultimately present in the systemic circulation. Chelation of this unbound fraction, to which iron toxicity is attributed, may not require large doses of DFO.

18. Explain the risks associated with DFO use.

Acute renal failure following DFO administration has been reported, particularly in patients with decreased intravascular volume from GI losses or shock. Hypotension may also occur with intravenous DFO, especially if volume contraction persists due to inadequate fluid resuscitation. Higher rates of infusion are associated with a greater risk for hypotension. Aggressive volume therapy combined with lower initial infusion rates may avoid these complications.

Substantial emphasis has been placed on the association between DFO infusion and the development of pulmonary toxicity, particularly the adult respiratory distress syndrome (ARDS). The mechanism by which this occurs is unclear but may involve the generation of free radicals during DFO therapy. Because ARDS tends to occur with prolonged infusions (> 24 hrs), use of higher initial doses of DFO with a shorter duration of infusion is becoming the preferred approach.

19. Which bacterial infection has been associated with DFO use?

Septicemia from *Yersinia enterocolitica* has been reported in patients following DFO therapy for iron toxicity. Ironically, it is the treatment of iron poisoning that predisposes to this complication. The uptake of iron, an essential growth factor, by *Yersinia* requires the presence of a siderophore (a compound that chelates iron and promotes its transport as a soluble complex). *Yersinia* lacks the ability to produce this necessary siderophore. DFO is a siderophore that is used clinically for its ability to chelate iron. Once DFO has been administered and the iron-DFO complex has formed, iron can be taken up by *Yersinia* and used for growth.

20. What is "vin rose" urine?

Rusty-red colored urine following treatment with DFO is classically referred to as the vin rose ("blush wine") urine change. This color change is due to the presence of ferrioxamine, the product of iron chelation with DFO. Previously, the absence of this color change following a DFO challenge was believed to exclude significant toxicity. However, numerous case reports of patients with negative DFO challenge tests despite known toxic serum iron concentrations disprove the clinical value of this maneuver. Thus, a lack of urine color change after initiating DFO does not obviate the need for continued antidotal treatment.

21. What is the end point for deferoxamine therapy?

Despite efforts to identify a simple, objective end point for chelation therapy, the decision to discontinue DFO remains one based largely on clinical parameters. Resolution of symptoms of toxicity, combined with normalization of the anion gap and clearing of acidosis, is the most widely accepted end point for DFO therapy.

22. Is DFO safe in pregnancy?

Yes. Animal studies have shown that while neither iron nor DFO concentrates in the fetal tissues, the fetus suffers significantly from the hemodynamic compromise that exists in the iron-poisoned mother. In addition to the overall higher risk for mortality seen in phase 3 of iron poisoning, pregnant patients at this stage are more likely to abort or deliver preterm. All known literature advocates aggressive treatment, because pregnant mothers and fetuses are far more likely to suffer from the effects of iron poisoning than from the risks of DFO. Successful chelation with DFO, as well as decontamination with WBI, has been reported in several pregnant patients.

Knowing the correct answer to this question is important, because iron is the second most common agent of overdose in pregnant women. Delaying appropriate therapy because of concern over DFO safety can lead to substantial and unnecessary risk to both the mother and her unborn child.

23. Can DFO be administered by other routes?

Intravenous infusion remains the superior route of DFO administration. Traditionally, DFO chelation in chronic iron overload states (e.g., hemochromatosis) was performed with intramuscular injections. Research involving acute iron overdose, however, suggests that IV infusion results in an increased urinary excretion of iron.

DFO also effectively chelates iron when administered orally, but the resultant ferrioxamine is readily absorbed. Thus, the amount of iron absorbed is actually increased, leading to ferrioxamine toxicity. Deferiprone is an oral chelator used to treat chronic iron overload states. It has shown early promise in animal models of acute iron overdose but has not yet been used in humans in this setting.

24. A 3-year-old boy is brought to the ED by his mother who had found him playing on the floor with an open bottle of multivitamins. The child had been unsupervised for 15 minutes. She isn't sure how many tablets were missing. Over the next 6 hours you obtain a KUB without opacities and a normal complete blood count and serum glucose. Throughout his stay, the child remains playful and active, without vomiting. You have not yet received the child's serum iron level from the laboratory, but the mother now believes that he is "fine," and requests discharge from the ED. At what point can this child be safely discharged home?

Because this child has remained completely asymptomatic throughout an extended ED observation (6 hours), the likelihood of significant ingestion is remote. Discharge at this point is appropriate even without a serum iron level. Of note, the absence of opacities on KUB, leukocytosis, or hyperglycemia, while consistent with the overall clinical picture of a nontoxic ingestion, does not exclude toxicity with any reliability. Parental education regarding safe storage of medications in the home should be done prior to discharge.

BIBLIOGRAPHY

1. Berkovitch M, Livne A, Lushkov G, et al: The efficacy of oral deferiprone in acute iron poisoning. Am J Emerg Med 18:36–40, 2000.
2. Chyka PA, Butler AY, Holley JE: Serum iron concentrations and symptoms of acute iron poisoning in children. Pharmacotherapy 16:1053–1058, 1996.
3. Everson GW, Oudjhane K, Young LW, Krenzelok EP: Effectiveness of abdominal radiographs in visualizing chewable iron supplements following overdose. Am J Emerg Med 7:459–463, 1989.
4. Litovitz TL, Klein-Schwartz W, Caravati EM, et al: 1998 Annual report of the American Association of Poison Control Centers Toxic Exposure Surveillance System Am J Emerg Med 17:435–487, 1999.
5. Mills KC, Curry SC: Acute iron poisoning. Emerg Med Clin North Am 12:397–413, 1994.
6. Mofenson HC, Caraccio TR, Sharieff N: Iron sepsis: Yersinia enterocolitica septicemia possibly caused by an overdose of iron. N Engl J Med 316:1092–1093, 1987.
7. Palatnick W, Tenenbein M: Leukocytosis, hyperglycemia, vomiting, and positive x-rays are not indicators of severity of iron overdose in adults. Am J Emerg Med 14:454–455, 1996.
8. Perrone J: Iron. In Goldfrank LR, Flomenbaum NE, Lewin NA, et al (eds): Goldfrank's Toxicologic Emergencies, 6th ed. Stamford, CT, Appleton & Lange, 1998, pp 619–627.
9. Siff JE, Meldon SW, Tomassoni AJ: Usefulness of the total iron binding capacity in the evaluation and treatment of acute iron overdose. Ann Emerg Med 33:73–76, 1999.
10. Tenenbein M: Whole bowel irrigation in iron poisoning. J Pediatr 111:142–144, 1987.
11. Tenenbein M, Kowalski S, Sienko A, et al: Pulmonary toxic effects of continuous desferrioxamine administration in acute iron poisoning. Lancet 339:699–701, 1992.
12. Tran T, Wax JR, Philput C, et al: Intentional iron overdose in pregnancy: Management and outcome. J Emerg Med 18:225–228, 2000.

IX. Chemicals

42. HYDROCARBONS

Manish M. Patel, M.D.

1. Why should I have to learn about hydrocarbons?

Aside from being one of the most common causes of fatality from ingestion in children younger than age 5, hydrocarbons are ubiquitous products that are easily accessible and result in high morbidity when ingested or aspirated. The annual incidence of hydrocarbon exposures in the United States is approximately 65,000; 95% of these are unintentional, and about 60% involve children. Children under age 5 years also disproportionately account for 90% of the reported deaths attributed to hydrocarbon poisoning. Through education, morbidity and mortality associated with these accidents can be reduced significantly.

2. Define hydrocarbon.

Any compound primarily consisting of hydrogen and carbon molecules is classified as a hydrocarbon. For many medical professionals, hydrocarbons are a source of confusion. Many of the ingested hydrocarbon products are compounds resulting from distillation of petroleum or crude oil. Other sources of hydrocarbons, including coal, animal fats, plants, and flowers (e.g., turpentine is derived from pine oil) are organic. The different arrangements of the hydrogen and carbon molecules are responsible for their physical and chemical properties. These products can be **aliphatic**, **aromatic**, or **halogenated** but often are mixtures of over 100 different hydrocarbon compounds. Some hydrocarbons pose unique risks because they have halogen side chains (e.g., carbon tetrachloride) or other inherently toxic compounds, such as heavy metals and insecticides.

3. What common products contain hydrocarbons?

The most common hydrocarbon product exposures reported to poison control centers are gasoline (33%), freon and propellants (11%), mineral spirits or paint thinner (9%), lubricating and motor oils (7%), lighter fluid or naphtha (7%), and kerosene (5%). The table lists common household products containing hydrocarbons.

Household Products Containing Hydrocarbons

Adhesives (glues)	Laxatives	Paste wax
Baby oil	Lighter fluid	Petroleum jelly
Car wax	Liquid solder	Pine oil
Cod liver oil	Liquid steel	Plastic cement
Contact cement	Mineral oil	Solvents
Furniture polish*	Mineral seal oil*	Stain remover
Furniture refinisher	Mineral spirits	Sterno fuel
Gasoline	Mothballs	Stoddard solvent
Home heating fuel	Motor oil	Turpentine
Kerosene	Naphtha	Typewriter correction fluid
Kitchen wax	Paint remover	Varnish remover
Lacquer	Paraffin	Wax

* Products with high aspiration potential
(Adapted from Shih RD: Hydrocarbons. In Goldfrank LR, Flomenbaum NE, Lewin NA, et al (eds): Toxicologic Emergencies, 6th ed. Stamford, CT, Appleton & Lange, 1998, p 1384.)

4. What different routes of hydrocarbon exposure lead to toxicity?

Ingestion, inhalation, and dermal absorption. Typically, a patient presents after unintentional ingestion of a household compound. Inhalation abuse of volatile hydrocarbons (e.g., "huffing" or "bagging") can also result in high morbidity and mortality, but one rarely gets a chance to intervene in the acute phase of intoxication. Dermal exposure to hydrocarbons (e.g., hot tar or high-pressure gun injection injury) or occupational inhalation exposures occasionally occur but are rarely life threatening. Infrequently, one may encounter a patient who has intentionally ingested or injected a hydrocarbon in a suicide attempt.

5. After ingestion of a hydrocarbon, what are the most common clinical signs and symptoms?

For ingested hydrocarbons, the most common and worrisome symptoms involve the pulmonary, central nervous, and gastrointestinal systems.

Pulmonary. Patients can present with complaints of cough, shortness of breath, and hemoptysis. Most hydrocarbon-toxic patients, especially children, do not have complaints, and signs of respiratory distress may be subtle with slight tachypnea, nasal flaring, coughing, retractions, wheezing, or rales. In cases of severe toxicity, worsening respiratory distress, hypoxia, and occasionally even cyanosis can be seen.

Central nervous system (CNS). Patients may present with drowsiness and decreased level of consciousness. Occasional cases of seizures and coma have been reported.

Gastrointestinal. Most commonly, patients report nausea and vomiting attributed to the local irritant effects, with rare hematemesis.

Other. Mild hemolysis has been reported following hydrocarbon ingestion. Interestingly, a majority of admitted patients (> 50%) are febrile and exhibit a leukocytosis on admission, raising the controversy of administering antibiotics (see question 16).

6. Is gastrointestinal absorption of ingested hydrocarbons responsible for the pulmonary and CNS toxicity?

No. Pulmonary toxicity is a result of aspiration of ingested hydrocarbon. Pulmonary toxicity is avoided after gastric instillation of hydrocarbon compounds in animals with surgically transected and ligated esophagi. Several mechanisms contribute to end-organ damage in these cases. After initial aspiration, hydrocarbons disrupt the surfactant layer of alveoli, resulting in early bronchospasm, ventilation-perfusion mismatch, and hypoxemia. Further direct lung contact leads to capillary and alveolar damage and promotion of interstitial inflammation, alveolar edema and hemorrhage, and possibly pulmonary necrosis. The definitive mechanism of hydrocarbon-induced CNS toxicity is unknown. Animal evidence suggests that large amounts of gastrointestinal hydrocarbon absorption must occur prior to CNS symptoms, supporting the hypothesis that pulmonary toxicity and hypoxia may contribute to these symptoms.

7. What is the clinical course of patients with hydrocarbon poisoning?

After hydrocarbon ingestion, patients follow one of three routes:

1. **Asymptomatic**. Overall, a majority of patients (> 80%) will be asymptomatic after hydrocarbon ingestion and can be followed at home without examination by a health care provider. A poison control based study of 120 initially asymptomatic patients followed at home found no progression of symptoms at 18-hour telephone follow-up.

2. **Initial symptoms**. An initial episode of coughing, gagging, choking, or vomiting within 30 minutes of ingestion should raise suspicion of pulmonary aspiration even when the patient is asymptomatic upon presentation to the health care provider. Based on pediatric literature, half of these patients will have abnormal findings on chest x-ray and approximately 10–15% of patients will have progression of symptoms over the initial 6 hours after ingestion.

3. **Persistent symptoms**. Greater than 90% of patients with persistent symptoms on initial examination will remain symptomatic 6 hours after ingestion and will have abnormal findings on chest x-ray.

8. Who needs to be admitted to the hospital after hydrocarbon ingestion?

Those patients who have never developed symptoms after hydrocarbon exposure can be followed at home—with children requiring close parental observation—for at least 6 hours. All other patients with initial or persistent symptoms should be referred to the emergency department, where an initial chest x-ray should be obtained, followed by a 6-hour observation period and a repeat chest x-ray. Patients who remain symptomatic or those with an abnormal chest x-ray should be admitted. Only approximately 10–15% of all hydrocarbon ingestions reported to poison control centers require admission. A majority of these (> 90%) have no progression of their pulmonary disease and are discharged within 72 hours. A small percentage of patients will have progressively worsening respiratory distress requiring mechanical ventilation.

9. What are the radiographic findings of hydrocarbon aspiration?

Bilateral perihilar infiltrates, bibasilar infiltrates, consolidated infiltrates, and enhanced bronchovascular markings are present in the majority of patients with respiratory signs and symptoms upon presentation following hydrocarbon exposure. Although most patients have abnormal chest radiographs within 4 hours and beginning as early as 30 minutes after ingestion, a small percentage will have progressively worsening findings over 24 hours. Right-sided infiltrates are more commonly reported, but bilateral findings are often present. Clinical improvement is usually seen prior to radiographic resolution but may take several days to weeks. Most of these findings occur as a result of lung surfactant destruction by the hydrocarbon.

10. Do the physical and chemical properties of hydrocarbon compounds impart any clinically relevant information to toxicology?

Viscosity, surface tension, and volatility are the physical properties of hydrocarbons that dictate their aspiration potential. Viscosity is the tendency of a compound to resist flow. Surface tension describes the cohesiveness between the molecules of the hydrocarbon, and volatility is the tendency of a liquid to become a gas. Thus, compounds with the lowest viscosity and surface tension tend to have the highest aspiration potential. Highly volatile compounds when aspirated or inhaled may be responsible for transient hypoxia as a result of displacing alveolar oxygen. The chemical side chains of these agents include heavy metals (e.g., arsenic), halogens (e.g., carbon tetrachloride), and aromatic hydrocarbons (e.g., toluene), all of which increase the risk of systemic toxicity (see Table). Hydrocarbon products with inherent systemic toxicity (apart from aspiration potential) can be remembered with the mnemonic CHAMP:

C Camphor
H Halogenated hydrocarbons
A Aromatic hydrocarbons
M Metals
P Pesticides

Examples of Hydrocarbons with Systemic Toxicity

EXAMPLE	SYSTEMIC EFFECT
Toluene (aromatic petroleum distillate)	Renal tubular acidosis
Benzene (aromatic petroleum distillate)	Aplastic anemia, leukemia
Methylene chloride (halogenated hydrocarbon)	Carbon monoxide poisoning
Carbon tetrachloride (halogenated hydrocarbon)	Hepatorenal toxicity

11. Aside from the physical properties of the hydrocarbon, are there any other risk-stratifying criteria I need to know?

As one might imagine, patients who ingest larger amounts of hydrocarbons (> 30 ml) are more likely to develop pulmonary and CNS complications. However, patients ingesting smaller amounts of highly volatile hydrocarbons (e.g., mineral seal oil) can still develop life-threatening pulmonary toxicity. Several studies and anecdotal reports suggest that victims with spontaneous initial vomiting are more likely to be at risk for aspiration. Also, because a majority of fatalities associated with hydrocarbons involve children with occasionally delayed progression of disease, one should consider extended observation of these patients in a health care facility.

12. Can hydrocarbons be intentionally abused?

Deep inhalation of a volatile hydrocarbon from a container ("sniffing"), a fabric ("huffing"), or plastic or paper bag ("bagging") with the intent of "getting high" is common in many parts of the world. Paints and adhesives (toluene), gasoline, cigarette lighter fluid (butane), typewriter correction fluids and thinners (trichloroethane), and amyl and butyl nitrates are some of the commonly misused hydrocarbons. The major risks associated with volatile substance abuse are cardiac arrhythmias and sudden death. High concentrations of hydrocarbons sensitize the heart to circulating catecholamines, placing the patient at increased risk for arrhythmias precipitated by sudden alarm, exercise, or sexual activity. CNS symptoms from these chemicals range from euphoria and disinhibition to dangerous delusions, hallucinations, stupor, agitation, or seizures at higher toxic doses.

13. Are hydrocarbons toxic to the skin?

Dermal exposure to tar or asphalt hydrocarbons can cause thermal burns and usually dry on contact, making them difficult to remove. Mechanical debridement of the product may result in worsening injury. Hydrocarbon ointments such as De-Solv-it, Polysorbate 80, and Tween-80 help dissolve tar and asphalt on skin. Other readily available products for this task include mineral oil, petroleum jelly, and antibiotic ointments. Burn injuries should be treated conventionally. Some hydrocarbon solvents can also damage subcutaneous fat if absorbed, leading to a "defatting dermatitis."

14. Is there an antidote for hydrocarbon poisoning?

No. Supportive care is the mainstay therapy for hydrocarbon toxicity, and emphasis should be placed on airway and breathing. Respiratory compromise from aspiration should be recognized early and treated appropriately with oxygen. Patients occasionally require mechanical ventilation. Pulmonary disease from these products is similar to that of acute respiratory distress syndrome (ARDS) and may require use of high levels of positive end-expiratory pressure (PEEP) and oxygen to counteract the large ventilation-perfusion mismatch. Data regarding use of inhaled beta agonists (e.g., albuterol) for bronchospasm are lacking. Anecdotal evidence suggests their use to be safe unless the patient is at risk for cardiotoxicity from sensitization following acute inhalational exposure. Cardiac arrhythmias from inhalational exposure should be treated conventionally, but blocking beta adrenergic receptors on heart muscle with beta blocking drugs such as propranolol or esmolol may be efficacious in terminating tachyarrhythmias.

15. What is the role of gastric decontamination in hydrocarbon ingestions?

Because most life-threatening clinical effects from hydrocarbons result from aspiration, gastric decontamination is rarely indicated. The risk of vomiting and possible aspiration must be weighed against the benefit of rapid removal of the hydrocarbon from the stomach.

Because vomiting seems to be a risk factor for aspiration pneumonitis, **syrup of ipecac** should not be used in a patient with hydrocarbon ingestion.

Gastric lavage (GL) has been advocated as a better choice for decontamination, but the procedure can also induce emesis. Furthermore, studies evaluating GL for poisoning in general have found only equivocal results, making it unwise to recommend it as a routine procedure. Patients ingesting hydrocarbons in large quantities or substances with high systemic toxicity (see CHAMP mnemonic in question 10) may benefit from lavage if the individual is awake with intact airway reflexes or is intubated and paralyzed.

Activated charcoal is not useful in decreasing hydrocarbon absorption.

16. Should every patient with hydrocarbon toxicity get steroids and antibiotics?

Current literature does not support the use of corticosteroids for hydrocarbon pneumonitis. Corticosteroids do not hasten the improvement of aspiration pneumonitis, and one animal study showed an increased risk of bacterial superinfection after their use with or without antibiotics. The use of antibiotics has two potential purposes in patients with hydrocarbon aspiration:

1. **Prophylactic.** Several animal models could not substantiate the use of prophylactic antibiotics in preventing superinfection in this situation. Therefore, blindly instituting antibiotics in every patient with pulmonary toxicity from hydrocarbon ingestion is of no benefit.

2. **Treatment of superinfection.** Patients with hydrocarbon pneumonitis frequently develop fever, leukocytosis, and an infiltrate from inflammation early in the course of their illness, making it difficult to assess for possible bacterial superinfection. Severely poisoned patients, febrile patients, and patients who have a leukocytosis after the initial period of poisoning (> 24 hours after ingestion) may require antibiotics.

17. *Extra credit:* **Turpentine intoxication is treated like any exposure to hydrocarbons, but what factor makes turpentine different from such a group?**

It is not a component of crude oil but is distilled from pine trees.

18. *Extra credit:* **We know that petroleum hydrocarbons are pervasive throughout society and can be toxic, but what popular humorist said, "We are the first nation in the history of the world to go to the poorhouse in an automobile"?**

Will Rogers.

BIBLIOGRAPHY

1. Anas N, Namasonthi V, Ginsburg CM: Criteria for hospitalizing children who have ingested products containing hydrocarbon. JAMA 246:840–843, 1981.
2. Flanagan RJ, Ruprah M, Meredith TJ, et al: An introduction to the clinical toxicology of volatile substances. Drug Saf 5:359–383, 1990.
3. Goldfrank LR, Flomenbaum NE, Lewin NA, et al (eds): Goldfrank's Toxicologic Emergencies, 6th ed. Norwalk, CT, Appleton & Lange, 1998.
4. Litovitz TL, Felberg L, White S, et al: 1995 annual report of the American Association of Poison Control Centers Toxic Exposure Surveillance System. Am J Emerg Med 14:487–537, 1996.
5. Machado B, Cross K, Snodgrass WR: Accidental hydrocarbon ingestion cases telephoned to a regional poison center. Ann Emerg Med 17:804–807, 1988.
6. Marks MI, Chicoine L, Legere G, et al: Adrenocorticosteroid treatment of hydrocarbon pneumonia in children: A cooperative study. J Pediatr 81:366–369, 1972.
7. Press E: Cooperative kerosene poisoning study: Evaluation of gastric lavage and other factors in the treatment of accidental ingestion of petroleum distillate products. Pediatrics 29:648–674, 1962.
8. Truemper E, Reyes de la Rocha SR, et al: Clinical characteristics, pathophysiology and management of hydrocarbon ingestion: Case report and review of the literature. Pediatr Emerg Care 3:187–193, 1987.
9. Wolfe BM, Brodeur AE, Shields JB: The role of gastrointestinal absorption of kerosene in producing pneumonitis in dogs. J Pediatr 76:867–873, 1970.
10. Zucker AR, Berger S, Wood LDH: Management of kerosene-induced pulmonary injury. Crit Care Med 14:303–304, 1986.

43. CAUSTICS AND BUTTON BATTERIES

Fred Harchelroad, M.D.

1. What are caustics?

Caustics is a generic term for any corrosive substance. Classically, a caustic was an alkaline substance; however, it now refers to both acid and alkaline products. Similarly, some agents not traditionally considered alkaline or acid are classified as caustics. Examples include detergents and hydrocarbons that may cause severe burns following exposure to mucous membranes.

ALKALIS (CAUSTICS)	ACIDS (CORROSIVES)	HYDROCARBONS THAT CAUSE CHEMICAL BURNS
Calcium carbides	Acetic acid	Ethylene dichloride
Calcium hydroxide	Copper chloride	Ethylene glycol monobutyl ether
Calcium oxide	Copper sulfate	Ethylene glycol monoethyl ether acetate
Caustic potash	Ferric chloride	Formaldehyde
Caustic soda	Hydrochloric acid	Gasoline
Diethylene triamine	Hydrofluoric acid	Isopropyl alcohol
Isopropylamine	Nitric acid	Naphthalene
Isopropylaminoethanol	Oxalic acid	Perchloroethylene
Lime	Phosphoric acid	Phenol
Potassium carbonate	Zinc chloride	Pine oil
Potassium hydroxide	Zinc sulfate	Turpenes
Potassium oxide		Turpentine
Sodium carbonate		Xylene
Sodium hydroxide		
Sodium metasilicate		
Sodium oxide		
Sodium silicate		
Sodium tripolyphosphate		
Trisodium phosphate		

2. What household products contain caustics?

Toilet bowl cleaners
Car batteries
Metal cleaning products
Cement cleaning products
Drain cleaners
Soldering flux
Swimming pool and hot tub disinfectant and and cleaning products
Automatic dishwashing detergents
Hair relaxers
Cement
Bleaches

3. Describe the mechanism by which caustics burn.

Caustic agents cause tissue injury by altering the structure of the dermis or mucous membrane, which affects the ionized state and disrupts covalent bonds. In water solutions, the hydronium ion (H^+) produces the main effect of acids, whereas the hydroxide ion (OH^-) produces the toxic effect for alkali substances. Tissue injury by liquefactive necrosis (saponification of fats and solubilization of proteins) is pathognomonic of **alkali exposure**. Cell death occurs from emulsification and disruption of cellular membranes. The hydroxide ion of the alkali reacts rapidly with collagen, causing it to become edematous. Small venous and arterial vessel thrombosis occurs. Severe life-threatening injury may occur with exposures of < 1 minute, depending on the potency of the caustic exposure. The most severely injured tissues from alkali exposure include the squamous epithelial cells of the oropharynx and esophagus. Historically, the stomach is involved only 20% of the time after intentional oral ingestion of alkali substances.

Acid exposures cause tissue injury by coagulation necrosis (desiccation or denaturation of proteins of superficial tissue) with the eventual formation of eschar or coagulum. This effect limits the extent of injury. Unlike alkali exposures, the squamous epithelium of the oropharynx and esophagus are somewhat more resistant to injury from acids. The stomach is much more frequently involved in intentional oral ingestions of liquid acids.

Hydrocarbon caustics are less likely to cause significant injury to the oropharynx, esophagus, or stomach. However, these chemicals will cause irritation and chemical burns to the skin following prolonged exposure because they penetrate into the dermis and cause adipose necrosis. The outer stratum corneum layer of the skin functions as a barrier against some chemical agents, whereas other agents, such as the hydrocarbons, readily penetrate skin. Chemicals may produce burns, dermatitis, allergic reaction, thermal injury, or systemic toxicity. Pathophysiologically, burns produced by all chemicals are similar. Tissue damage is determined by strength and concentration of the agent, manner of contact, quantity of agent, duration of contact, mechanism of action, and extent of penetration.

4. Describe the symptoms of caustics exposure.

After an **accidental exposure** to a small amount of caustic to either the skin or the mucous membranes, some patients complain of severe burning and irritation. Mucous membrane exposure will result in lacrimation or sialorrhea consistent with the inflammatory response. Likewise, there may be complaints of difficulty breathing or swallowing, depending on the amount and viscosity of the substance swallowed. Usually, however, the volumes are small and frequently do not cause significant problems. Accidental exposure of caustics to the eyes may cause severe pain and blindness if not treated immediately. The special case of hydrofluoric acid exposure to the skin causes severe pain, usually several hours after the exposure. The discomfort is delayed because hydrofluoric acid is able to penetrate skin prior to dissociation of the fluoride ion from hydrogen. This is in contrast to the more immediate pain caused by exposure to other caustic agents with more rapid dissociation such as potassium hydroxide or hydrochloric acid.

Intentional exposure to caustics almost always involves oral ingestion of strong alkali or acids. These patients typically present several minutes or hours after ingestion, when the oropharyngeal and esophageal pain and swelling become severe. They frequently have a muffled voice and sit in the classic "sniffing" position because of airway compromise. Patients complain of severe sore throat and substernal and esophageal pain.

5. What are the physical findings of caustics exposure?

Deep **inhalational injuries** from many caustics are rare because most aerosol particles are filtered out in the upper airways. Thus, there is limited irritation of the lung parenchyma. Nevertheless, this can occur, and physical findings include an increased respiratory rate, anxiety (usually caused by hypoxemia), and cyanosis. Tachycardia may be observed secondary to discomfort and hypoxemia. In rare instances, pulmonary edema will be noted with rales on auscultatory examination of the lungs.

Ocular exposure to caustics cause severe conjunctival injection and corneal burns. This develops rapidly with alkali exposures, but it can occur even with acid and hydrocarbon exposures.

Dermal exposure to caustics manifests with the classic symptoms of thermal injury: erythema, blistering, and full-thickness skin loss. An acute injury may be deceptively mild, only to be followed by extensive skin damage and systemic toxicity. Chemical burns of the skin generally are much slower to heal than thermal injuries.

Physical findings noted to the **mucous membranes** of the mouth and esophagus include marked sialorrhea and tachypnea secondary to airway obstruction. Glottic edema is frequent and worrisome. Granular solid caustics, such as many toilet bowl cleaners, will cause significant injury to the oropharynx and esophagus because the granules embed themselves in the mucous membranes.

6. Which caustic agents cause systemic toxicity?

Exposure to specific caustic agents that cause systemic toxicity is rare. Profound hypocalcemia accompanied by hyperkalemia may be seen with both hydrofluoric acid and oxalic acid exposures. These may result in death. Tannic acid, chromic acid, formic acid, picric acid, and phosphorus may cause hepatic necrosis and nephrotoxicity. Cresol is associated with methemoglobinemia and massive hemolysis. Sodium nitrate and potassium nitrate may cause severe methemoglobinemia. Gasoline exposures in conjunction with inhalational injury may result in severe pulmonary and neurologic complications.

7. What is the initial management of caustic exposures?

Exposures to the skin or eyes should be treated immediately with water irrigation. If large amounts of solid alkali such as lime remain on the skin, they should be brushed off prior to water irrigation because a significant thermal burn may be generated from contact of the solid alkali with water. Because alkalis penetrate the skin and eye for a prolonged period, irrigation should continue for at least 15 minutes after initial debridement. Irrigation of the eye should be maintained even longer if pH testing of tears demonstrates a persistent alkaline pH. Prolonged irrigation with water following exposure to acids is generally not needed.

Oral ingestion of caustics is a life-threatening exposure. Any evidence of airway obstruction following a caustic ingestion, whether from acid or alkali, should be treated with emergent endotracheal intubation. There is little reason to attempt decontamination after an oral ingestion because in almost all instances the exposure would have occurred in a time frame that would have allowed injury to already occur. If arterial blood gases show a pH ≤ 7.2, surgical intervention is needed.

8. Which patients can be discharged safely from the emergency department after oral exposure to a caustic?

If there is no evidence of edema, erythema, or burns on thorough oropharyngeal examination and if no symptoms develop over 4 hours after the exposure, it is unlikely that significant exposure occurred. Other symptoms to consider are alterations of phonation, inability to tolerate swallowing, and severe esophageal pain. In cases where the patient has significant substernal discomfort and burning following a liquid caustic exposure but there is no evidence of oropharyngeal irritation, emergent endoscopy may be required. If endoscopy reveals evidence of only grade I burns to the esophagus or stomach, outpatient management is indicated.

9. What is so important about button batteries?

Children frequently ingest button batteries, which become lodged in the gastrointestinal tract. Button batteries range in size from 8 to 25 mm, with the larger sizes being more prone to esophageal impaction. Burns to the esophagus have been known to occur as soon as 4 hours after ingestion. Lithium-containing button batteries have a higher incidence of adverse outcomes.

If it is known that a button battery has been swallowed, and the airway is not compromised, radiographs of the body should be obtained to determine the battery's location. If the button battery has passed through the esophagus, it need not be retrieved in the asymptomatic patient. However, if it is lodged in the esophagus and more than 4 hours has elapsed since ingestion, the battery should be removed endoscopically.

Because parents may not be aware that their toddler swallowed a battery, any child with dysphagia and vomiting should be questioned, and radiographic evaluation of the body should be considered if there is likelihood of such an ingestion.

10. Is there an absolute or consistent way to treat caustic oral ingestions?

No. Some patients with caustic ingestions can be discharged safely following initial evaluation in the emergency department. Others will come in with life-threatening airway compromise from massive edema of the upper airway, which is usually the case with alkali ingestions. However, in all patients with caustic oral ingestion, airway compromise is the most frequent early cause of death. In addition, all patients with significant evidence of caustic burns, whether to the skin or mucous membranes, can sequester large amounts of fluid in the extracellular space and become significantly hypotensive and dehydrated as a result. Therefore, all patients should be treated with appropriate quantities of intravenous fluid. Delayed causes of death following oral ingestions of caustics include perforation of the esophagus, resulting in mediastinitis or significant gastrointestinal bleeding from tissue necrosis.

Appropriate surgical consultation should be obtained early in these cases. Patients who survive significant alkali or acid oral ingestions may have severe chronic disabilities related to esophageal stricture formation. Some studies recommend emergent esophageal resection with intestinal anastomosis to provide a conduit for food.

11. What other treatment modalities can be used for patients with oral caustic ingestions?

There is inconclusive evidence that treatment with H_2 blockers, proton pump inhibitors, or steroids will alleviate delayed complications such as esophageal or gastric perforation or strictures. Theoretically, prophylactic antimicrobials may benefit patients with computed tomographic evidence of severe esophageal burns or gas within the musculature of the esophagus. The reasoning is that, if gas can penetrate through the severely injured esophageal muscular layer, bacteria can also, potentially causing life-threatening mediastinitis.

12. Are nasogastric tubes contraindicated in patients following oral caustic exposure?

Yes. Placing a nasogastric tube blindly following a severe caustic exposure is not recommended because of the risk of perforating the esophagus or stomach. However, if exposure to the caustic occurred within 1–2 hours of the evaluation, sufficient time probably has not elapsed to allow significant esophageal tissue necrosis to develop and enable easy perforation. If peritonitis or mediastinitis is not present on examination, the risk of perforation with nasogastric tube placement is minimal. Nevertheless, if emergent endoscopy is going to be performed, a nasogastric tube can be placed under direct observation during this procedure. The reason for such placement is to maintain a tract into the stomach and help prevent severe stricture and obliteration of the esophagus. Newer modalities to protect esophageal patency include esophageal stents that are placed by interventional radiologists.

13. *Extra credit:* What famous Italian singer spent years paying extortion to the Black Hand criminal organization, who threatened to harm him by putting lye (sodium hydroxide) into his drinks to ruin his voice?

Enrico Caruso.

14. *Extra credit:* A popular writer for children and adults wrote some rather tasteless verbiage (from a toxicologic point of view) on caustics. An example is: "L is also for Lye. Do you want a nice red lollipop? Go pour all the lye into the toilet. Now tell Mommy you have eaten the lye (that is a fib or a white lye). Mommy will take you to the doctor in a taxi cab. After the doctor pumps your stomach, he will give you a nice red lollipop." Who was the author of this supposedly humorous passage from *Uncle Shelby's ABZ Book*?

Shel Silverstein.

BIBLIOGRAPHY

1. Anderson KD, Rouse T, Randolph JG: A controlled trial of corticosteroids in children with corrosive injury of the esophagus. N Engl J Med 323:637–640, 1990.
2. Berkovits RN, Bos CE, Wijburg FA, Holzki J: Caustic injury of the esophagus: Sixteen years' experience, and introduction of a new model of esophageal stent. J Laryngol Otolaryngol 110:1041–1045, 1996.

3. Berthert B, Castellani P, Brioche MI, et al: Early operation for corrosive injury to the upper gastrointestinal tract. Eur J Surg 162:951–953, 1996.
4. Blais BR: Treating chemical eye injuries. Occup Health Saf 65:23–26, 1996.
5. Gaudreault P, Parent M, McGuigan M, et al: Predictability of esophageal injury from signs and symptoms: A study of caustic ingestion in 378 children. Pediatrics 71:767–770, 1983.
6. Gorman RL, Khin-Maung-Gyi MT, Klein-Schwartz W, et al: Initial symptoms as a predictor of esophageal injury in alkaline corrosive ingestions. Am J Emerg Med 10:189–194, 1992.
7. Graundis A, Burns MJ, Aaron CK: Regional intravenous infusion of calcium gluconate for hydrofluoric acid burns of the upper extremities. Ann Emerg Med 30:604–607, 1997.
8. Homan CS, Singer AJ, Henry MC, Thode HC: Thermal effects of water and milk for acute injury of the esophagus. Acad Emerg Med 4:27–32, 1997.
9. Litovitz T, Schnitz BF: Ingestion of cylindrical and button batteries: An analysis of 2382 cases. Pediatrics 89:747–757, 1992.
10. Zargar SA, Kochhar R, Mehta SK: The role of fiberoptic endoscopy in the management of corrosive ingestion and modified endoscopic classification of burns. Gastrointest Endosc 37:165–169, 1991.

44. METHEMOGLOBIN

Saralyn R. Williams, M.D.

1. What is methemoglobin?

Methemoglobin is an abnormal hemoglobin in which the iron moiety of unoxygenated hemoglobin is in the ferric (Fe^{3+}) state rather than the ferrous (Fe^{2+}) state. When hemoglobin contains a ferric iron, it is unable to carry oxygen or carbon dioxide.

2. How does methemoglobin affect oxygen-carrying capacity?

Hemoglobin contains a tetramer of peptide (globin) chains. In adult hemoglobin, the most common peptides are two α chains and two β chains. Each of the globin chains encloses a heme molecule in a hydrophobic pocket. Each heme molecule is capable of carrying oxygen when the iron moiety is in the reduced (ferrous) state. The α and β chains can undergo a conformational change so that the hemoglobin molecule can vary its oxygen affinities. As oxygen binds to the heme molecule, the affinity for additional binding increases, giving the oxyhemoglobin dissociation curve a sigmoidal shape. The binding and release of oxygen vary with temperature, level of 2,3-biphosphoglycerate, and pH of the serum. As the temperature increases, pH decreases or levels of 2,3-biphosphoglycerate increase, and the sigmoid curve shifts to the right, facilitating the release of oxygen and binding of carbon dioxide.

Methemoglobin reduces the oxygen-carrying capacity of the blood by two mechanisms. First, methemoglobin is unable to carry oxygen molecules. Second, the presence of methemoglobin shifts the oxyhemoglobin dissociation curve to the left. This shift increases the affinity of the remaining hemoglobin to oxygen. The remaining hemoglobin is able to bind oxygen molecules more efficiently; however, it is less able to release oxygen to tissues.

3. What are normal methemoglobin levels?

In adults with no hereditary methemoglobinemia, the baseline methemoglobin level is approximately 1% of total hemoglobin.

4. How is methemoglobin reduced or eliminated in the body?

The red blood cell has two mechanisms for reduction of methemoglobin. The dominant pathway uses reduced nicotine adenine dinucleotide (NADH). NADH results from the metabolism of glucose to pyruvate during glycolysis. NADH then becomes the electron donor to the ferric iron of methemoglobin. Originally, one enzyme was thought to be involved in this reaction and was named NADH methemoglobin reductase. More recently, two enzymes have been identified in this reduction process: cytochrome b_5 and cytochrome b_5 reductase. In vivo, this dual enzyme system is capable of > 95% of the methemoglobin reduction activity.

The second mechanism for methemoglobin reduction requires the presence of reduced nicotine adenine dinucleotide phosphate (NADPH), which is produced by the hexose monophosphate shunt. The enzymatic conversion of glucose-6-phosphate (G-6-P) to 6-phosphogluconate occurs by the enzyme glucose-6-phosphate dehydrogenase (G-6-PD). With this conversion, $NADP^+$ is reduced to NADPH. NADPH uses NADPH methemoglobin reductase to reduce the ferric iron to a ferrous state. This enzymatic system is less efficient and accounts for < 5% of the methemoglobin-reducing capacity of the red blood cell.

5. What is the difference between acquired methemoglobinemia and congenital methemoglobinemia?

Acquired methemoglobinemia is the most common form of methemoglobinemia and most often results from exposure to drugs or toxins that oxidize ferrous iron. Hereditary forms of methemoglobinemia do occur and are usually due to one of two conditions, hemoglobin M or NADH methemoglobin reductase deficiency. Hemoglobin M is a variant in which the iron is stabilized in the oxidized (Fe^{3+}) state. One type of this autosomal dominant mutation results from the replacement of a histidine by a tyrosine on either the α or β subunit of the hemoglobin molecule.

The other form of congenital methemoglobinemia occurs from a deficiency in the NADH methemoglobin reductase enzyme system. A deficiency could occur with either enzyme cytochrome b_5 or cytochrome b_5 reductase. Because this trait is autosomal recessive, patients who are homozygous for this deficiency may have clinical cyanosis from elevated methemoglobin levels.

6. Describe common causes for acquired methemoglobinemia.

One of the most common classes of drugs responsible for acquired methemoglobinemia is local anesthetics. Three of the local anesthetics that are most notorious are benzocaine, prilocaine, and lidocaine. Benzocaine-induced methemoglobinemia from topical mucosal membrane application is associated with endoscopy, bronchoscopy, and transesophageal echocardiography. Benzocaine is also found in many over-the-counter products such as hemorrhoid creams and teething gels.

Nitrites are another major class of agents that cause methemoglobinemia. Therapeutic induction of methemoglobin for cyanide poisonings utilizes nitrites. Methemoglobin from ingestion of well water results from contamination by nitrates that are converted to nitrites in vivo.

Other well-known inducers of methemoglobin include sulfonamide antibiotics, phenazopyridine, dapsone, aniline dyes, chloroquine, and primaquine. Benzene derivatives, dinitrophenol, chlorates, and other oxidizing chemicals may also produce methemoglobinemia as well as ingestion of *Gyromitra* mushrooms. Nitroethane, found in many artificial fingernail removers, also has been reported to cause delayed methemoglobinemia when ingested.

7. What are the signs and symptoms of methemoglobinemia?

One of the first clues is generalized cyanosis. Application of oxygen does not improve the cyanosis. Symptoms may be quite variable depending on the level of the methemoglobin and the patient's ability to handle the loss of the oxygen-carrying capacity. Early symptoms include anxiousness and dizziness, with fatigue and confusion occurring at higher levels. Tachycardia may be seen at lower levels along with cyanosis. With higher levels, tachypnea, altered mental status, dysrhythmias, and acidosis may occur. Death can occur at methemoglobin levels > 70% of the total hemoglobin.

8. What level of methemoglobin is required for a patient to appear cyanotic?

Methemoglobin is usually reported as a percent of hemoglobin in the methemoglobin form. The absolute amount of hemoglobin that must be in the ferric state to cause cyanosis is 1.5 gm/dl. Provided that hemoglobin levels are in normal range (12–15 mg/dl), 1.5 gm/dl would account for 10–15% of the hemoglobin. If a patient is anemic, 1.5 gm/dl will account for a larger percentage of net hemoglobin. Therefore, a larger percentage of the hemoglobin will need to be in the methemoglobin state for the patient to be cyanotic. For example, if a male patient with renal failure has a hemoglobin of only 8 mg/dl, then 1.5 gm/dl would account for approximately 19% of his hemoglobin. Thus, the methemoglobin level in this patient would be at least 19% before he would appear cyanotic.

9. How is the diagnosis of methemoglobinemia made in a cyanotic patient?

The most important bedside clue is persistent cyanosis after the administration of high-flow oxygen. The pulse oximeter will read abnormally low saturations in these patients, although the low reading does not correspond with the level of methemoglobin. In addition, methemoglobin-containing blood does not turn bright red with the exposure of oxygen. A drop of the patient's blood placed onto filter paper will appear chocolate colored instead of bright red.

Another clue to the diagnosis of methemoglobinemia is the presence of a normal partial pressure of oxygen (pO_2) on an arterial blood gas (ABG) sample. The ABG measures the partial pressure of dissolved oxygen in the serum. It does not measure the oxygen-carrying capacity of the hemoglobin. Methemoglobin does not interfere with the diffusion of oxygen from the lungs, so the pO_2 is usually normal. The reported number for oxygen saturation on an ABG is calculated, not measured. The calculation assumes normal hemoglobin and is based on the standard oxygen-hemoglobin saturation curve.

To directly measure methemoglobin, a heparinized blood sample (venous or arterial) should be sent for analysis by a co-oximeter. The co-oximeter determines the actual level or percent of methemoglobin in the blood sample.

10. What is the treatment for methemoglobinemia?

Treatment of the patient with methemoglobinemia begins with supportive care. Oxygen supplementation is initiated using a non-rebreather face mask. Decontamination with activated charcoal may be necessary if the condition is the result of an ingestion of a long-acting substance such as dapsone. In a patient with significant symptoms or signs, reduction of the methemoglobin level by administration of methylene blue should be considered. Methylene blue is administered intravenously, 1 mg/kg, over 3–5 minutes. The dose of methylene blue may be repeated in 30 minutes if cyanosis does not improve. The methemoglobin level should be significantly reduced within an hour of the infusion of methylene blue.

11. How does methylene blue enhance the reduction of methemoglobin?

Methylene blue acts as a cofactor that accelerates the efficiency of the NADPH methemoglobin reductase. Instead of accounting for the usual 5% of the reduction capacity of the erythrocyte, the addition of methylene blue allows this pathway to become the predominate mechanism for reduction of methemoglobin. Methylene blue is converted to leukomethylene blue, which is actually colorless. Leukomethylene acts as an electron donor to the ferric iron, reducing it back to the ferrous state.

12. Are there contraindications to the administration of methylene blue?

The primary contraindication to the administration of methylene blue is G-6-PD deficiency. G-6-PD is an enzyme used in the first step of the hexose monophosphate shunt. This enzymatic reaction reduces $NADP^+$ to NADPH. NADPH is used by methemoglobin reductase for the reduction of methylene blue. In the absence of G-6-PD, the secondary pathway using NADPH methemoglobin reductase to reduce methemoglobin is useless because no NADPH is created. In this setting, red cells may be subject to hemolysis because methylene blue can create oxidative stress.

13. What is the differential diagnosis if the administration of methylene blue does not reverse the methemoglobinemia?

The primary element in the differential is G-6-PD deficiency. Additional causes include NADPH methemoglobin reductase deficiency or sulfhemoglobinemia.

14. What is sulfhemoglobin?

Sulfhemoglobin results from the incorporation of a sulfur atom into the porphyrin ring of hemoglobin. Sulfhemoglobin will cause the patient to appear cyanotic and may be incorrectly interpreted by co-oximeters as methemoglobin. Sulfhemoglobin also is unable to carry oxygen molecules; however, the patient usually tolerates sulfhemoglobinemia better. Only 0.5 gm/dl of hemoglobin must be sulfhemoglobin in order to cause cyanosis. Sulfhemoglobin also shifts the oxygen dissociation curve to the right, thus allowing oxygen to be more easily released into tissues.

Sulfhemoglobin lasts for the life cycle of the individual red blood cell. It is not reversed by the administration of methylene blue because the sulfuration process is permanent. Detection of sulfhemoglobin requires spectrophotometric techniques.

15. What is the treatment for methemoglobinemia when methylene blue is contraindicated or is not working?

Exchange transfusions or infusions of packed red blood cells may be used in a patient who has G-6-PD deficiency or in whom methylene blue is not reducing the methemoglobin. This treatment is reserved for patients with very high concentrations of methemoglobin or very low total hemoglobin concentrations.

16. Is there any indication for a continuous infusion of methylene blue?

Recurrence of methemoglobinemia has been reported with longer acting oxidizing agents such as dapsone, nitroethane, and aniline dyes. In these cases, repetitive dosing of methylene blue or possibly an infusion drip may be required to keep the hemoglobin in the reduced state.

17. *Extra credit:* In 1947, Berton Roueche, a writer for *The New Yorker* magazine, wrote of the medical detective work involved in a classic 1944 incident, in which a group of men suffered from methemoglobinemia when sodium nitrite was accidentally added to their oatmeal instead of table salt. What is the title of this now classic toxicologic story?

"Eleven Blue Men."

BIBLIOGRAPHY

1. Curry S: Methemoglobinemia. Ann Emerg Med 11:214–221, 1982.
2. Dinneen SF, Mohr DN, Fairbanks VF: Methemoglobinemia from topically applied anesthetic spray. Mayo Clin Proc 69:886–888, 1994.
3. Hansen DG, Challoner KR, Smith DE: Dapsone intoxication: Two case reports. J Emerg Med 12:347–351, 1994.
4. Mansouri A, Lurie AA: Concise review: Methemoglobinemia. Am J Hematol 42:7–12, 1993.
5. Park CM, Nagel RL: Sulfhemoglobinemia clinical and molecular aspects. N Engl J Med 310:1579–1584, 1984.
6. Shepherd G, Grover J, Klein-Schwartz W: Prolonged formation of methemoglobin following nitroethane ingestion. Clin Toxicol 36:613–616, 1998.
7. Wright RO, Lewander WJ, Woolf AD: Methemoglobin: Etiology, pharmacology, and clinical management. Ann Emerg Med 34:646–656, 1999.

X. Pesticides

45. INSECTICIDES: ORGANOPHOSPHATES AND CARBAMATES

Summon Chomchai, M.D.

1. What are organophosphates and carbamates?

Organophosphates and carbamates are two of the most commonly used classes of insecticides. Both compounds are inhibitors of carboxylic ester hydrolases, including acetylcholinesterase (AChE) and pseudocholinesterase. AChE is found in the human nervous system and plays a crucial role in controlling neurotransmission at synapses.

2. What is their mechanism of toxicity?

Acetylcholine is a neurotransmitter at the neuromuscular junction, pre- and postganglionic parasympathetic synapses, preganglionic sympathetic synapses, and central nervous system (CNS) cholinergic synapses. When the nerve terminal is stimulated by an action potential, acetylcholine is released into the synapse and binds its postsynaptic receptors. AChE immediately hydrolyzes acetylcholine and terminates its action to prevent continuous stimulation of the receptors, which could lead to eventual paralysis of the synapse.

Inhibition of AChE results in accumulation of acetylcholine at synapses and excessive stimulation of the autonomic and somatic nervous systems. This overstimulation produces the main toxic effects of organophosphates and carbamates.

3. In what respect is organophosphate poisoning different from that of carbamates?

1. Carbamates cause reversible inhibition of AChE as opposed to the irreversible inhibition caused by organophosphates. Carbamates bind with the active site on the AChE molecule by carbamoylation. The carbamoylated enzyme can degrade spontaneously within minutes to hours to reactivate the enzyme. Therefore, carbamate poisoning usually resolves within 24–48 hours. In contrast, organophosphates and AChE form a phosphorylated complex that degrades over days to weeks. However, within 24–48 hours after phosphorylation, the enzyme complex loses an alkyl group in a process called **aging**, after which the enzyme can no longer spontaneously regenerate. New enzyme molecules must then be produced for physiologic activity to return.

2. Unlike organophosphates, carbamates poorly penetrate the blood-brain barrier, resulting in limited CNS effects.

4. How significant is organophosphate and carbamate poisoning? How are people exposed to these agents?

Organophosphates and carbamates are widely used as insecticides for agricultural and household purposes. Poisoning by these substances is still common worldwide. In the United States, over 10,000 cases of poisoning from these insecticides occur annually, and deaths from these exposures occur every year. Morbidity and mortality rates are much higher in developing countries, where use, storage, and sales are not well regulated. A person may be exposed to these compounds through gastrointestinal, dermal, and respiratory routes. Modes of exposure include suicide attempts, food contamination, and accidental occupational exposures.

5. What are the clinical manifestations of acute organophosphate and carbamate poisoning?

1. Stimulation of **muscarinic receptors** produces a clinical picture best remembered by the mnemonic DUMBBELS:

Diarrhea
Urinary incontinence
Miosis
Bradycardia
Bronchospasm and bronchorrhea
Emesis
Lacrimation
Salivation

In addition to bradycardia, cardiac conduction disturbances can result from augmented vagal tone.

2. Stimulation of **nicotinic receptors** at the neuromuscular junction causes muscle weakness, fasciculations, and paralysis. Effects at ganglionic nicotinic receptors result in diaphoresis, mydriasis, tachycardia, and hypertension, which most often appear early in the course of poisoning.

3. **CNS effects** include anxiety, restlessness, lethargy, confusion, psychosis, coma, and seizures.

Deaths from organophosphate and carbamate poisoning occur secondary to respiratory failure and cardiovascular collapse.

6. What are the differences between presentations of acute cholinesterase inhibitor organophosphate and carbamate poisoning in children as opposed to adults?

From studies in relatively large groups of patients aged 3 months to 8 years, signs and symptoms of organophosphate and carbamate poisoning in children are related mainly to the CNS. Children usually present with lethargy, stupor, or coma in addition to hypotonia, muscle weakness, and miosis. Other signs of cholinergic syndrome such as excessive salivation and tearing, cool and diaphoretic skin, gastroenteritis, muscle fasciculations, and bradycardia are seen less often in children than in adults. Therefore, the possibility of cholinesterase-inhibitor poisoning should not be excluded in children with CNS depression, even in the absence of classic muscarinic effects.

7. In addition to acute cholinergic syndrome, what are other manifestations of organophosphate and carbamate poisoning?

1. **Acute pancreatitis** with hyperamylasemia and hyperglycemia

2. A **prolonged QT interval** on ECG with or without torsades de pointes. This finding is believed to be a result of intense and unequal sympathetic stimulation of myocardial fibers. This dysrhythmia has been treated successfully with ventricular pacing and isoproterenol; magnesium also may be effective.

3. **Hydrocarbon pneumonitis**. Patients who ingest and aspirate the petroleum distillate vehicle of the insecticide may develop hydrocarbon pneumonitis.

8. How is organophosphate or carbamate poisoning diagnosed?

Diagnosis is made by history of exposure to an insecticide, manifestations of excessive cholinergic stimulation, and depressed cholinesterase levels. In most cases, treatment needs to begin before the cholinesterase level returns. Response to atropine and pralidoxime therapy help confirm the diagnosis.

9. How is organophosphate or carbamate poisoning treated?

Caregivers should wear adequate protective gear. Latex and vinyl gloves are not adequate for protection; neoprene or nitrile gloves should be used until the patient is completely decontaminated. Contaminated clothing, including shoes, should be removed and treated as toxic waste. Skin should be cleaned with large amounts of water and soap. Activated charcoal can be given for gastrointestinal decontamination.

After airway stabilization, synaptic cholinergic overstimulation and cholinesterase blockade should be corrected with atropine and pralidoxime.

10. How is a cholinesterase level interpreted? Other than organophosphate and carbamate poisoning, what else can lower cholinesterase levels?

Two types of cholinesterase can be measured in clinical practice: red blood cell (RBC) cholinesterase and plasma cholinesterase. Generally, organophosphates and carbamates affect both. RBC cholinesterase correlates with nervous system AChE better than plasma cholinesterase. Thus, RBC cholinesterase is more specific for organophosphate and carbamate poisoning. However, there are limitations in interpretation of its result. A single level may not help in diagnosis except when very low; normal values of cholinesterase vary among the general population, and in most cases a patient's baseline level is not known. In acute poisoning, symptomatic patients usually have more than 50% of cholinesterase inhibited. The rate of enzyme depression is also important. Patients with small repeated exposures to these chemicals may have very low enzyme levels with few symptoms. Moreover, other factors depress RBC and plasma cholinesterase levels. RBC cholinesterase is lower in disorders that shorten the circulating life of the red cell such as hemoglobinopathies and hemolytic anemia. Plasma cholinesterase levels are lower in liver cirrhosis, malnutrition, and pregnancy and can vary genetically. Therefore, other clinical parameters must be considered when interpreting cholinesterase levels.

11. How does atropine work in cholinesterase inhibitor poisoning? When and how much should be given?

Atropine is a competitive antagonist of acetylcholine at muscarinic receptors, both in the peripheral nervous system and CNS. Atropine can be helpful in drying excessive secretions and increasing the heart rate of cholinergic patients. It has no effect on nicotinic receptors or muscle weakness.

In adults with muscarinic symptoms, an initial dose of atropine of 1–2 mg can be given intravenously. This dose can be doubled every 5–10 minutes thereafter until symptoms are relieved. The end point of atropine treatment is clearing of bronchial secretions. Tachycardia is not a contraindication for atropine treatment. Once bronchial secretions are controlled, continuous infusions or repeated boluses of atropine may be required for 24 hours or more. Atropine should be tapered before being discontinued.

12. What is pralidoxime? When, how, and how much should be used in victims of anticholinesterase poisoning?

Pralidoxime is the only oxime available in the U.S. It works primarily by attaching onto the phosphorylated enzyme and removing the phosphate moiety of the organophosphate-enzyme complex to regenerate AChE. The process can occur only before the complex has aged. In addition, pralidoxime may act as a scavenger for remaining organophosphate molecules. These enzyme-regenerating effects occur at nicotinic, muscarinic, and possibly CNS receptors. Pralidoxime therapy should be initiated as early as possible after the diagnosis of organophosphate poisoning is made and whenever atropine is required because their therapeutic effects may be synergistic. From animal studies, the minimum therapeutic concentration of pralidoxime is a serum level of 4 µg/L. Intravenous bolus dosing fails to maintain pralidoxime levels above this threshold, and continuous intravenous infusion is therefore recommended. In adults, the initial dose is 1–2 gm, given intravenously over 30 minutes. After the initial dose, a continuous infusion of 500 mg/hour is sufficient to maintain serum levels in most cases. Side effects of pralidoxime are minimal with recommended doses. At higher doses or rapid administration, respiratory and cardiac arrest, diastolic hypertension, dizziness, and blurred vision have been reported.

Generally, pralidoxime is not indicated in carbamate poisoning because aging does not occur. However, when it is impossible to exclude a mixed poisoning with an organophosphate, pralidoxime should be considered.

13. What is the intermediate syndrome (IMS)?

IMS is a clinical illness that starts 24–96 hours after the onset of organophosphate poisoning. It is characterized by weakness of muscles innervated by cranial nerves (facial, external ocular, and palatal), neck flexor muscles, proximal extremity muscles, and respiratory muscles, especially the diaphragm. IMS can be found in poisonings by any organophosphate pesticide and nerve agent. IMS was first described as a distinct clinical entity of organophosphate poisoning after recovery from acute cholinergic crisis. However, later reports and case series reveal that this syndrome may be associated with muscarinic effects and prolonged cholinesterase inhibition. Electromyographic studies of IMS suggest combined pre- and postsynaptic dysfunctions of neuromuscular transmission. Although the exact mechanism is still unknown, IMS appears to be the result of excess accumulation of acetylcholine at the neuromuscular junction, and its occurrence correlates with severity of preceding acute cholinergic crisis and a high level of exposure to organophosphates. IMS is not very responsive to atropine or pralidoxime therapy, but early and adequate treatment by pralidoxime after the onset of poisoning may prevent the syndrome. With effective supportive care and respiratory support, the outcome from IMS is favorable, and most cases recover within 14–28 days.

14. Describe organophosphate-induced delayed neuropathy (OPIDN).

OPIDN is a delayed complication of organophosphate poisoning that begins 1–3 weeks after exposure. Symptoms begin with leg cramping, symmetric lower extremity weakness, and glove and stocking paresthesias followed by similar symptoms in the upper extremities. Sensory changes begin as numbness and tingling in the feet and may progress to the hands. Electromyographic studies reveal a denervation pattern. Consequences of OPIDN include wasting of small hand and peroneal muscles, with foot drop as a common result. Prognosis of OPIDN ranges from irreversible to slowly reversible over 6–15 months. After the peripheral neuropathy subsides, a spastic paresis from involvement of long tracts in the spinal cord or upper motor neurons may persist. The onset of OPIDN has been correlated with inhibition of a neuronal enzyme, termed **neurotoxic esterase** (NTE), and is not necessarily associated with inhibition of cholinesterase. In addition to NTE inhibition, aging or dealkylation of the enzyme complex is needed to induce OPIDN. Some of the organophosphates reported to cause OPIDN in humans include tri-ortho-cresyl phosphate (TOCP), parathion, chlorpyriphos, dichlorvos, leptophos, methamidophos, mipafox, omethoate, trichlorfon, trichlornat, 4-nitrophenyl phenylphosphonothionate (EPN), and various war nerve gas agents. There is no specific antidote for OPIDN, and treatment is supportive.

15. What are nerve agents?

Nerve agents (sarin, tabun, soman, and VX) are organophosphate compounds developed for war. Their primary mechanism of action is cholinesterase inhibition with phosphorylation and aging of the enzyme similar to that of organophosphate insecticides. Major routes of exposure are inhalation and percutaneous contact. Onset of toxicity after inhalation is immediate, but skin exposure may delay symptom onset. Clinical effects include overstimulation of muscarinic, nicotinic, and CNS receptors resembling those of related cholinesterase-inhibiting insecticides.

16. What is the treatment for patients suffering from nerve agent toxicity?

All rescue personnel must wear personal protective equipment. Exposed skin should be decontaminated with large amounts of water and alkaline soap. Atropine and pralidoxime should be started as soon as possible after the onset of symptoms. Asymptomatic exposed patients should be observed for at least 18 hours for possible delayed effects from skin exposure.

17. Is there any interaction between organophosphates or carbamates and other drugs?

The reports of prolonged and potentiated neuromuscular blockade from succinylcholine in patients with organophosphate and carbamate poisoning can be explained by two mechanisms. First, hydrolysis of succinylcholine by plasma cholinesterase is delayed because the enzyme is inhibited by the insecticide. Second, increased levels of acetylcholine at neuromuscular junctions may contribute to the neuromuscular blocking effect. Therefore, succinylcholine should be avoided in cases of organophosphate and carbamate poisoning.

A significant portion of cocaine is also metabolized by plasma cholinesterase to its major metabolite, ecgonine methyl ester. Patients with organophosphate and carbamate poisoning may therefore have an increased vulnerability to the toxic effects of this drug.

18. *Extra credit:* **The condition known as "orange-picker's flu" is caused by low-level chronic exposure to what type of pesticides?**

Organophosphates.

19. *Extra credit:* **The trade name of what carbamate insecticide sounds like a cardinal number?**

Sevin, generically named carbaril.

BIBLIOGRAPHY

 1. Aaron CK, Howland MA: Insecticides: Organophosphates and carbamates. In Goldfrank LR, et al (eds): Goldfrank's Toxicologic Emergencies, 6th ed. Stamford, CT, Appleton & Lange, 1998, pp 1429–1444.
 2. Bardin PG, van Eeden SF, Moolman JA, et al: Organophosphate and carbamate poisoning. Arch Intern Med 154:1433–1441, 1994.
 3. Bleeker JD, Neucker KVD, Willems J: The intermediate syndrome in organophosphate poisoning: Presentation of a case and a review of the literature. J Toxicol Clin Toxicol 30:321–329, 1992.
 4. Bleeker JD, Neucker KVD, Willems J: Neurological aspects of organophosphate poisoning. Clin Neurol Neurosurg 94:93–103, 1992.
 5. Brown MA, Brix KA: Review of health consequences from high-, intermediate-, and low-level exposure to organophosphorus nerve agents. J Appl Toxicol 18:393–408, 1998.
 6. Ecobichon DJ: Toxic effects of pesticides. In Klaassen CD (ed): Casarett & Doull's Toxicology: The Basic Science of Poisons, 5th ed. New York, McGraw-Hill, 1995, pp 643–689.
 7. Frederick BC, Simpson WM, Haddad LM: The organophosphates and other insecticides. In Haddad LM, Shannon MW, Winchester JF (eds): Clinical Management of Poisoning and Drug Overdose, 3rd ed. Philadelphia, W.B. Saunders, 1998, pp 836–845.
 8. Holstege CP, Kirk M, Sidell FR: Chemical warfare. Crit Care Clin 13:923–942, 1997.
 9. Karalliedde L, Senanayake N: Organophosphorus insecticide poisoning. Br J Anaesth 63:736–750, 1989.
10. Karalliedde L: Organophosphorus poisoning and anaesthesia. Anaesthesia 54:1073–1088, 1999.
11. Marrs TC: Organophosphate poisoning. Pharm Ther 58:51–66, 1993.
12. Minton NA, Murray VSG: A review of organophosphate poisoning. Med Toxicol 3:350–375, 1988.
13. Schenker MB, Louie S, Mehler LN, Albertson TE: Pesticides. In Rom WN (ed): Environmental and Occupational Medicine, 3rd ed. Philadelphia, Lippincott-Raven, 1998, pp 1157–1172.
14. Tafuri J, Roberts J: Organophosphate poisoning. Ann Emerg Med 16:193–202, 1987.

46. INSECTICIDES: CHLORINATED HYDROCARBONS, PYRETHRINS, AND DEET

Timothy E. Albertson, M.D., Ph.D., and Thomas J. Ferguson, M.D., Ph.D.

1. What are chlorinated hydrocarbon pesticides?

This group of cyclic organic chlorinated compounds was once widely used in agriculture, structural pest control, red fire ant control, and mosquito abatement. Starting with DDT in 1972, most of these agents have been banned in the United States and many other countries. Most organochlorines have long-lasting environmental effects and concentrate in certain species. In addition, the high lipid solubility of these compounds results in prolonged half-lives in humans. Lindane (the gamma isomer of benzene hexachloride) is still used topically for control of ticks, scabies, and lice in human and veterinary medications and is also used as a general garden insecticide.

Chlorinated Hydrocarbon Pesticides

COMPOUND	TOXICITY	STATUS
Endrin	High	Banned in the U.S.
Aldrin	High	Banned in the U.S.
Endosulfan	High	Banned in the U.S.
Dieldrin	High	Banned in the U.S.
Chlordane	Moderate	Banned in the U.S.
DDT (dichlorodiphenyltrichloroethane)	Moderate	Banned in the U.S.
Heptachlor	Moderate	Banned in the U.S.
Kepone (chlordecone)	Moderate	Banned in the U.S.
Lindane	Moderate	Wide use
Mirex	Moderate	Banned in the U.S.
Toxaphene	Moderate	Limited or restricted use
Ethylan	Low	Limited or restricted use
Hexachlorobenzene	Low	Banned in the U.S.
Methoxychlor	Low	Limited or restricted use

2. What is the clinical toxicity of chlorinated hydrocarbon pesticides?

Toxic doses of chlorinated pesticides vary even though symptoms are similar. Because lindane is still widely used, it will serve as the class prototype. Medical formulations of lindane are usually a 1% concentration as a cream, shampoo, or lotion. Lindane crosses the placental barrier, into breast milk, and into the brain. It is concentrated in fat. Lindane is well absorbed by inhalation and ingestion. It is less well absorbed dermally unless skin contact is prolonged, the surface area is large, or the skin is damaged. Lindane is metabolized by the liver and removed in the feces, urine, and breast milk. Fatal doses in adults range from 10 to 48 gm. Seizures have been reported after ingestion of 1.6–392 gm and after some extensive dermal applications. After topical exposure, peak levels are seen in 6 hours with a half-life of about 48 hours. The mechanism of neurotoxicity is most likely from blockade of gamma aminobutyric acid (GABA) mediation of neural chloride ion uptake associated with barbiturate and benzodiazepine receptors. The loss of inhibitory effect leads to neurotoxic symptoms, including apprehension, irritability, confusion, dizziness, tremors, paresthesias, coma, and seizures. Respiratory failure, arrhythmias, vomiting, hepatic damage, renal compromise, agranulocytosis, and aplastic anemia have all been reported after large lindane exposures. Aspiration can cause cough, wheezing, and rales, usually from the hydrocarbon vehicle. From 1985 to 1990, over 20,000 poisonings and 6 deaths were reported from chlorinated hydrocarbons in the U.S.

3. How are chlorinated hydrocarbon pesticide poisonings treated?

Treatment of lindane poisoning begins with decontamination of skin with soap and water and removal of contaminated clothing. Gastric lavage and activated charcoal should be considered for ingestions. Symptomatic and supportive care is indicated for respiratory, renal, and hepatic failure. Arrhythmias from the myocardial irritant effect of chlorinated hydrocarbon pesticides can be treated with intravenous lidocaine or beta-receptor antagonists. Seizures should be controlled with benzodiazepines (diazepam or lorazepam) or barbiturates such as phenobarbital. Daily oral mineral oil can be used to reduce fat levels of lindane, and oral cholestyramine can reduce the toxicity of the persistent organochlorine pesticide chlordecone.

4. Is there a difference between pyrethrins and pyrethroids?

The insecticide pyrethrum is derived from the ground, dried flowers of *Chrysanthemum cineriifolium*. Pyrethrum is made up of six active chemicals called pyrethrins. Pyrethroids are synthetic derivatives of these compounds developed because of the relatively high cost, high biodegradability, and light instability of natural pyrethrum. The pyrethroids are divided into two functional toxicity classes. Allethrin, permethrin, and cismethrin are examples of type I pyrethroids, and type II pyrethroids include fenvalerate, deltamethrin, and cypermethrin. Products using both pyrethrins and pyrethroids are usually combined with synergistic compounds such as piperonyl butoxide and *n*-octyl bicycloheptane dicarboximide to inhibit enzymatic degradation of the pyrethroids in insects. The mixed function oxidase metabolism in humans of pyrethrins and pyrethroids can also be affected by these additives. Many commercial household pesticide products include organophosphate or carbamate pesticides along with pyrethrins and pyrethroids. The pyrethrins or pyrethroids provide the rapid paralytic or "knockdown" effect of household pesticides on flying insects, whereas the longer acting carbamate or organophosphate pesticides ensure lethality.

Synthetic Pyrethroids

Allethrin	Cypermethrin	Furamethrin
Barthrin	Decamethrin	Permethrin
Bioallethrin	Deltamethrin	Phthaltrin
Bioresmethrin	Dimethrin	Resmethrin
Cismethrin	Fenothrin	Supermethrin
Cymethrin	Fenvalerate	Tetramethrin

Type I pyrethrins cause repetitive nerve axon discharge in insects by delaying sodium channel inactivation. Type II pyrethroids cause an even longer prolongation of the sodium influx along the axon leading to persistent nerve depolarization and blockage of axonal conduction. The type II pyrethroids also may block inhibitory pathways through binding and altering GABA receptor-mediated chloride channels. Pyrethrum and pyrethroids are available as sprays, liquids, and dusts, usually in a hydrocarbon vehicle. Little mammalian toxicity to these chemicals has been described. The synthetic pyrethroid permethrin is effective against mosquitoes, flies, ticks, and chiggers. It is poorly absorbed through the skin of mammals and is rapidly inactivated by ester hydrolysis. Unlike the pyrethrins, permethrin is resistant to degradation by heat, sun, and immersion in water. It can be applied to clothing or tents but not directly to skin.

5. What human toxicity can be seen after exposure to pyrethrins and pyrethroids?

Although these compounds can be absorbed across intact skin, intestinal mucosa, and the lungs, bioavailability is poor. Pyrethrins and pyrethroids are less toxic to mammals than most other classes of insecticides. The toxic dose is usually greater than 100–1000 mg/kg with lethal doses estimated to be 10–100 gm in humans. A death was reported in a man who ingested beans cooked in 10% cypermethrin. Hypersensitivity or allergic reactions and direct irritant effects are the most commonly reported symptoms. Natural pyrethrum, its pyrethrin derivatives, and particularly crude extracts contain dermal and respiratory allergens. Frequent effects include contact dermatitis, cough, rhinitis, and asthma. Pyrethrin-associated anaphylactic or anaphylactoid responses have been reported only rarely. The synthetic pyrethroids may have some direct irritant effects but are less allergenic than the crude extracts of pyrethrum. Corneal irritation has been reported after eye exposure. Ingestion of large amounts of pyrethrins or pyrethroids causes nausea, vomiting, diarrhea, and abdominal cramping. Vague neurologic effects have also been noted after large exposures. Massive type I pyrethroid (permethrin) exposures have demonstrated increasing limb tremors and body temperature. Large exposures to type II (deltamethrin) agents result in pronounced salivation, course whole body tremors, choreoathetosis, vomiting, diarrhea, seizures, and, in rare cases, death. One report of a young woman who ingested 750 mg (30 ml) of 2.5% deltamethrin described convulsions. A unique burning paresthesia has been seen after cutaneous exposure to the type II agent fenvalerate. Symptoms usually last between 12 and 18 hours. Paresthesias resulting from these chemicals are thought to be secondary to chemical activity on cutaneous sensory nerve endings. The toxicity seen after large-scale exposure to pyrethroid commercial pesticides is often complicated by the other synergistic chemicals and vehicles included in these products.

6. Describe the treatment for pyrethrin or pyrethroid toxicity.

The majority of pyrethroid and pyrethrin exposures are benign. Symptomatic and supportive measures may be required for bronchospasm and anaphylaxis. Decontamination of the eyes and the skin is suggested. Oral or topical antihistamine and corticosteroid administration can be used for pyrethrin-associated dermatitis. The cutaneous paresthesia associated with type II pyrethroid exposure is reported to be modulated by topical vitamin E oil preparations. In a large series of pyrethroid poisonings, 1 patient died and 8 patients became intoxicated from large doses of atropine administered for the salivation and tremors that were misdiagnosed as acute organophosphate poisoning. Benzodiazepines and barbiturates are effective in animal models in controlling pyrethroid-induced tremors and seizures.

7. What is DEET?

DEET is the 95% *m*-isomer of *N,N*-diethyl-3-methylbenzamide (diethyltoluamide). It is a colorless or amber liquid available in gels, impregnated towelettes, aerosol and pump sprays, creams, and lotions in concentrations between 5% and 100% as a broad-spectrum repellent effective against chiggers, fleas, ticks, biting flies and mosquitoes. A 35% slow-release DEET, polymer-based product is the repellent given to U.S. military personnel and is as effective as a 75% alcohol-based DEET preparation. Between 5% and 9% of an applied dose of DEET is absorbed through the skin, reaching peak blood levels in about 1–2 hours. The plasma half-life is 2.5 hours, with about 10–15% of each dose eliminated unchanged in the urine. DEET undergoes enterohepatic recirculation with hepatic oxidation by cytochrome P450 enzyme systems. DEET and its metabolites can be found in the urine for several weeks and in the skin and adipose tissue for several months after use.

8. What are the symptoms of DEET poisoning?

Excessive topical use of DEET has resulted in < 20 case reports of central nervous system toxicity marked by lethargy, confusion, acute manic psychosis, headaches, ataxia, tremors, encephalopathy, and convulsions. Oral ingestions of 50 ml or more of 50–90% DEET have resulted in seizures, hypotension, and coma within 1 hour followed by death in 3 of 6 patients. Bradycardia has also been noted after extensive topical DEET exposure. Allergic reactions leading to anaphylactic shock and death have been reported from DEET. In a series of more than 9000 cases of DEET exposure reported to poison control centers in the U.S., the most common symptoms were related to irritation when the compound was sprayed into the eyes. Urticaria, hemorrhagic bulla, contact dermatitis, conjunctivitis, and exacerbations of seborrhea and acne have been noted. DEET has a remarkably high degree of safety considering the millions of yearly exposures since it was patented by the U.S. Army in 1946.

9. How is DEET toxicity treated?

High concentrations and prolonged exposures to DEET products should be avoided, especially in infants and young children. Preventive application of DEET to the hands and fingers of infants and children will limit oral exposures. DEET should be applied only to the outside layer of clothing and to exposed skin. For oral ingestions, gastric lavage can be considered for early presentations, and activated charcoal can be administered once the airway is secure. Dermal exposure decontamination should include removing exposed clothing and washing the exposed skin with soap and water. Supportive, symptomatic care and controlling seizure activity with benzodiazepines or barbiturates are indicated. Specific treatment for cerebral edema including intracranial pressure monitoring should be considered in some encephalopathic patients.

10. *Extra credit:* What chemical can be synthesized in the laboratory but occurs naturally in the mineral sassolite and can be used as an herbicide, an insecticide, a flame retardant, and an antiseptic?

Boric acid.

11. *Extra credit:* It is believed that, some 2000 years ago, the ancient Chinese used the first insecticide for fleas. What plant source was used?

Powdered chrysanthemums.

BIBLIOGRAPHY

1. Cohn WJ, Boylan JJ, Blanke RV, et al: Treatment of chlordecone (Kepone) toxicity with cholestyramine. Results of a controlled clinical trial. N Engl J Med 398:243–248, 1978.
2. Fischer TF: Lindane toxicity in a 24-year-old woman. Ann Emerg Med 24:972–974, 1994.
3. Flannigan SA, Tucker SB: Variation in cutaneous sensation between synthetic pyrethroid insecticides. Contact Dermatitis 13:140–147, 1985.
4. Fradin MS: Mosquitoes and mosquito repellents: A clinician's guide. Ann Intern Med 128:931–940, 1998.
5. He F, Wang S, Liu L, et al: Clinical manifestations and diagnosis of acute pyrethroid poisoning. Arch Toxicol 63:54–58, 1989.
6. Insect repellents: Med Lett Drugs Ther 31:45–47, 1989 [published erratum appears in Med Lett Drugs Ther 31:68, 1989].
7. Klein Schwartz W, Smith GS: Agricultural and horticultural chemical poisonings: Mortality and morbidity in the United States. Ann Emerg Med 29:232–238, 1997.
8. Osimitz TG, Murphy JV: Neurological effects associated with use of the insect repellent *N,N*-diethyl-*m*-toluamide (DEET). J Toxicol Clin Toxicol 35:435–441, 1997.
9. Paton DL, Walker JS: Pyrethrin poisoning from commercial-strength flea and tick spray. Am J Emerg Med 6:232–235, 1988.
10. Schenker MD, Louie S, Mehler LN, et al: Pesticides. In Rom WN (ed): Environmental and Occupational Medicine, 3rd ed. Philadelphia, Lippincott-Raven, 1998, pp 1157–1172.
11. Telch J, Jarvis DA: Acute intoxication with lindane (gamma benzene hexachloride). Can Med Assoc J 126:662–663, 1982.
12. Tenenbein M: Severe toxic reactions and death following the ingestion of diethyltoluamide-containing insect repellents. JAMA 258:1509–1511, 1987.

47. RODENTICIDES

Chulathida Greethong, M.D.

1. By what mechanism do anticoagulants act as rodenticides?

Warfarins and "superwarfarins" alter the synthesis of coagulation factors in the liver by interfering with vitamin K-mediated gamma carboxylation of precursor coagulation factor proteins. The factors affected are II, VII, IX, and X. However, for the anticoagulation effect to become clinically evident, vitamin K stores in the body must be depleted. Once this occurs, factor VII, with the shortest half-life of 7 hours, will disappear most rapidly. For the prothrombin time (PT) to be affected, clotting factor levels must fall to less than 25% of their original values. This requires approximately two to three half-lives; thus, the earliest onset of anticoagulation may not be evident until 21 hours after exposure.

2. Describe the difference between warfarin and the so-called superwarfarin rodenticides.

Superwarfarins (brodifacoum, indanedione) are so named because they are designed to be effective against even warfarin-resistant rodents. Although their mechanism of action is identical to warfarin, superwarfarins can be lethal to rodents after just one dose as opposed to the estimated 21 days of feeding needed with warfarin. This occurs because superwarfarins have much higher lipid solubility and are more selectively concentrated in hepatic cells. In addition, superwarfarins have the ability to saturate hepatic enzymes at much lower serum levels, resulting in a half-life of 156 hours, compared with warfarin's plasma half-life of about 37 hours. Brodifacoum is, therefore, a more efficient rodenticide because it is able to exert its effect in smaller amounts and eliminate the need for frequent feedings.

3. What is the clinical course of accidental versus intentional ingestion of anticoagulant rodenticides?

Accidental ingestion of anticoagulant rodenticides usually involves children. Several reported cases and case series involving superwarfarin poisoning in children suggest that most victims remain asymptomatic and require no treatment. Coagulation profiles of these patients rarely become abnormal. An estimated 25 gm of 0.005% brodifacoum (one entire packet) is needed to produce appreciable changes in coagulation of a 10-kg child. However, most accidental childhood ingestions involve no more than one or two grains of rodent bait.

On the other hand, **intentional ingestion** of brodifacoum is associated with a much higher risk of complication, probably because of the greater dose ingested. Patients intentionally ingest brodifacoum for two main reasons: to simulate an illness in order to obtain medical attention (Munchausen's syndrome) and to attempt suicide. Most patients with deliberate superwarfarin ingestion have an abnormal PT, and a majority develop bleeding complications such as easy bruisability, epistaxis, hematuria, bloody stools, and intracranial hemorrhage.

4. How should patients with anticoagulant-rodenticide ingestion be evaluated?

For children with acute, accidental exposure, gastric decontamination is often unnecessary if less than a box of pellets has been ingested. Syrup of ipecac is recommended in children whose acute exposure is within 1 hour of their presentation, although this practice has recently been questioned.

Because anticoagulant rodenticides have a delayed onset of action, baseline coagulation studies often are not useful in determining the need for treatment. However, initial coagulation studies should be done if chronic ingestion cannot be ruled out. Measurement of the PT should be performed 24–36 hours after exposure to identify patients at risk for coagulopathy. Prophylactic vitamin K should not be given on the initial visit because it can prevent the natural decline of vitamin K and delay the onset of coagulopathy, which might lead to an incorrect assumption that the patient's coagulation was not affected by the ingestion. In addition, because of the long half-life of superwarfarin, its prolonged effect on the coagulation profile is unlikely to be eliminated merely by giving one or two doses of vitamin K.

In contrast to those with acute, unintentional ingestions, patients with deliberate anticoagulant poisoning are always presumed to be at risk for severe coagulopathy. Because these patients often do not seek medical care until many days after the acute ingestion, gastric emptying usually is not indicated. If they present within an hour or two of ingestion, activated charcoal can be of benefit, and a single dose should be administered if not contraindicated. These patients should be placed in an environment where they are protected from trauma and evaluated with coagulation studies every 12 hours for about 36 hours.

5. What is the treatment for anticoagulant-rodenticide ingestion?

The goal of therapy for anticoagulant-rodenticide ingestions is to reverse the coagulopathy and replace blood loss. Fresh frozen plasma is the treatment of choice when there is active bleeding. Vitamin K administration is required if long-term anticoagulation is anticipated.

Vitamin K_1 is the only form of vitamin K that should be used to reverse anticoagulant-induced prolongation of PT. Not only is this form more active, thus requiring a smaller dose, but it also works more rapidly than other vitamin K preparations (i.e., K_3 and K_4). Vitamin K can be given orally, subcutaneously, or intravenously (IV). IV administration of vitamin K is slightly faster than oral dosing at correcting a prolonged PT. However, the IV route is also associated with an increased risk of cardiorespiratory depression, possibly because of anaphylaxis or an anaphylactoid reaction. Therefore, its use should be reserved for cases when the oral route is not feasible and the required dose exceeds the maximum of 5 cc, which is the usual dose for subcutaneous administration.

6. How do patients become exposed to strychnine-containing rodenticides?

Strychnine is a tasteless, odorless crystal that is extremely bitter tasting in its powder form. It has been in use since the 16th century as a vermicide and rodenticide. Strychnine continues to be used today as a minor component of some cathartics and tonics available in health food stores. Strychnine exposure should be suspected in the following circumstances:

- Accidental ingestion of proprietary tonics by children
- Suicide attempts using a rodenticide or veterinary products
- Use of adulterated illicit drugs (e.g., cocaine, heroin)

Strychnine poisoning should also be considered in the differential diagnosis of patients who present with major motor seizure-like activity who otherwise appear awake and show no postictal phase.

After exposure, strychnine is absorbed rapidly from gastrointestinal (GI), intravenous, or nasal routes. Toxicity usually occurs promptly. Strychnine competes with the neurotransmitter glycine within the brain stem, spinal cord, and higher centers. Because glycine mediates polysynaptic inhibition, strychnine poisoning leads to an increase in motor neuron stimulation, an effect that predominates in the spinal cord.

7. What are the typical symptoms of strychnine ingestion?

The onset of symptoms usually begins within 15–30 minutes after ingestion or within 5 minutes of inhalation exposure. Symptoms include:

- Generalized hyperreflexia and hypersensitivity to stimuli
- Severe and recurring diffuse muscle contractions that last anywhere from 30 seconds to 2 minutes
- Opisthotonic posturing
- Jaw spasms
- Risus sardonicus ("sardonic smile"—a twisted stretching of the facial muscles into a grimace)
- Consciousness with clear sensorium until hypoxia supervenes

Complications from strychnine poisoning occur as the direct result of the duration and intensity of convulsion. Profound lactic acidosis, rhabdomyolysis, and hyperthermia have all been observed. Most deaths occur from respiratory muscle paralysis.

8. What is the treatment of strychnine poisoning?

Treatment of strychnine poisoning should focus on adequate oxygenation and ventilation of patients. Prophylactic intubation should be considered in significant acute ingestions, because fatalities most often result from respiratory compromise. Aggressive control of muscle activity is the key to successfully reduce other complications, such as rhabdomyolysis and acute renal failure. Diazepam and other benzodiazepines are used to provide sedation and reduce muscle spasms caused by external stimuli. Neuromuscular paralysis and assisted ventilation may be necessary for severe cases.

9. Name some sources of barium.

In addition to its use as a rodenticide, barium and its salts have uses in a variety of industries including the manufacture of ceramic glaze, glass, and dyeing of textiles. In insoluble salt, barium sulfate is not absorbed and is used extensively as a contrast material for radiologic procedures. Other barium salts are water soluble and are poisonous because of their conversion to barium chloride by stomach acid.

10. What is the mechanism of barium toxicity?

It is postulated that barium causes a reduction in K^+ efflux from cells. As a result, K^+ accumulates inside cells, leading to hyperpolarization, with associated depression of cardiac conduction and skeletal muscle weakness. Extracellular potassium depletion leads to the characteristic finding of profound systemic hypokalemia. Patients with barium poisoning present with a multitude of symptoms, including vomiting, diarrhea, and abdominal cramping. Barium also has direct stimulatory effects on skeletal and cardiac muscles, causing myoclonus, rigidity, and ventricular tachyarrhythmias. Muscle paralysis often follows, secondary to hypokalemia.

11. How is barium poisoning treated?

Many therapies for toxic barium ingestion have been postulated. Gastric lavage may be of benefit for recent ingestions. Oral administration of magnesium or sodium sulfate can precipitate ingested barium into the insoluble barium sulfate salt, thus preventing its absorption. However, the mainstay of therapy still remains the aggressive administration of potassium, which has been shown to improve cardiac, GI, and neurologic symptoms.

12. Vacor (*N*-3-pyridylmethyl-*N*-*p*-nitrophenyl urea or PNU), a highly effective rodenticide, was withdrawn from the market in 1979 because of its lethality to human. Why does Vacor poisoning continue to be reported each year?

Vacor was originally introduced to the U.S. market in 1975. It was promoted as an ideal rodenticide because it was believed that the LD_{50} for humans was much higher than that of rodents. In addition, because its mechanism of action was mediated through the interference of niacinamide metabolism, it was presumed that niacinamide could serve as an effective antidote should human or livestock poisoning occur. During its availability on the supermarket shelf as a rodenticide, numerous cases of accidental and intentional poisoning were reported. Patients who ingest Vacor develop elevated blood glucose and ketone levels resembling diabetic ketoacidosis (DKA) within a few hours. In addition, autonomic dysfunction follows, and patients develop severe postural hypotension, bladder atony, and GI hypomotility.

Because of the severe morbidity associated with its product, the manufacturer of Vacor voluntarily withdrew it from the market in 1979. However, there was no public recall, and Vacor continues to be available in older garages, as well as in other countries, resulting in sporadic cases of poisoning each year.

13. Is there an antidote for Vacor poisoning?

Yes and no. Niacinamide is an effective antidote and should be given to all patients with suspected Vacor ingestion. It can be given every 4 hours once exposure has been established, and the frequency should be increased to every 2 hours if the patient becomes symptomatic. Unfortunately, niacinamide is no longer commercially available in this country, and although nicotinic acid (niacin) had been recommended for use as a substitute, it is not as effective. The majority of Vacor-poisoned patients who develop DKA continue to require insulin replacement on a long-term basis.

14. What is the phosphide group of rodenticides? How do they cause toxicity?

The phosphide group of rodenticides includes zinc and aluminum phosphide. Use of these potent rodenticides has been severely restricted in the U.S. because of the potential for lethality. The most common route of phosphide intoxication is oral ingestion, but phosphide also can be inhaled as a dust or absorbed through broken skin. Toxicity of these agents is mediated by phosphine gas, which is generated when the phosphides come in contact with weak acids. The liberation of phosphine gas gives the rat bait its characteristic fish odor. This odor is exuded by the poisoned subject as well when phosphide comes in contact with gastric acid.

15. List the symptoms of phosphide rodenticides.

Early symptoms:	*Late symptoms:*
Fatigue	Shock
Nausea	Hypocalcemia
Cough	Pulmonary edema
Headache	Convulsion
Dizziness	Coma
Tachypnea (suggestive of more serious intoxication)	
Dyspnea (suggestive of more serious intoxication)	
Tremulousness	
Hypotension	
Fishy odor	

16. How is phosphide poisoning treated?

The treatment of phosphide poisoning includes gastric lavage, neutralization of stomach acids with sodium bicarbonate, and administration of activated charcoal (although its benefit in these cases is unknown). Induction of emesis with syrup of ipecac is discouraged because phosphides can cause direct esophageal irritation and burns. Cardiorespiratory support is of paramount importance in phosphide poisoning. This includes maintaining adequate perfusion and oxygenation as well as early endotracheal intubation and mechanical ventilation in the event of pulmonary edema.

Patients who die from phosphide poisoning succumb within the first 30 hours of presentation. Pulmonary edema and cardiovascular collapse are the two most common causes, both of which appear to result from direct effects of phosphine on end organs.

17. *Extra credit:* The classic toxic manifestation of this chemical, once used as a rodenticide, is hair loss. Name the chemical.

Thallium.

BIBLIOGRAPHY

1. Clarkson TW: Inorganic and organic pesticides. In Hayes WJ, Laws ER (eds): Handbook of Pesticide Toxicology. San Diego, Academic Press, 1991, pp 497–583.
2. Flomenbaum NE: Rodenticides. In Goldfrank LR, Flomenbaum NE, Lewin NA, et al (eds): Goldfrank's Toxicologic Emergencies, 6th ed. Stamford, CT, Appleton & Lange, 1998, pp 1459–1474.

3. Gallanosa AG, Spyker DA, Curnow RT: Diabetes mellitus associated with autonomic and peripheral neuropathy after Vacor rodenticide poisoning: A review. Clin Toxicol 18:441–449, 1981.
4. Johnson CH, Van Tassell VJ: Acute barium poisoning with respiratory failure and rhabdomyolysis. Ann Emerg Med 126:1138–1142, 1991.
5. Katona B, Wason S: Superwarfarin poisoning. J Emerg Med 7:627–631, 1989.
6. Kruse JA, Carlson RW: Fatal rodenticide poisoning with brodifacoum. Ann Emerg Med 21:331–336, 1992.
7. Mulkey JP, Oehme FW: A review of thallium toxicity. Vet Hum Toxicol 35:446–453, 1993.
8. Pelfrene AF: Synthetic organic rodenticides. In Hayes WJ, Laws ER (eds): Handbook of Pesticide Toxicology. San Diego, Academic Press, 1991, pp 497–583.
9. Pont A, Rubino JM, Bishop D, Peal R: Diabetes mellitus and neuropathy following Vacor ingestion in man. Intern Med 139:185–189, 1979.
10. Rodenberg HD, Chang CC, Watson WA: Zinc phosphide ingestion: A case report and review. Vet Human Toxicol 31:559–562, 1989.
11. Smith BA: Strychnine poisoning. J Emerg Med 8:321–325, 1990.

48. HERBICIDES

Thomas J. Ferguson, M.D., Ph.D., and Timothy E. Albertson, M.D., Ph.D.

1. What are herbicides?

By definition, herbicides are chemical compounds capable of killing or injuring plants. Herbicides may be classified by mechanism of action or chemical derivative. These chemicals are widely used in agriculture and account for approximately 60% of all pesticide sales in the United States. **Nonselective herbicides** affect all plants, whereas **selective herbicidal agents** are used against certain target weeds. **Contact herbicides** affect plant parts that are touched by the chemical. **Translocated herbicides** are absorbed by the plant and act at distant sites. Most significant herbicide exposures are related to intentional ingestion, although occupational exposures do occur during mixing or application accidents. The most common groups of herbicides are chlorophenoxyacetic acid derivatives (e.g., 2,4-dichlorophenoxyacetic acid, 2,4,5-trichlorophenoxyacetic acid), bipyridyl derivatives (e.g., paraquat, diquat), and glyphosate (e.g., Roundup). Less commonly used herbicides are benzonitrile derivatives (ioxynil, bromoxynil).

2. What are some examples of chlorophenoxy herbicides?

Chlorophenoxy herbicides are plant-growth regulators that are translocated by the plant and cause stimulation of abnormal growth and the ultimate demise of most broadleaf plants. The most common agents are 2,4-dichlorophenoxyacetic acid (2,4-D), 2,4,5-trichlorophenoxyacetic acid (2,4,5-T), and 2-methyl-4-chlorophenoxyacetic acid (MCPA).

3. How are patients likely to be exposed to chlorophenoxy herbicides?

The most common exposure is intentional ingestion. Despite widespread use and availability, human fatalities are rare. Absorption of these herbicides across intact skin is relatively minimal, and skin contamination can be removed effectively using soap and water. The chlorophenoxy herbicides degrade rapidly in the environment so contamination of water supplies has not been a major problem.

4. What is "agent orange"?

During the Vietnam conflict, over 11 million gallons of a mixture of 2,4-D and 2,4,5-T were applied to the jungle as a defoliant (Operation Ranchhand). It was later determined that the mixture was contaminated with low levels of dioxin (less than 50 µg/gm) during manufacture. Because dioxin has been associated with birth defects and cancer in animal studies, there was concern that the personnel handling or exposed to this mixture would experience adverse health effects. The epidemiologic studies of veterans from New Zealand, Australia, and the U.S. provided inconclusive evidence of health effects. Some studies demonstrated an increase in soft tissue sarcomas, but recent analysis has challenged those conclusions. Thus, despite claims of health effects attributed to exposure to dioxin-contaminated herbicides, various studies have provided inconclusive evidence that low-level exposure to dioxin caused long-term human health effects.

5. *Extra credit:* Where did agent orange get its colorful nickname?

It was derived from the color of the bands painted around the center of the 55-gallon drums that contained the herbicide.

6. Which acute health effects are expected following ingestion of chlorophenoxy herbicides?

These herbicides are typically mixtures, and stock solutions may have significant concentrations of petroleum distillates or other organic solvents. Therefore, ingestion of concentrated solutions of these herbicides likely will result in significant exposure to petroleum distillate as well as the chlorophenoxy compound. Acute oral ingestions have been reported to cause anorexia, mucous membrane irritation, gastrointestinal (GI) ulceration, nausea, vomiting, diarrhea, and fatigue. High-level exposure may uncouple oxidative phosphorylation, leading to pyrexia, tachycardia, hyperventilation, and severe agitation. Central nervous system (CNS) effects following massive ingestion include muscle fasciculation, ataxia, and coma. Demyelination of peripheral nerves has been reported.

7. What other health effects have been reported following exposures to chlorophenoxy herbicides?

Respiratory complaints and dermatitis have been reported among people who apply these herbicides. None of these herbicides is absorbed significantly across intact skin. Peripheral neuropathies have been reported following exposure in some cases.

8. How should acute exposures to chlorophenoxy herbicides be managed?

Most patients ingesting these products who are without CNS involvement may be managed conservatively. The risk of fatality or long-term sequelae is low. Activated charcoal and other absorptive agents (Fuller's Earth) have been recommended, but controlled studies are lacking. It is reasonable to obtain serum chemistries and an electrocardiogram (ECG) and closely follow mental and respiratory status. Remember that these herbicides may contain petroleum distillates or other organic solvents. Alkaline diuresis has been demonstrated to increase elimination of these weakly acidic compounds in noncontrolled studies. The use of hemodialysis and resin hemoperfusion for removal of 2,4-D in severe poisoning has been described, but these chemicals are rapidly cleared in the urine if renal function is normal.

9. Are the benzonitrile derivative herbicides (ioxynil and bromoxynil) toxic?

Yes. The principal toxic action of these compounds in humans is to uncouple oxidative phosphorylation. Exposure to these herbicides has been associated with fatalities secondary to cardiac arrest. Acute effects include excessive sweating, thirst, pyrexia, anxiety, tachycardia, and hyperventilation. Note that these chemicals may be contained in mixtures with chlorophenoxy herbicides.

10. What is the treatment for benzonitrile poisoning?

Benzonitrile ingestions require monitoring in an intensive care unit. Decontamination with activated charcoal is reasonable because it may diminish absorption. Hyperpyrexia should be monitored carefully and treated aggressively.

11. Describe the effects of glyphosate (Roundup) exposure.

Glyphosate, an isopropylamine derivative of the amino acid glycine, is used as a nonselective herbicide to control many grasses, broadleaf weeds, and other brush species. It is typically marketed as a 40% mixture of glyphosate and surfactant. It has skin-irritant properties that are likely related to the surfactant, and massive intentional ingestions of concentrated solutions of glyphosate have been associated with severe GI tract erosions and occasional deaths. Overall, the human toxicity of this product is much less than that of other herbicides.

12. What are paraquat and diquat?

Paraquat is a bipyridyl contact herbicide that is licensed for use in the U.S. only by certified pesticide applicators. Diquat is similar to paraquat in chemical characteristics but does not have the same human toxicity profile. Paraquat and diquat are often combined in commercial products, and some manufacturers have added colored dyes and emetics in an attempt to limit poisonings.

13. How do human poisonings secondary to bipyridyl derivatives occur?

Although some exposure may occur through contact with skin or mucous membranes, almost all fatalities have occurred following intentional ingestion. Chronic occupational exposure to paraquat does not appear to cause pulmonary toxicity.

14. What are the clinical consequences of paraquat ingestion?

Ingestion of concentrated solutions of paraquat is associated with severe GI symptoms including esophageal ulceration and upper GI tract bleeding and ulceration. Approximately 10% of an ingested dose is absorbed. Although approximately 90% of the absorbed dose of paraquat is eliminated within 24 hours, there is selective concentration in lung and renal tissue. Biochemical studies have demonstrated uptake of paraquat by alveolar cells, which then undergoes nicotinamide adenine dinucleotide phosphate (NADPH)–dependent reduction to produce a free radical capable of forming a reactive paraquat cation and reactive oxygen that ultimately contributes to cellular membrane damage. Thus, paraquat causes an acute alveolitis followed by an inflammatory response, collagen deposition, and ultimately lung fibrosis.

15. What are the degrees of paraquat intoxication?

Vale and associates have described three degrees of paraquat toxicity that are based on ingested dose:

GROUP	DESCRIPTION	CLINICAL MANIFESTATIONS	EXPECTED OUTCOME
I	Mild poisoning following ingestion of 20 mg/kg paraquat	Asymptomatic or vomiting and diarrhea	Full recovery
II	Moderate to severe poisoning following ingestion of 20–40 mg/kg	Diarrhea, vomiting, systemic toxicity, pulmonary fibrosis	Possible recovery, but death occurs in a majority of cases Death may be delayed for 2–3 weeks
III	Acute fulminant poisoning following ingestion of > 40 mg/kg	Marked ulceration of the oropharynx with multiorgan failure	Mortality typically within 24 hours and always within 1 week

16. How well is paraquat absorbed following an occupational exposure?

Paraquat is poorly absorbed across intact skin, but damage to the skin or prolonged skin contact could contribute to systemic absorption. Respiratory absorption is also poor because most aerosolized particles have a diameter larger than respirable size.

17. How should paraquat poisonings be managed?

Paraquat poisonings should always be managed as medical emergencies. Efforts should be made to obtain early endoscopy to determine the extent of GI tract injury. Gastric fluid and serum should be collected for determination of levels that may be prognostic of outcome. If ingestion occurred within 1 hour of initial evaluation, gastric lavage may be beneficial. Administration of absorptive agents such as activated charcoal or Fuller's Earth may be useful, because some reports indicate that paraquat may be deactivated after coming in contact with such absorptive materials. However, their use may complicate the ability to assess the upper GI tract by endoscopy. Hydration should be maintained, and renal and hepatic function followed closely. Avoidance of high-flow oxygen is probably reasonable because it accelerates oxidative lung damage from paraquat in animal models; nonetheless, this must be tempered to the need to treat hypoxia. Elimination enhancement using hemodialysis or hemoperfusion has been suggested, but paraquat disappears from the serum relatively rapidly after ingestion, making this endeavor of limited use except in unusual circumstances. Thus, supportive care and measures to ensure patient comfort are the mainstays of therapy.

18. If death from paraquat poisoning is secondary to respiratory failure, why not perform urgent lung transplantation?

Lung transplant has been suggested for treatment of respiratory failure following paraquat poisoning in patients with single organ failure. However, attempts at transplant demonstrated that the transplanted lung is at risk for injury from residual circulating paraquat. Of more promise is the development of paraquat-specific antibody preparations that, given early in the course of ingestion, could trap circulating paraquat before it could react in pulmonary tissue. Unfortunately, preliminary rodent studies have demonstrated limited usefulness of this therapy because of the volume of antibody needed to react with a typical human ingestion.

19. Is paraquat-treated marijuana dangerous?

Concern about the potential health effects of paraquat-treated marijuana was raised when marijuana fields were sprayed as part of a marijuana eradication program in Mexico. A subsequent study demonstrated that human toxicity was not likely because of the limited half-life of the chemical and its destruction by pyrolysis.

20. Is diquat as toxic as paraquat?

Diquat has similar properties to paraquat but does not selectively concentrate in lung tissue, so respiratory failure is much less likely. However, severe GI effects have been noted following diquat ingestion, and there are some reports of chronic neurologic effects in these patients.

21. Can diquat ingestion cause Parkinson's syndrome?

There has been at least one report of a persistent Parkinson's-like syndrome within a few days of exposure to diquat solution. It was postulated that this was related to the chemical similarity between diquat and 1-methyl-4-phenyl-1,2,3,6-tetrahydropyridine (MPTP), a "designer drug" that is known to cause Parkinson's symptoms from destruction of dopaminergic neurons.

22. *Extra credit:* The ingestion of what potent herbicide precludes treatment by the administration of oxygen?

Paraquat.

BIBLIOGRAPHY

1. Cooper JD: The Toronto Lung Transplant Group: Sequential bilateral lung transplantation for paraquat poisonings case report. J Thorac Cardiovasc Surg 89:734, 1985.
2. Dickey W, McAleer JJ, Callender ME: Delayed sudden death after ingestion of MCPP and ioxynil: An unusual presentation of hormonal weed killer intoxication. Postgrad Med J 64:681–682, 1988.
3. Durakovic Z, Durakovic A, Durakovic S, Ivanovic D: Poisoning with 2,4-dichlorophenoxyacetic acid treated by hemodialysis. Arch Toxicol 66:518–521, 1992.
4. Eriksson M, Hardell L, Adami HO: Exposure to dioxins as a risk factor for soft tissue sarcoma: A population-based case-control study. J Natl Cancer Inst 82:486–490, 1990.
5. Fingerhut MA, Halperin WE, Marlow DA, et al: Cancer mortality in workers exposed to 2,3,7,8-tetrachlorodibenzo-p-dioxin. N Engl J Med 324:212–218, 1991.
6. Flanagan RJ, Meredith TJ, Ruprah M, et al: Alkaline diuresis for acute poisoning with chlorophenoxy herbicides and ioxynil. Lancet 335:454–458, 1990.
7. Hampson ECFM, Pond SM: Failure of haemoperfusion and haemodialysis to prevent death in paraquat poisoning: A retrospective review of 42 patients. Med Toxicol Adverse Drug Exp 3:64–71, 1988.
8. Kline JN, Darden IL, Lohne E, Larson RK: Pulmonary function of San Joaquin Valley agricultural laborer with occupational paraquat exposure. Chest 98:65S, 1990.
9. Landrigan P, Powell K, James LM, Taylor PR: Paraquat and marijuana: Epidemiologic assessment. Am J Public Health 73:784–788, 1983.
10. Maibach HI: Irritation, sensitization, photoirritation and photosensitization assays with glyphosate herbicide. Contact Dermatitis 15:152–156, 1986.
11. Meredith T, Vale J: Treatment of paraquat poisoning in man: Methods to prevent absorption. Hum Toxicol 6:49–59, 1987.
12. Sechi GP, Agnetti V, Piredda M, et al: Acute and persistent parkinsonism after use of diquat. Neurology 42:261–263, 1992.
13. Vale JA, Meredith TJ, Buckley BM: Paraquat poisoning: Clinical features and immediate general management. Hum Toxicol 6:41–47, 1987.
14. Wright AF, Green TP, Daleyyat P, Smith LL: Monoclonal antibody does not protect mice from paraquat toxicity. Vet Human Toxicol 29(suppl 2):102, 1987.

XI. Gases

49. TEAR GAS AND PEPPER SPRAY

Stephen W. Munday, M.D., M.P.H., M.S.

1. What is tear gas and how is it used?

Tear gas, also known as crowd control, lacrimating, or harassing agents, is a chemically diverse group of compounds used to control violent or potentially violent individuals or groups.

2. How were these agents developed and selected?

Chemical agents have been used in war since ancient times when sulfur vapors were used to incapacitate an enemy. However, scientific study of these compounds only began just before World War I. At the same time that blistering agents and pulmonary toxicants (e.g., chlorine, phosgene, and nitrogen mustards and nerve gases) were being developed and used, less toxic but highly irritating agents were being produced. Although the use of chemical warfare has declined, law enforcement agencies have begun to use crowd control agents on rioters and dangerous individuals to avoid the use of potentially life-threatening force.

3. What chemicals are used as tear gas and what are their common toxicities?

Like nerve agents, lacrimating agents are sometimes identified by letters:

CA   bromobenzylcyanide
CS   *ortho*-chlorobenzylidenemalononitrile
CR   dibenoxapine
CN   2-chloroacetophenone
CNC   chloroacetophenone in chloroform
CNS   chloroacetophenone and chloropicrin in chloroform
Others include:
Bromoacetone
Benzyl bromide
Ethyl bromoacetate

These agents all share the ability to cause severe ocular and upper respiratory burning and discharge, blepharospasm, and, in some individuals, bronchospasm and shortness of breath. Some are also irritating to intact skin. Additional toxicity can occur from the agent's delivery system; for example, explosive shrapnel or pyrotechnics can cause injury and burns.

4. What are some unique features of the acute toxicities of CN and CS, the most commonly used agents?

CN is a highly lipid-soluble powder that is dissolved in an organic solvent (e.g., chloroform) to allow effective aerosol delivery. It has an estimated minimally tolerated airborne concentration of 0.3 mg-min/m^3 and an estimated LC$_{50}$ of 10,000 mg-min/m^3. It is the active ingredient in **Mace** and is generally delivered at a concentration of 0.9–1.2%. CN has caused many cases of contact dermatitis, some of them allergic, and has caused permanent corneal injury—although this is due in part to the explosive charge that delivers the chemical. Pulmonary edema can occur for up to 18 hours after a prolonged CN exposure; there have been at least six deaths due to acute respiratory failure associated with use of CN in confined spaces. However, these cases are complicated by extenuating circumstances such as concurrent illicit drug use or extreme physical agitation during the attempted takedown by law enforcement personnel.

CS was developed to be a more effective but less toxic lacrimating agent. It has a lower minimally tolerated dose of 0.004 mg-min/m^3 but a higher LC_{50} of 60,000 mg-min/m^3; therefore, it is often referred to as **super tear gas**. It is a white crystalline powder, delivered by grenade or by burning a mixture of the powder with fuel. CS causes less severe ocular toxicity than CN. Even though CS is more irritating to the skin than CN, it has not been reported to cause allergic contact dermatitis.

5. Are there populations who are more susceptible to the toxicity of CN and CS? Is there any chronic toxicity?

Although persons with cardiovascular disease might be more susceptible to these agents, other sensitive groups (e.g., asthmatics) have not been identified. There is no current evidence to suggest that chronic pulmonary disease occurs as a result of exposure. Although some assays suggest that these agents might be mutagenic, there is no evidence of increased risk of cancer in exposed people.

6. How is exposure to these agents treated?

Initial treatment should address the ABCs (airway, breathing, circulation). Decontamination should take place as soon as possible and simply requires removal of clothing and showering. The eyes should be irrigated, and local anesthetic may be necessary to allow adequate access. In addition, 5% $NaHCO_3$ can be used on the skin to decompose CN if necessary.

7. What is pepper spray and how is it used?

Pepper spray (oleoresin capsicum) is an oily extract of pepper plants of the genus *Capsicum*. This extract consists of a number of phenols known as capsaicinoids. Capsaicin (trans-8-methyl-*N*-vanilly-6-noneamide) and dihydrocapsaicin are the most potent capsaicinoids, and they constitute 80–90% of the total pepper spray mixture.

The extracts are used with a spraying device as a deterrent by law enforcement and corrections personnel to obviate the need for lethal force. Private citizens also use pepper spray for personal protection. The potency of specific sprays varies widely among manufacturers.

8. Can pepper spray be used to season food?

No! Although the substance in pepper spray is found in chili peppers, it can lead to severe gastroenteritis if consumed in excess.

9. What is the acute toxicity of pepper spray?

Capsaicin is a natural product contained in food that millions of people eat every day, whereas lacrimatory agents are actually synthesized compounds. Although this might seem favorable toxicologically, the most toxic substance known, botulism toxin, is also a natural product.

10. Compare and contrast pepper spray and lacrimating agents.

Like lacrimating agents, pepper spray causes chemical irritation of the eyes, mucous membranes, and intact skin; symptoms include burning and irritation. However, pepper spray is believed to cause pain by stimulating C fibers and nociceptors by release of substance P. This process leads to neurogenic inflammation with increasing vascular permeability, bronchoconstriction, mucous secretion, and neutrophil chemostasis. Repeated stimulation depletes the neurotransmitter and leads to tolerance and a decreased pain threshold. This has led to the topical use of capsaicin for pain relief. Unlike lacrimating agents, pepper spray does not cause corneal ulceration or skin damage.

11. Are there populations with increased sensitivity to pepper spray?

Pepper spray sensitivity (like that of lacrimating agents) does not appear to be increased in asthmatics. Acute pulmonary edema is extremely rare. Two cases have been reported in children: treatment for one child was delayed 4 hours after exposure, and the second occurred after a 1-month-old infant was accidentally sprayed in the face. Pulmonary edema following capsaicin exposure in adults has never been demonstrated. However, one reported death is possibly related to pepper spray. A man was sprayed 10–15 times by authorities attempting to subdue him, and postmortem analysis showed lung epithelial damage.

12. Does pepper spray have any chronic effects?

Although some in vivo tests on capsaicin have demonstrated mutagenicity, others have not. The doses required to induce mutagenicity were quite large and would not be expected to be applicable to human exposures. There are also conflicting data on tumor-promoting activity.

13. How is pepper spray exposure treated?

Treatment begins with the ABCs. Decontamination should take place as soon as possible in the form of removal of clothing and showering. The eyes should be irrigated copiously; local anesthetic can be applied as needed. Some patients report worsening of symptoms with irrigation and rubbing.

The use of Bioshield Chemical Agent Decontaminate (Roce Group, Inc., Chesaning, MI), a towelette product used to wipe the exposed part, successfully decontaminated 5 exposed adults in one report. Although the report noted immediate relief of symptoms upon use, clinical experience in more recent studies failed to show dramatic pain relief.

14. *Extra credit:* The term *tear gas* is really a misnomer. What is wrong with the term?

Tear gas is actually an aerosolized solid.

15. *Extra credit:* The first riot control agent, ethyl bromoacetate, was used in 1912. In what major European city was it used?

Paris, France.

BIBLIOGRAPHY

1. Beswick FW: Chemical agents used in riot control and warfare. Hum Toxicol 2:247–256, 1983.
2. Billmire DF, Vinocur C, Ginda M, et al: Pepper-spray–induced respiratory failure treated with extracorporeal membrane oxygenation. Pediatrics 98:961–963, 1996.
3. Busker RW, van Helden HPM: Toxicological evaluation of pepper spray as a possible weapon for the Dutch police force. Am J Forensic Med Pathol 19:309–316, 1998.
4. Chapman AJ, White C: Death resulting from lacrimatory agents: A case report. J Forensic Sci 23:527–530, 1978.
5. Danto BL: Medical problems and criteria regarding the use of tear gas by police. Am J Forensic Med Pathol 8:317–322, 1997.
6. Hu H, Fine J, Epstein P, et al: Tear gas: Harassing agent or toxic chemical weapon? JAMA 262:660–663, 1989.
7. Lee BH, Knopp R, Richardson ML: Treatment of exposure to chemical protection agents. Ann Emerg Med 13:123–124, 1984.
8. Leopold IH, Lieberman TW: Chemical injuries of the cornea. Fed Proc 30:92–95, 1971.
9. Miller RSL: Pepper spray exposure during a carjacking attempt: A case review. J Emerg Nursing 22:390–392, 1996.
10. Smith CG, Stopford W: Health hazards of pepper spray. N C Med J 60:268–273, 1999.
11. Steffee CH, Lantz PE, Flannagan LM, et al: Oleoresin capsicum (pepper) spray and "in-custody deaths." Am J Forensic Med Pathol 16:185–192, 1995.
12. Stewart CE, Sullivan JB: Military munitions and antipersonnel agents. In Sullivan JB, Krieger GR (eds): Hazardous Materials Toxicology: Clinical Principles of Environmental Health. Baltimore, Williams & Wilkins, 1992, pp 986–1014.
13. Vaca FE, Myers JH, Langdorf M: Delayed pulmonary edema and bronchospasm after accidental lacrimator exposure. Am J Emerg Med 11:402–405, 1996.
14. Wheeler H, MacLehose R, Euripidou E, Murray V: Surveillance into crowd control agents. Lancet 352:991–992, 1998.

50. SIMPLE ASPHYXIANTS AND PULMONARY IRRITANTS

Frederick Fung, M.D., M.S.

1. What are simple asphyxiants?

Simple asphyxiants are gases that are physiologically inert. In contrast, chemical asphyxiants such as carbon monoxide, hydrogen sulfide, and cyanide cause cellular hypoxia by altering oxygen-carrying capacity or causing biochemical changes in respiratory enzymes. Simple asphyxiants do not suppress or alter the physiologic functions or anatomic integrity of the living organism. They produce asphyxiation only when present in sufficiently high concentrations to lower the percent of the oxygen in inspired air. This results in a fall in oxygen saturation and inadequate oxygen delivery to tissues and cells.

2. What is the toxic pathophysiology of oxygen deficiency?

Normal atmospheric air contains about 21% oxygen, 78% nitrogen, 0.9% argon, and 0.04% carbon dioxide along with trace helium, xenon, krypton, radon, and hydrogen and varying concentrations of ozone, ammonia, and water vapor. Mammalian cells require oxygen for mitochondrial-based energy production. Asphyxiation simply refers to insufficient cellular oxygenation.

3. What are the common simple asphyxiants and the symptoms of asphyxiation?

Common simple asphyxiants include carbon dioxide, hydrogen, helium, methane, ethane, nitrogen, and inert gases. There are generally no symptoms associated with oxygen concentrations between 16% and 21% in the presence of simple asphyxiants. When the oxygen concentration decreases below 16%, tachypnea, tachycardia, and slight incoordination appear. When the oxygen concentration drops between 10% and 12%, emotional lability and exhaustion with minimal exertion occur. When the oxygen content is 6–10%, nausea, vomiting, lethargy, and unconsciousness results. Breathing air with less than 6% oxygen produces convulsions, apnea, and cardiac arrest. These symptoms occur more rapidly during exertion in an oxygen-deficient environment. The duration and severity of the symptoms also depend on the degree and duration of hypoxia and tissue injury.

4. What are the characteristics and exposure sources of simple asphyxiants?

1. **Carbon dioxide** (CO_2) is a colorless, odorless, slightly acid-tasting gas with a vapor density of 1.5. Inhaling CO_2 stimulates the respiratory center of the brain. At air levels of 2%, CO_2 causes an increase in tidal volume. At 5%, it produces an increase in minute ventilation. CO_2 is toxic as a simple asphyxiant but also can produce the clinical entity of **carbon dioxide narcosis** with symptoms of unconsciousness when inhaling concentrations that exceeds 10% for less than 1 minute. Sources of CO_2 include the end product of respiration by animals and humans, fermentation of carbohydrates, volcanic activities, combustion, dry ice, and **afterdamp**. Afterdamp is CO_2 gas resulting from the explosion of "firedamp" in mines. **Blackdamp**, which is also found in coal mines, is a simple asphyxiant containing 87% nitrogen and 13% CO_2. Because it is heavier than air, when large amounts of CO_2 are present, the CO_2 accumulates in the lowest lying area.

2. **Methane** (CH_4) is a member of the saturated aliphatic hydrocarbon series also known as **paraffins**. It is a colorless, odorless, tasteless, inflammable gas with a vapor density of 0.55. Methane emanates from decaying organic matter such as marshes ("marsh gas"). **Firedamp** is a combination of methane and air found in mines. Because methane is lighter than air, it accumulates in the upper region of an enclosed space. Therefore, losing consciousness and collapsing onto the floor may be therapeutic if the lower air contains no other contaminants and is better oxygenated.

3. **Nitrogen** (N_2) is a colorless, odorless gas that is toxic only when it displaces oxygen. N_2 bubbles are responsible for decompression sickness, although the gas itself has no toxic effects. Decompression sickness is due to the mechanical presence of nitrogen bubbles in tissues and blood vessels, which produces local ischemia.

5. Discuss pulmonary irritants and their toxic pathophysiology.

Pulmonary irritants are a diverse group of chemicals and gases. When inhaled, they result in mucous membrane irritation with nonspecific inflammation. The pathophysiology of injury from these agents varies from oxidation-reduction reactions (ozone, chlorine) to acid-base alterations (ammonia, hydrogen chloride, hydrogen fluoride). The degree and severity of injury produced by pulmonary irritants depend largely on the chemical's physical characteristics (particle size), concentration, and water solubility. Water solubility and concentration determine the location of injury. The pathogenesis involves a direct cytotoxic effect on mucosal cells. This is followed by a release of inflammatory mediators, increases in mucus production, and impairment in mucociliary clearance. When the clearance mechanism for pulmonary secretions is compromised, mucus retention increases the risk of secondary infections. Pathologically, in addition to inflammation, denudation of bronchial and alveolar epithelium and intravascular thrombosis can be seen. Highly water-soluble compounds such as ammonia and hydrogen chloride produce injury in the upper airways. Insoluble gases such as nitrogen dioxide and ozone enter into deeper lung tissues, causing alveolar injuries. These pulmonary irritants produce a chemical burn that results in rapid collection of fluid in the interstitial spaces and alveoli (pulmonary edema). Significant inflammation resulting from mucous membrane irritation may produce an increased susceptibility to nonspecific irritants and infections. Additionally, inflamed mucous membranes may create an enhanced route of absorption for other chemicals and gases.

6. What general health effects are caused by pulmonary irritants?

The upper airways extend from nose to larynx. This portion of the pulmonary system functions as an air-conditioning and filtration system. In addition, mucus produced by airway linings provides a scrubbing mechanism for water-soluble irritants. Odors of gases and chemicals are perceived by the olfactory nerve. Sensations of irritation are carried by the trigeminal nerve. Therefore, when an individual is exposed to pulmonary irritants, mucosal inflammation, sensory nerve irritation, increased mucus production, airway narrowing, and other nonspecific responses may occur. The reaction usually takes place within minutes to hours after the exposure. The degree of the immediate response can be modified, enhanced, or diminished by exposures that occur in the recent past or by preexisting underlying medical conditions. Nasal irritation produces a burning sensation in the nasal passages, nasal congestion, rhinorrhea, and sneezing. Pharyngeal irritation causes sore throat. Larynx irritation causes hoarseness and laryngeal edema. Coughing with chest tightness, chest pain, wheezing, and dyspnea may occur when irritants gain access to deeper lung tissues.

7. List the clinically important pulmonary irritants and their sources.

- **Acrolein**, a by-product of petroleum combustion, is used in the manufacturing of plastic, rubber, resin, and textiles.
- **Acrylonitrile** is used in manufacturing of synthetic fiber, acrylic resin, and fire retardants. Acrylonitrile may be metabolized in the liver to cyanide.
- **Ammonia** is used to make explosives, plastics, synthetic fibers, and petroleum products. It is also used as a refrigerant and fertilizer. Many household cleaners contain ammonia compounds.
- **Arsine** is generated during smelting and refining of petroleum products and is used as doping agent in electronic industry. In addition to irritation, it causes hemolysis and renal failure.
- **Carbon disulfide** is used in the manufacture of rayon and cellophane, electroplating, sulfur processing, and degreasing operations. Carbon disulfide can cause altered mentation and peripheral neuropathy.

- **Chlorine** is found in bleach, household cleaners, and swimming pools and is used in the manufacture of chlorinated compounds.
- **Formaldehyde** is used as a disinfectant, as an embalming agent, and in the paper and photography industry. Formaldehyde has been shown to produce allergic-type asthma.
- **Hydrogen chloride** is used in the production of chlorinated compounds and organic polymers. It also is used in the production of fertilizers, dye products, petroleum products, textiles, and rubber products.
- **Hydrogen fluoride** is used as an insecticide, bleaching agent, and fluoridating agent in drinking water and is used for glass polishing and etching and metal refining.
- **Hydrogen sulfide** is found in natural gas and is used in the paper industry and sewer and oil refining.
- **Metal fumes** are generated during welding, braising, alloy making, and foundry operations. Exposure to metal fumes may cause metal fume fever with flu-like symptoms.
- **Nitrogen oxides** result from welding, farming, and fertilizing activities. Nitrogen oxides may produce a delayed onset of pulmonary edema, methemoglobinemia, and bronchiolitis obliterans.
- **Ozone** is generated in arc welding, sewage and water treatment, and laser and photocopying machines.
- **Phosgene** is used as an intermediary chemical for organic compounds such as isocyanates. It is formed by the interaction of ultraviolet light (arc welding) and vapors of chlorinated hydrocarbon solvents such as trichloroethane.
- **Phosphine** is formed when zinc phosphide, used as a rodenticide, reacts with water or acid.
- **Sulfur oxides** are used in bleaching and papermaking and are found as outdoor air pollutants.
- **Zinc chloride** is used in battery making, soldering, welding flux, and smoke screens.

8. Which common diseases are caused by pulmonary irritants?

The ability of a pulmonary irritant to produce pathology and disease depends on the chemical and physical properties of the agent, its water solubility, concentration, and duration of exposure. Because the target tissue of pulmonary irritants is the mucous membrane of the respiratory tract, chemical rhinitis and conjunctivitis occur initially upon exposure to these agents. With increasing concentrations in the environment and duration of exposure, chemical sinusitis and laryngitis may occur. With further exposure, symptoms can progress to chemical bronchitis, pneumonitis, and eventually pulmonary edema. The first clinical indication of impending pulmonary edema is usually progressive dyspnea and oxygen desaturation several hours after exposure.

9. List the four most commonly encountered pulmonary irritants and their toxic effects.

1. **Ammonia** is a colorless, alkaline, highly water-soluble gas. It has a characteristic pungent odor and is typically transported as a gas or liquid. It has an odor threshold between 40 and 50 ppm. Ammonia reacts rapidly with water on mucous membranes to form ammonium hydroxide, producing liquefaction necrosis. Low-dose exposure produces local irritation symptoms of the eyes and upper airways. High-dose and prolonged exposure may result in nausea, vomiting, hoarseness, cough, shortness of breath, and bronchospasm. Acute massive exposure can produce hemoptysis and adult respiratory distress syndrome. Residual effects of ammonia exposure include bronchiectasis with frequent infections and reactive airway dysfunction syndrome (RADS). There is currently no evidence that chronic, low-concentration ammonia exposure causes adverse health effects.

2. **Chlorine** is a greenish-yellow gas with a distinct odor. It is moderately soluble in water, with an odor threshold of around 3 ppm. Levels exceeding 25 ppm are regarded as immediately dangerous to life and health. Low-level chlorine exposure typically produces irritating symptoms in the eyes and upper airways. Additional exposure produces nasal, pharyngeal, and laryngeal inflammation. Severe exposure produces chemical bronchitis, pneumonitis, and pulmonary edema. Symptoms in massive exposure include coughing, chest pain, shortness of breath, and bronchial spasms. In general, if the patient recovers from an acute massive chlorine exposure, there are usually no significant long-term residuals.

3. **Hydrogen fluoride** is a colorless, nonflammable gas that forms hydrofluoric acid in aqueous solution. Inhaling hydrofluoric acid mist or vapor produces immediate onset of eye irritation, burning throat, headache, and shortness of breath. Objectively, there is a decrease in FEV_1 on spirometry, hypoxia, and hypocalcemia. Hypocalcemia may produce cardiac dysrhythmias. Other symptoms of respiratory tract irritation include hoarseness, epistaxis, laryngoedema, chemical bronchitis, pneumonitis, and pulmonary edema.

4. **Phosgene** is a colorless gas with a musty hay odor. It is heavier than air and is poorly water soluble. In addition to mild upper respiratory tract irritation, phosgene can cause delayed (24 hours) pulmonary edema.

10. What are the principles of evaluation and treatment for patients who have suffered pulmonary irritant exposure?

Most pulmonary irritants cause symptoms that are readily perceived by patients. As a natural protective behavior, the exposed individual will avoid further exposure by leaving the area (if possible). Most patients arrive at the health care facility conscious but with discomfort. If the patient is in acute distress, obtaining baseline tests such as arterial blood gases (ABG) and chest radiographs should follow an initial focused examination. Physical examination should center on mucous membranes such as the conjunctiva and nasal and oral cavities for evidence of erythema, edema, and discharge. Mucosal surfaces should be examined for evidence of chemical burns and soot. Respiratory examination should be performed to check for abnormal lung sounds such as wheezing and use of accessory muscles for breathing. The patient should be reevaluated periodically, preferably every 1–2 hours during the initial 4 hours. If there is evidence of clinical deterioration, additional tests such as serial ABG, carboxyhemoglobin, spirometry, electrocardiograms, and other pertinent laboratory studies may be needed. However, if the patient does not exhibit any respiratory distress and the clinical status is stable, observation for 4–6 hours should be adequate. Precautions and instructions for any delayed symptoms should be provided to the patient upon discharge from the health care facility.

In cases where exposure to water-soluble gases has occurred but the patient is not in acute distress, observation for 4–6 hours is sufficient. For exposure to water-insoluble gases, observation for 24 hours may be necessary. Treatment for acute pulmonary irritant exposure includes immediate removal from exposure, decontamination with simple water irrigation, vigorous bronchial hygiene measures, oxygen, bronchodilators, ventilator support, and other supportive measures for other organ systems (if indicated). The value of nebulized sodium bicarbonate, prophylactic steroids, and antibiotics has not been proven in double-blinded studies. Some authors recommend nebulized calcium solutions for hydrofluoric acid exposures.

11. What are the potential long-term health effects after acute pulmonary irritant exposure?

Survivors of acute pulmonary irritant exposure typically improve slowly over several weeks. The pathologic response of the lung to irritant gases ranges from an acute exudative phase to a subacute proliferation phase to a chronic fibrosing phase. Depending on the severity of the exposure, recurrence of pneumonitis may appear 2–3 weeks after the initial insult. After 3–4 weeks, most patients will undergo a gradual recovery, which may take up to 1–2 years. Most patients will recover without long-term residual effects. However, a small percentage of patients will suffer prolonged pulmonary function abnormalities, RADS, and, rarely, bronchiolitis obliterans. These individuals typically have underlying host factors or premorbid lung disease, such as asthma or atopy, or a history of cigarette smoking.

12. *Extra credit:* From December 3–5, 1930, meteorologic conditions in the Meuse River Valley promoted the concentration of factory smoke that resulted in 65 deaths. This was the first significant industrial air pollution disaster. Near what city and in what country did this toxic event occur?

Liege, Belgium.

13. *Extra credit:* **Because of its ability to cause rapid unconsciousness, this toxic gaseous compound is sometimes known as "knockdown gas"? Name this gas.**

Hydrogen sulfide.

14. What are the characteristics of RADS?

RADS is secondary to a massive, acute, high-level irritant exposure resulting in a nonallergic inflammatory response. Almost all pulmonary irritants are capable of inducing RADS. The symptoms and signs of RADS are similar to bronchial asthma. This condition develops without a preceding latent period and occurs shortly after the exposure. The physiologic manifestation of this syndrome is persistent nonspecific airway hyperreactivity. Typically, the individual does not have a history of atopy or asthma. Bronchial biopsy shows nonspecific airway inflammation without eosinophilia. The criteria for diagnosing RADS include:

- A high level exposure to a massive, typically accidental, concentration of irritant
- A rapid onset of symptoms (within minutes to hours)
- A nonspecific, inflammatory, nonallergic mechanism
- An unbroken train of illness (no "honeymoon" period between the immediate onset of symptoms and the disease)
- No other reasonable explanation for this disease, such as childhood asthma or significant underlying allergy

BIBLIOGRAPHY

1. Arwood R, Hammond J, Ward GG: Ammonia inhalation. J Trauma 25:444–447, 1985.
2. Blanc PD, Galbo M, Hiatt P, Olsen KR: Morbidity following acute irritant inhalation in a population-based study. JAMA 266:664–669, 1991.
3. Brooks SM, Weiss MA, Berstein IL: Reactive airways dysfunction syndrome (RADS). Persistent asthma syndrome after high level irritant exposure. Chest 88:376–384, 1985.
4. Finnegan MJ, Hodson ME: Prolonged hypoxemia following inhalation of hydrogen chloride vapor. Thorax 44:238–239, 1989.
5. Guidotti TL: An international registry for toxic inhalation and pulmonary edema: notes from work in progress. Int Arch Occup Environ Health 68:380–386, 1996.
6. Hedges JR, Morrissey WL: Acute chlorine gas exposure. J Am Coll Emerg Physicians 8:59–63, 1979.
7. Jones RN, Hughes JM, Glindmeyer H, Weill H: Lung function after acute chlorine exposure. Am Rev Respir Dis 134:1190–1195, 1986.
8. Moore BB, Sherman M: Chronic reactive airway disease following acute chlorine gas exposure in an asymptomatic atopic patient. Chest 100:855–856, 1991.
9. Robinson FR, Runnels LJ, Conrad DA, et al: Pathologic response of the lung to irritant gases. Vet Hum Toxicol 32:569–572, 1990.
10. Schwartz DA, Smith DD, Lakshminarayan S: The pulmonary sequelae associated with accidental inhalation of chlorine gas. Chest 97:820–825, 1990.
11. Substances for which proposed limits are based on avoidance of sensory irritation. Federal Register 29 CFR, Part 1910. Air Contaminants; Final Rule. Book 2:2434–2478, 1989.
12. Summer W, Haponik E: Inhalation of irritant gases. Clin Chest Med 2:273–287, 1981.
13. Wegman DH, Eisen EA: Acute irritants. More than a nuisance. Chest 97: 773–775, 1990.
14. Weiss SM, Lakshminarayan S: Acute inhalation injury. Clin Chest Med 15:103–116, 1994.
15. Wing JS, Sanderson LM, Brender JD, et al: Acute health effects in a community after a release of hydrofluoric acid. Arch Environ Health 46:155–160, 1991.

51. SMOKE INHALATION

Richard D. Gerkin, Jr., M.D.

1. What are the three mechanisms of injury in smoke inhalation?

1. **Asphyxiation.** Simple asphyxiants displace oxygen, such as nitrogen and methane, whereas tissue asphyxiants affect cellular metabolism, such as carbon monoxide, cyanide, and hydrogen sulfide.

2. **Thermal damage.** Thermal damage occurs from heat in gases, vapors, fumes, droplets, and particulates.

3. **Pulmonary irritation.** Pulmonary irritants injure tissue by direct contact due to alterations of pH, specific toxic effects, or nonspecific chemical reactions. Some examples of pulmonary irritants are ammonia, chlorine, acrolein, nitrogen dioxide, and phosgene.

2. List some of the main toxic products of combustion (TCPs).

PRODUCTS OF COMBUSTION	SOURCES
Acids/aldehydes	Cellulose acetate (film), cotton, paper, polystyrene, polyvinyl acetate, wood
Acrolein	Acrilan (carpet), acrylic, celluloid, cellulosics, polyolefins
Ammonia	Nylon, resins (melamine, phenolics), silk, wood
Carbon monoxide/dioxide	All organic material
Cyanide/hydrogen cyanide	Acrylonitrile, nylon, paper, polyurethane, nitrocellulose (film), resins, silk, wool
Halogen acids and gases (Br, F)	Halogenated hydrocarbon, films, resins, flame retardants/extinguishers
Isocyanates	Polyurethane
Nitrogen oxides	Celluloid, cellulose nitrate fabrics, paper, petroleum products, wood
Styrene	Polystyrene
Sulfur oxides/hydrogen sulfide	Hair, hides, meat, petroleum products, rubber, wool

From Linden CH: Smoke inhalation. In Harwood-Nuss A (ed): The Clinical Practice of Emergency Medicine, 2nd ed. Philadelphia, Lippincott-Raven, 1996, pp 1497-1500, with permission.

3. Which factors determine the site of deposition of TCPs and therefore site of injury?

Water solubility
Duration of exposure
Minute ventilation
Degree of adsorption to particulates (smoke)

Gases with high water solubility, such as acids, ammonia, and chlorine, tend to dissolve in the moisture of the upper airways. Those with lower solubility, such as aldehydes, isocyanates, phosgene, and oxides of nitrogen and sulfur, are deposited in smaller bronchi, bronchioles, and alveoli. As exposure lengthens, protective mechanisms such as breath-holding and laryngospasm play less of a role, and injury occurs more in the lower airways. Increasing minute ventilation and particulate adsorption (especially smaller size particles) add to lower airway damage.

4. Outline the basic steps in the evaluation of victims of smoke inhalation.

1. **History.** The nature of the exposure should be determined, including the length of exposure, the color of the smoke, whether it occurred in a confined space, and whether there was

steam (which is often associated with lower airway injury). Any recent use of alcohol or illicit drugs should be established.

    2. **Past history**. Past history of heart and lung disease affects the severity of injury and has implications for treatment.

    3. **Symptoms**. Loss of consciousness, chest pain, and respiratory difficulty are important symptoms.

    4. **Examination**. A trauma survey should be performed, vital signs should be assessed, and careful examination of mental status, skin, eyes, nose, pharynx, and chest should be done.

    5. **Other tests**. Arterial blood gas analysis (ABGs) or pulse oximetry, chest radiograph, and bedside spirometry help assess pulmonary status. An electrocardiogram (ECG) will detect some abnormalities relative to myocardial ischemia. A carboxyhemoglobin level gives some idea of exposure to carbon monoxide.

5. How can the physical examination help differentiate upper from lower airway injury?

Signs of upper airway injury:	*Signs of lower airway injury:*
Conjunctivitis	Carbonaceous sputum production
Lacrimation	Wheezing
Rhinitis	Rhonchi
Pharyngitis	Chest pain or burning
Dysphagia	Rales
Drooling	
Hoarseness	
Stridor	

6. What findings on examination are associated with a higher incidence of inhalation injury?

Burns over 15% of body surface area
Facial burns
Singed facial hair
Soot in the airways

7. Describe the role of pulse oximetry and carboxyhemoglobin determination.

Determining oxygen saturation using pulse oximetry is accurate in many instances. Unfortunately, if carboxyhemoglobin or methemoglobin is present, oxygen saturation may falsely be measured as normal because the abnormal hemoglobin is not carrying oxygen. Carboxyhemoglobin concentrations are helpful if they are significantly elevated but may be normal if measured later in the course of serious carbon monoxide poisoning.

8. What are the basic steps in treatment of smoke inhalation?

Decontamination should be performed if it has not already been done, and all patients should receive humidified oxygen. Inhaled beta agonists can be used for bronchospasm, and epinephrine should be given for stridor or respiratory distress. Fluid resuscitation should be instituted as needed for trauma or surface burns.

9. When should asymptomatic patients be observed and for how long?

Asymptomatic patients with any of the following features should be observed for at least 4 hours:
- Facial, oral, or nasal burns
- Increased carboxyhemoglobin level
- History of exposure to toxic fumes or exposure in a confined space

10. Are steroids and antibiotics useful in the treatment of smoke inhalation?

Systemic steroids can be used for refractory bronchospasm. However, they are not helpful and may be harmful when used for pulmonary parenchymal injury. Prophylactic antibiotics have not been shown to improve clinical outcome of inhalation injuries.

11. List the criteria for endotracheal intubation.

1. Decreased mental status
2. Laryngeal obstruction
3. Full-thickness burns of the face (nasolabial) or neck (circumferential)
4. $pO_2 < 60$
5. $pCO_2 > 50$

Recent reports have indicated that high-frequency percussive ventilation reduces morbidity from inhalation injury. Extracorporeal membrane oxygenation also has been used experimentally.

12. What is the correct way to use the cyanide antidote kit for smoke inhalation?

Cyanide poisoning, seen in 8% of fire victims, can complicate smoke inhalation and carbon monoxide poisoning. Signs of cyanide poisoning include coma, seizures, hypotension, and acidosis. Other concomitant conditions such as drug intoxication, hypovolemia, hypoxemia, carboxyhemoglobinemia, and methemoglobinemia may mimic cyanide toxicity. A serum lactate level > 10 mmol/L suggests a blood cyanide level of > 1 mg/ml.

The nitrites in the cyanide antidote kit, amyl nitrite and sodium nitrite, induce methemoglobin formation, which leads to preferential binding of cyanide to this nonoxygenated hemoglobin. Although this condition may help patients with cyanide poisoning, it is detrimental in concomitant carbon monoxide poisoning. The other component of the cyanide antidote kit, sodium thiosulfate, does not induce methemoglobin formation and may be used safely in these cases. Aggressive supportive care is needed to limit morbidity and mortality from severe cyanide poisoning.

13. What signs mandate hospital admission of a smoke-inhalation victim?

1. Decreased mental status
2. Respiratory symptoms (cough, tightness, dyspnea, hoarseness, wheezing)
3. History of coronary artery disease or chronic obstructive lung disease
4. Increased carboxyhemoglobin level
5. Carbonaceous sputum
6. Abnormal chest x-ray
7. Arteriovenous oxygen (AVO_2) difference > 100 mm
8. Bicarbonate level < 15
9. Confined space exposure > 10 minutes

14. *Extra credit:* In a famous hotel fire in 1980, 79 people died despite being far from the actual flames. Their deaths were due to inhalation of toxic smoke and fumes. What was the name of the hotel that burned?

The MGM Grand Hotel.

15. *Extra credit:* On October 30, 1938, CBS aired radio "reports" of a war waged with weapons that included a "poisonous black smoke" that was killing hundreds of innocent civilians. What war was being described?

Orson Welles' *The War of the Worlds* on *The Mercury Theater On the Air.*

BIBLIOGRAPHY

1. Barillo DJ, Goode R, Esch V: Cyanide poisoning in victims of fire: Analysis of 364 cases and review of the literature. J Burn Care Rehabil 15:46–57, 1994.
2. Clark WR: Smoke inhalation: Diagnosis and treatment. World J Surg 16:24–29, 1992.
3. Fitzpatrick JC, Cioffi WG Jr: Ventilatory support following burns and smoke-inhalation injury. Respir Care Clin North Am 3:21–49, 1997.
4. Linden CH: Smoke inhalation. In Harwood-Nuss A (ed): The Clinical Practice of Emergency Medicine, 2nd ed. Philadelphia, Lippincott-Raven, 1996, pp 1497–1500.
5. Morse LH, Pasternak G, Fujimoto G: Toxic hazards of firefighters. In Sullivan JB, Krieger GR (eds): Hazardous Materials Toxicology. Baltimore, Williams & Wilkins, 1992, pp 545–550.

6. O'Toole G, Peek G, Jaffe W, et al: Extracorporeal membrane oxygenation in the treatment of inhalation injuries. Burns 24:562–565, 1998.
7. Pruitt BA Jr, Cioffi WG: Diagnosis and treatment of smoke inhalation. J Intensive Care Med 10:117–127, 1995.
8. Wittram C, Kenny JB: The admission chest radiograph after acute inhalation injury and burns. Br J Radiol 67:751–754, 1994.

52. CARBON MONOXIDE

Kevin L. Wallace, M.D.

1. How common is carbon monoxide (CO) poisoning and how often is it fatal?

Of the 2,241,082 human exposures to drugs and chemicals reported to the American Association of Poison Control Centers in 1998, 17,480 involved CO poisoning; 31 resulted in fatal outcomes. A review of U.S. death certificates from the 9-year period between 1979 and 1988 revealed that CO exposure contributed to 56,133 deaths, roughly half of which were thought to be intentional.

2. What are some of the physical characteristics and reported sources and settings of CO exposure?

CO is a colorless, odorless gas—hence, its designation as a silent killer. It is the product of the incomplete combustion of an essentially limitless variety of carbon-containing compounds, including fuels burned for the production of heat, those used in internal combustion engines, and combustion products of structure fires. Peak incidence of human CO poisoning occurs during the fall and winter, roughly correlating with the use of space heaters. Intentional and unintentional exposure to CO in automotive exhaust and smoke from residential structure fires are other common causes of CO poisoning.

Methylene chloride, a solvent contained in paint stripping products, is a unique source of CO exposure. Production of CO occurs endogenously through hepatic metabolism of inhaled methylene chloride.

Sources and Settings of Toxic CO Exposure

- Smoke from burning organic materials (e.g., cigarettes)
- Faulty heating equipment (e.g., furnaces, space heaters, water heaters) using various fuels (e.g., wood, coal, oil, kerosene, propane, oil)
- Exhaust from internal combustion engines (e.g., gasoline, diesel, propane) used to power machinery (e.g., electric generators, automobiles, forklifts, ice rink resurfacing machines)
- Methylene chloride (e.g., paint stripper)

3. What are the major pathophysiologic mechanisms involved in CO poisoning?

CO exerts its pathologic effects through a number of different mechanisms. In susceptible tissues, these may include a combination of impaired O_2 delivery, O_2 utilization, and, possibly, oxidant stress injury. The high-affinity binding of CO to hemoglobin (200–250 times the affinity of oxygen for hemoglobin) results in (1) formation of carboxyhemoglobin (COHb), (2) displacement of oxygen from hemoglobin and lowered oxygen-carrying capacity, and (3) a leftward shift of the oxyhemoglobin dissociation curve. There is also evidence that CO binds to other heme-containing proteins, such as myoglobin and certain cytochromes, which play a critical role in meeting cellular energy requirements; it is unclear to what degree binding to proteins other than hemoglobin are clinically relevant. Recent experimental evidence suggests that relatively intense CO exposure can trigger a cascade of events, including brain lipid peroxidation, that leads to transient and irreversible neuronal dysfunction.

4. Describe the clinical features of acute carbon monoxide poisoning.

A high clinical index of suspicion is critical for diagnosing CO poisoning. Clinical presentations such as nonspecific viral complaints that occur during cold weather should prompt consideration of CO poisoning, especially when conditions such as widespread power outages occur secondary to damage from major storms. In addition, presentations involving multiple members from the same residential or work environment should raise suspicion about the potential sources and effects of CO exposure.

The clinical manifestations of CO poisoning depend on the magnitude and timing of exposure. Acute high-concentration exposure, such as might occur in a confined-space exposure to automobile exhaust, is more likely to result in severe toxicity (e.g., coma, seizures, cardiopulmonary arrest). More prolonged exposure at mildly or moderately elevated ambient levels of CO may lead to subtle symptoms. Patients with subacute and chronic CO poisoning caused by unrecognized heating system defects, for example, often present with nonspecific signs and symptoms such as headache, malaise, fatigue, and upper respiratory irritation. Often, these signs are overlooked by health care providers or are misdiagnosed as flu, occasionally with disastrous consequences.

In general, organs with relatively high metabolic demands, such as the brain and heart, are most sensitive to the effects of CO exposure. The severity and functional pattern of altered mental status in victims of CO poisoning ranges from almost undetectable behavioral changes to frank coma, depending on the intensity and duration of exposure. Clinical or electrocardiographic (ECG) evidence of myocardial dysfunction is more likely in individuals with underlying heart disease.

The table lists the clinical manifestations of acute exposure to CO at varying levels of intensity. Although cherry red skin and retinal hemorrhages have been described in severe cases of CO poisoning, they are not commonly seen in victims who survive to the point of health care facility presentation.

Initial Clinical Manifestations of Acute Carbon Monoxide Exposure

EXPOSURE INTENSITY	SYMPTOMS AND SIGNS
Mild	Headache, dizziness, weakness, nausea, malaise
Moderate	Confusion, lethargy, syncope, nystagmus, ataxia
Severe	Coma, seizures, pulmonary edema, myocardial infarction, cardiac arrest

5. What are the subacute clinical sequelae of CO exposure?

Persistent neurologic and myocardial dysfunction
Ischemic skin
Muscle and neural tissue injury resulting in bullous skin changes
Rhabdomyolysis
Peripheral neuropathy
Aspiration pneumonitis

6. What is CO-induced delayed neuropsychiatric syndrome (CO-DNS)?

Delayed-onset neurobehavioral dysfunction after apparent recovery from acute CO poisoning is the hallmark of CO-DNS. Onset occurs between several days and several weeks or even months following exposure. An estimated 10–30% of acute poisoning victims will develop CO-DNS. Clinical manifestations include decrements in cognitive function, personality changes, dementia, parkinsonism, and decerebrate rigidity. Most patients recover within 1 year.

7. How accurate and reliable are routine laboratory test findings in the diagnosis of CO poisoning?

The results of routine laboratory tests, including serum chemistries, hematologic assays, and arterial blood gas (ABG) determinations, are nonspecific indicators of CO poisoning and may actually mislead diagnostic efforts. Total hemoglobin and hematocrit are not affected to any significant extent by the presence of CO or COHb nor are the arterial blood concentrations of oxygen (PaO_2) or carbon dioxide ($PaCO_2$). An anion gap metabolic acidosis with elevated blood levels of lactate can occur with severe CO poisoning but is certainly not specific for this disorder.

Because blood gas analysis of the percentage of arterial blood oxygen-bound hemoglobin (SaO_2 or oxyhemoglobin) is commonly an indirect or calculated determination, it frequently fails to detect the decrease in actual SaO_2 that results from the high-affinity binding of CO to hemoglobin. Thus, routine blood gas determination of SaO_2 is often falsely elevated in victims of CO poisoning. Direct measurement of SaO_2 requires use of a blood gas cooximeter, which usually requires a special order and may not even be available at some health care facilities.

8. What is the value of measuring blood COHb levels in the evaluation and management of suspected CO poisoning?

Blood gas cooximetry not only provides a direct measurement of SaO_2, but also allows for the simultaneous direct measurement of blood levels of other hemoglobin species such as COHb and methemoglobin (metHb). If obtained within a short time of acute CO exposure, COHb levels correlate with severity of clinical intoxication. The sensitivity and prognostic value of COHb measurement is limited by a number of factors, including time delay and oxygen treatment after the patient is removed from the exposure. Cigarette smokers have CO levels in excess of 10% after recent direct exposure to tobacco smoke.

Repeat COHb-level determination in individuals with significantly elevated initial values may provide an objective means of assessing the effects of treatment, with a decline to normal levels (< 5%) serving as a targeted end point for therapy. Because there is no considerable difference in the affinity or degree of binding of CO to hemoglobin between arterial and venous blood, either specimen is suitable for COHb determination. The relative comfort and convenience of venipuncture over arterial blood collection make the former sampling method preferred in individuals who present with minimal to mild intoxication.

9. Is pulse oximetry useful in the diagnosis of CO poisoning?

No. Pulse oximetry fails to distinguish pathologic hemoglobin species (e.g., COHb and metHb) from oxyhemoglobin adequately. The value it provides for arterial blood oxyhemoglobin saturation frequently overestimates actual SaO_2 in the setting of significant CO intoxication or methemoglobinemia.

10. Are other diagnostic tests indicated in the evaluation of the victim of toxic CO exposure?

Most other tests, including electrophysiologic, radiologic, and neurobehavioral studies are of limited diagnostic sensitivity and specificity for CO poisoning. Plain-film radiography of the chest may reveal pulmonary edema and pulmonary aspiration. Other imaging modalities such as conventional computed tomography (CT), single photon emission CT (SPECT), and magnetic resonance imaging (MRI) of the brain may detect lesions of the globus pallidus and deep white matter regions in cases of severe CO poisoning. Many of these nonspecific, abnormal findings are detected late in the clinical course of CO poisoning and are of little value to its initial management. ECG often demonstrates evidence of myocardial ischemia or infarction; however, cardiac effects are more likely to occur in the moderate to severe CO-poisoned individual with underlying cardiac disease.

Formal tests of cognitive function (e.g., the Carbon Monoxide Neuropsychological Screening Battery), commonly referred to as psychometric tests, have been developed specifically for the assessment of suspected CO poisoning. These tests are sometimes employed in the acute and post-treatment assessment of CO-exposed patients. The usefulness of psychometric test results is limited by factors such as the lack of standardized, clinically validated testing methods, the absence of prior baseline test data, sources of test bias including the effect of repeated testing, and confounding factors such as sleep deprivation, drugs, alcohol, and major depressive illness. Therefore, the results of such testing are of limited diagnostic and prognostic value.

11. Who is at increased risk for mortality or morbidity from carbon monoxide toxicity?

- Individuals with underlying heart disease are at increased risk for CO-induced impairment of tissue oxygen delivery and use.

- Patients with chronic underlying pulmonary disease also may be at risk for more severe manifestations of toxicity.
- Pregnant women also warrant special consideration because the fetus exhibits a greater sensitivity to the harmful effects of CO. Fetal hemoglobin has a greater affinity for CO, causing prolonged and severe impairment in oxygen delivery to the hypoxia-sensitive fetal tissues.

12. What is the initial management of the CO poisoning victim?

Victims of CO poisoning should always be evaluated for other etiologies of altered consciousness, including toxicity from central nervous system (CNS) depressant agents such as ethanol or opioid analgesics, CNS infections, metabolic derangements, trauma, and cerebrovascular accidents. Initial management should include:

- Careful attention to the possibility of cervical spine injury
- Early evaluation and aggressive management of the upper airway
- Volume and electrolyte replacement as indicated
- Rapid blood glucose determination and supplemental dextrose administration, if needed
- Administration of naloxone and thiamine if history or examination indicates the possibility of opioid intoxication or thiamine deficiency
- The performance of other diagnostic testing such as chest x-ray, ECG, head CT, and lumbar puncture, as indicated by history or examination

13. Should patients be given oxygen?

As soon as possible after he or she is removed from exposure, the CO-poisoned victim should be placed on high-flow supplemental oxygen. This treatment decreases the circulating COHb half-life from 4–5 hours on room air to < 1 hour at an FiO_2 (fractional concentration of oxygen in inspired gas) of 100%. High-flow supplemental oxygen therapy should be continued until the COHb level falls to within the normal range. High-risk individuals may require longer treatment. Treatment of pregnant women with significant CO exposure should be continued well beyond the point where maternal COHb values return to normal, because the half-life of fetal COHb is longer than that of maternal COHb.

14. How does cyanide exposure affect treatment?

Cyanide (CN) exposure from the smoke of some burning materials such as polyurethane foam, nitrocellulose, and silk may complicate CO poisoning and cause early treatment failure with high-flow oxygen. If concomitant CO and CN toxicity is suspected, cautious use of the CN antidote kit may be warranted. CN-specific treatment should be limited to administration of sodium thiosulfate because nitrite-induced methemoglobinemia may impair tissue oxygen delivery further.

15. Name additional complications of CO poisoning.

Subsequent management of severe CO poisoning may require attention to complications such as:

Aspiration pneumonia
Adult respiratory distress syndrome
Myocardial infarction and congestive heart failure
Rhabdomyolysis and myoglobinuric renal tubular injury
Skin necrosis
Secondary infections

16. When is hyperbaric oxygen therapy (HBO) indicated in the management of CO poisoning?

Theoretically, tissue delivery of oxygen increases, and the half-life of COHb declines further, from an average of approximately 1 hour during treatment with 100% normobaric oxygen (NBO) to less than half an hour on 100% oxygen at 3 atmospheres of pressure. Improvement in clinical outcome after CO poisoning, including decline in mortality, enhanced recovery from acute effects, and decreased incidence of CO-DNS, has not yet been adequately demonstrated. Advocates of the liberal application of HBO often recommend this therapy for the loss of consciousness associated with CO exposure. Evidence for this therapy is largely anecdotal, with few reported side effects. Only a handful of clinical studies on human CO poisoning have incorporated design features such as randomization and blinded control intervention, and results from such trials are mixed. Health care providers must weigh the pros and cons of HBO therapy on a case-by-case basis. Although persistent severe neurologic dysfunction or fetal distress despite aggressive supportive care and NBO therapy might be compelling indications for HBO treatment, the efficacy of this therapy in less severe cases is much less clear. The length of time required for transfer of the patient to an institution with an HBO chamber and the hemodynamic stability of the patient must be factored into all treatment decisions.

17. When should CO-poisoned individuals be admitted to the hospital?
  • Persistent clinical signs and symptoms of poisoning despite oxygen therapy
  • Evidence of complications of CO poisoning such as ongoing myocardial ischemia
  • Other injuries (e.g., thermal burns) for which hospitalization is indicated
  • Suboptimal social disposition, including a high-risk environment for repeated exposure

18. What measures may prevent further occurrences of CO poisoning?
The diagnosis of CO poisoning should prompt investigation into the possibility of repeated exposure or other individuals who may be at risk. Local law enforcement, fire departments, and heating company personnel may assist in assessment of this risk.

Education regarding potential sources of CO, such as home heating and automotive engine exhaust systems, helps to prevent exposure. The proper installation and use of ambient CO detectors, especially those equipped with electronically activated alarm systems, may prevent serious, potentially life-threatening exposure to CO.

19. *Extra credit:* In 1929, a fire at the Cleveland Clinic precipitated the deaths of 97 workers from carbon monoxide and hydrogen cyanide intoxication and 26 delayed fatalities from fumes of nitrous oxides. What was the specific source of these toxic fumes?
The burning of 50,000 nitrocellulose x-ray films.

20. *Extra credit:* "I feel sick. My head is splitting. No, don't you see the dog is sick, too. We are both ill. It must be something we have eaten. It will pass away. Let us not bother them." On September 28, 1902, these were the final words of what famous French writer, who was to succumb to the effects of carbon monoxide poisoning from a faulty stove in his Paris apartment?
Emile Zola, as said to his wife.

BIBLIOGRAPHY

1. Cobb N, Etzel RA: Unintentional carbon monoxide-related deaths in the United States, 1979 through 1988. JAMA 266:659–663, 1991.
2. Hampson NB, Norkool DM: Carbon monoxide poisoning in children riding in the back of pickup trucks. JAMA 267:538–540, 1992.
3. Hampson NB: Pulse oximetry in severe carbon monoxide poisoning. Chest 114:1036–1041, 1998.
4. Hardy KR, Thom SR: Pathophysiology and treatment of carbon monoxide poisoning. Clin Toxicol 32:613–629, 1994.
5. Olson KR, Seger D: Hyperbaric oxygen for carbon monoxide poisoning: Does it really work? Ann Emerg Med 25:535–537, 1995.
6. Scheinkestel CD, Bailey M, Myles PS, et al: Hyperbaric or normobaric oxygen for acute carbon monoxide poisoning: A randomized, controlled clinical trial. Med J Aust 170:203–210, 1999.
7. Seger D, Welch L: Carbon monoxide controversies: Neuropsychologic testing, mechanism of toxicity, and hyperbaric oxygen. Ann Emerg Med 24:242–248, 1994.

8. Thom SR, Taber RL, Mendiguren II, et al: Delayed neuropsychologic sequelae after carbon monoxide poisoning: Prevention by treatment with hyperbaric oxygen. Ann Emerg Med 25:474–480, 1995.
9. Tibbles PM, Perrotta PL: Treatment of carbon monoxide poisoning: A critical review of human outcome studies comparing normobaric oxygen with hyperbaric oxygen. Ann Emerg Med 24:269–276, 1994.
10. Weaver LK: Carbon monoxide poisoning. Crit Care Clin 15:297–317, 1999.
11. Weaver LK: Hyperbaric oxygen in carbon monoxide poisoning: Conflicting evidence that it works. BMJ 319:1083–1084, 1999.

53. CYANIDE AND HYDROGEN SULFIDE

Lynn Bui, M.D.

1. What are the sources of cyanide exposure?

Cyanide ranks among the most potent poisons known. It is used as a reagent in numerous **industrial chemical processes** including electroplating, precious metal extraction, photography, laboratory analysis, and fumigation. Cyanide commonly exists in its salt forms: sodium cyanide, potassium cyanide, or calcium cyanide. Its gaseous state, HCN, is colorless and is released from the combustion of plastic, wool, silk, and many synthetic products.

Thousands of **botanical sources** of cyanide (e.g., amygdalin, cyanogenic glycosides) are known. The more commonly known ones are pits of apricots and peaches; seeds of apple, pear, plum, and cherry; bamboo sprouts; cassava; and various nuts (bitter almond, macadamia).

In the **medical setting**, sodium nitroprusside and *l*-mandelonitrile-β-glucuronic acid (Laetrile; an unproven antineoplastic agent) are potential sources of cyanide exposure. Each molecule of sodium nitroprusside releases five molecules of cyanide when metabolized. When nitroprusside is infused at a rate faster than recommended, accumulation of cyanide can result. When an intravenous form of Laetrile (containing amygdalin) is ingested, the intestinal enzyme β-D-glucosidase can metabolize it to cyanide, benzaldehyde, and glucose.

Another source of cyanide that is commonly overlooked is acetonitrile, a component of some **artificial-nail glue removers**.

2. How does cyanide exert its toxicity?

Cyanide is an inhibitor of many enzymes. The most well-studied is cytochrome oxidase. In mitochondria, cyanide binds reversibly to cytochrome oxidase at the cytochrome aa3 portion of the enzyme, inhibiting oxidative phosphorylation. This inhibition results in ineffective energy production. Cells revert to anaerobic metabolism and lactic acid builds up, resulting in metabolic acidosis. **Arteriolization of venous blood** (increased oxygen saturation in venous blood) occurs from the inability of tissues to extract and use oxygen.

Under normal physiologic conditions, trace amounts of cyanide are detoxified by binding to small amounts of normally existing methemoglobin, preventing cyanide from binding with cytochrome oxidase enzymes. Cyanomethemoglobin is removed by forming a thiocyanate complex through the action of rhodanese enzyme, a sulfur transferase. Thiocyanate is eliminated by renal excretion. When this system is overwhelmed by introduction of exogenous cyanide, toxicity results. Antidotes for cyanide attempt to magnify endogenous pathways by supplying necessary agents, methemoglobin, and sulfate donors.

3. What is a toxic dose of cyanide?

In an adult, a lethal oral dose of cyanide is about 200 mg. Cyanide contains compounds that have a faint odor of bitter almonds; however, up to 40% of the population lack the ability to smell this odor. For hydrogen cyanide, a detectable smell occurs at 0.2–5.0 ppm. The workplace limit is 4.7 ppm. Fatalities have been reported at levels as low as 150–200 ppm. Toxicity from ingestion of seeds containing cyanide has been reported but is thought to be possible only when seeds have been chewed. Though delayed, severe toxicity has occurred following the ingestion of artificial-nail glue remover.

4. Describe the clinical presentations of cyanide-toxic patients.

In the acute setting, the onset of symptoms can be rapid and profound. Central nervous system symptoms include headache, confusion, agitation, coma, and convulsions. Respiratory symptoms range from dyspnea and pulmonary edema to respiratory arrest. Cardiovascular effects can present initially as hypotension with reflex tachycardia, followed by bradycardia. If ingested, cyanide can cause severe abdominal pain with nausea and vomiting. In high-dose exposure, death can occur in minutes.

5. What are some of the laboratory findings in cyanide-poisoned patients?

Whole blood cyanide levels of 0.5–1.0 mg/L are considered toxic. In cigarette smokers, levels of up to 0.1 mg/L are often measured. In clinical practice, cyanide levels are rarely available in enough time to aid in diagnosing and managing a suspected case of cyanide toxicity. More often than not, clinicians rely on a suggestive history of exposure, coma, acidosis, and sudden collapse. Other laboratory tests that can be useful are arterial blood gas (ABG), electrolytes, lactic acid, carbon monoxide, and methemoglobin level.

6. Describe the antidote for cyanide poisoning.

Previously known as the Lilly kit, the cyanide antidote kit is now packaged by Taylor Pharmaceutical and contains two parts.

The first part includes nitrites to induce methemoglobin. Cyanide preferentially binds to methemoglobin over cytochrome oxidase enzymes; this frees the enzyme from inhibition and allows oxidative phosphorylation to resume. If intravenous access is not available, **amyl nitrite pearls** should be used. One or two pearls should be crushed in gauze and placed under the patient's nose, face mask, or endotracheal tube port for 30-second intervals each minute. Each pearl lasts for 2–3 minutes, and there are 12 pearls in a kit. Amyl nitrite can only induce a methemoglobin level of about 3%.

Once intravenous access is obtained, **sodium nitrite** should be used. Sodium nitrite can generate up to 14% methemoglobin. In adults, 300 mg of sodium nitrite (10 ml of 3% solution) is administered intravenously over 3–5 minutes. Peak methemoglobin levels should be reached 30 minutes after a dose of sodium nitrite. If there is no response, half of the original dose can be repeated. In children, care should be taken in dosing sodium nitrite. If the hemoglobin level is known, dosing is according to hemoglobin level (see Table). However, if clinically indicated, sodium nitrite should be given without waiting for a hemoglobin level. Empiric dosing for sodium nitrite in children ranges from 0.15 to 0.33 ml/kg to a maximum dose of 10 ml. If anemia is suspected, a lower dose can be given. As in adults, half the initial dose can be readministered if needed. Adverse affects of nitrites include potentially life-threatening levels of methemoglobin and hypotension.

Sodium Nitrate Dosing in Cyanide Poisoning

HEMOGLOBIN (gm/dl)	INITIAL DOSE (mg/kg)	INITIAL DOSE OF 3% SODIUM NITRITE (ml/kg)
7	5.8	0.19
8	6.6	0.22
9	7.5	0.25
10	8.3	0.27
11	9.1	0.3
12	10	0.33
13	10.8	0.36
14	11.6	0.39

The second part of the antidote kit is the sulfur donor, **thiosulfate**. Through the reaction catalyzed by rhodanese, thiosulfate binds with cyanide (from the cyanohemoglobin complex) to form a relatively nontoxic complex, thiocyanate, which is eliminated by renal excretion.

Thiosulfate should be infused immediately after sodium nitrite administration. In adults, 12.5 gm (50 ml of 25% solution) of thiosulfate is administered intravenously at 2.5–5.0 ml/min.

The pediatric dose is 400 mg/kg (1.6 ml/kg of 25% solution) up to 50 ml. If there is no response in 30 minutes, half the original dose can be given.

Experimental evidence suggests that other detoxification pathways might exist. There is evidence documenting the efficacy of nitrites in the absence of methemoglobin. It is postulated that nitrite is converted to or releases the potent vasodilator nitric oxide, a compound that may have some detoxification effect on cyanide.

7. When should the cyanide antidote be used?

In clinical practice, cyanide blood levels are rarely available in time for diagnosis. In most serious cases of cyanide poisoning, rapid and fatal clinical progression of patients occurs in minutes. Clinicians must rely on a suggestive history and clinical symptoms to dictate antidote use. In many cases, this is a difficult decision because the antidote itself is toxic and may jeopardize some already critically ill patients.

Because thiosulfate does not have some of the significant side effects of nitrites, it can be used alone, without nitrite, in cases of moderate clinical suspicion or in cases where the patient's oxygenation capacity is limited, such as in victims of structure fires. Thiosulfate has also been used concomitantly with sodium nitroprusside to avoid cyanide toxicity. For this indication, it is normally given in doses at 10 mg for every milligram of sodium nitroprusside infused.

8. What are other antidotes for cyanide toxicity?

In Europe, **4-methylaminophenol** (4-DMAP) is used instead of sodium nitrite. 4-DMAP produces a higher and more rapid formation of methemoglobin, with peak levels of up to 30% in 5 minutes.

Hydroxycobalamin is a synthetic form of vitamin B_{12}. It binds with cyanide to form nontoxic cyanocobalamin (another form of vitamin B_{12}). Because the required ratio of hydroxycobalamin to cyanide is 50:1 for complete neutralization, an impractically large dose of hydroxycobalamin is needed for most cases. Empiric dosing of 4 gm (50 mg/kg) of hydroxycobalamin is therefore recommended. In the U.S., hydroxycobalamin has not been approved by the Food and Drug Administration (FDA) for the treatment of cyanide toxicity. In Europe, hydroxycobalamin is available as a 2-gm/ml solution.

Dicobalt EDTA (Kelocyanor) is a cyanide chelator that only binds to cyanide in circulation. Its efficacy is questionable because it does not bind to intracellular cyanide.

Hyperbaric oxygen has also been reported anecdotally to successfully treat cyanide poisoning; however, other treatments such as nitrite and thiosulfate were administered concomitantly in these case reports. Therefore, hyperbaric oxygen should not take precedence over supportive care, normobaric oxygen, nitrite, and thiosulfate.

9. How should cyanide toxic patients be decontaminated?

Cyanide can be absorbed through many routes. When inhalation exposure is suspected, first responders must wear a self-contained breathing apparatus before entering the contaminated area to rescue victims. For dermal exposure, clothes should be removed and skin flushed with water. In oral ingestion, gastric lavage, when appropriate, and activated charcoal should be administered. Despite its low binding to charcoal (1:35 ratio), only 80 gm of charcoal is needed for optimal absorption of a potentially lethal oral cyanide dose of 200 mg.

10. What are some of the long-term sequelae of acute and chronic cyanide intoxication?

After recovery from an acute overdose, patients may develop permanent neurologic damage. The most commonly reported persistent clinical symptoms are similar to Parkinson's disease. The basal ganglia are thought to be the site of damage, but whether this injury is a direct result of cyanide or secondary to hypoxia is still debatable.

Subacute exposure to cyanide is involved in tobacco amblyopia and tropical ataxic neuropathy. Tobacco amblyopia is a gradual loss of vision in smokers. Cyanocobalamin and thiosulfate levels are low in these patients, thus implicating a relative deficiency in the detoxification pathway.

In some victims, cessation of smoking and treatment with hydroxycobalamin improve symptoms. Tropical ataxic neuropathy is a demyelinating disease endemic to some third-world populations, especially in certain parts of Africa where cassava is a main dietary component. An increased level of thiocyanate is found in these patients. Removal of cassava from their diet and administration of vitamin B_{12} seems to reverse most symptoms completely. In Leber hereditary optic atrophy, the insidious onset of visual loss is thought to occur in individuals with a deficiency in rhodanese. Smoking is hypothesized by some to be the inciting event in these patients; however, vision loss can also occur in individuals who do not smoke.

11. What are sources of hydrogen sulfide (HS) exposure?

HS is a colorless and highly toxic gas. It is produced from the decomposition of sulfur-containing organic materials found in sewage, gas wells, liquid manure, volcanoes, and sulfur hot springs. Industrial processes in petroleum refineries, synthetic rubber, leather making, and roofing asphalt also generate large amounts of HS as by-products.

12. Explain the mechanism of toxicity of HS.

Like cyanide, HS causes cellular hypoxia. It inhibits cytochrome oxidase at the cytochrome aa3 portion of the enzyme, blocking normal cellular respiration, which leads to metabolic acidosis. HS is also thought to enhance potassium-mediated hyperpolarization and other neuronal inhibitory mechanisms. HS is highly lipid soluble and is rapidly absorbed after inhalation, affecting brain stem respiratory centers and resulting in abrupt onset of unconsciousness. For this reason, it is known as a "knockdown gas."

13. What are toxic levels of HS?

HS LEVEL	CHARACTERISTIC
0.02–0.13 ppm	Signature rotten egg smell is detectable
10 ppm for an 8-hour shift	Average allowable workplace limit
50–100 ppm	Respiratory and cutaneous irritation
100–150 ppm	Olfactory paralysis
200–300 ppm	Pulmonary edema
> 700 ppm	Rapid death

14. How do HS-toxic patients present?

At low levels, irritant effects predominate. Symptoms include keratoconjunctivitis ("gas eyes") and upper airway irritation with coughing. At higher levels, systemic effects such as nausea, vomiting, confusion, headache, dizziness, and coma are seen. At very high levels, respiratory arrest leading to cardiovascular collapse and death can occur in minutes.

15. What are some clues for bedside diagnosis of HS exposure?

A history of rapid and profound onset of symptoms of cellular hypoxia and sudden collapse in a suggestive location may help. Patients may have a rotten egg smell. Finding blackened coins or blackened jewelry on the victim is a helpful clue. Because of the instability of HS in vitro, specific levels are not available. Other laboratory tests such as electrolytes, ABG, carbon monoxide, and methemoglobin levels may be useful.

16. How should patients with HS toxicity be managed?

Rescuers should wear a self-contained breathing apparatus before entering a contaminated area. Patients should be moved into fresh air immediately. Oxygen and supportive care should be given. Because the mechanism of toxicity of HS and cyanide is similar, the use of nitrites has been advocated. It has been hypothesized that methemoglobin may bind to sulfide to form sulfidehemoglobin, a less-toxic compound. The effectiveness of this practice is still not well supported. Although there are anecdotal reports of success in using hyperbaric oxygen to treat HS poisoning, there is no study demonstrating its efficacy.

17. *Extra credit:* **The 1997 novel by Frank Freudberg describes a man who, dying of cancer, plants hundreds of packages of cyanide-poisoned cigarettes in stores, offices, and restaurants around the country in order to discredit the tobacco industry. What is the title of this disturbing work?**

Gasp! A Novel of Revenge.

18. *Extra credit:* **What is unique about cyanide in space exploration?**

Cyanide was one of the first polyatomic molecules discovered in interstellar space.

BIBLIOGRAPHY

1. Abuye C, Kelbessa U, Wolde-Gebriel S: Health effects of cassava consumption in south Ethiopia. East Afr Med J 75:166–170, 1998.
2. Agency for Toxic Substances and Disease Registry: Cyanide toxicity. Am Fam Physician 48:107–114, 1993.
3. Ballantyne B: Artifacts in the definition of toxicity by cyanides and cyanogens. Fund Appl Toxicol 3:400–408, 1983.
4. Beauchamp RO Jr, Bus JS, Popp JA, et al: A critical review of the literature on hydrogen sulfide toxicity. Crit Rev Toxicol 13:25–97, 1984.
5. Gonzales S: Cyanide poisoning: Pathophysiology and current approaches to therapy. Int J Artificial Organs 12:347–355, 1989.
6. Gregorakos L, Dimopoulos G, Liberi S, Antipas G: Hydrogen sulfide poisoning: Management and complications. Angiology 46:1123–1131, 1995.
7. Johanning RJ: A retrospective study of sodium nitroprusside use and assessment of the potential risk of cyanide poisoning. Pharmacotherapy 15:773–777, 1995.
8. Rainey PM, Roberts WL: Diagnosis and misdiagnosis of poisoning with the cyanide precursor acetonitrile: Nail polish remover or nail glue remover? Am J Emerg Med 11:104–108, 1993.
9. Reiffenstein RJ, Hulbert WC, Roth SH: Toxicology of hydrogen sulfide. Annu Rev Pharmacol Toxicol 32:109–134, 1992.
10. Wilson J: Cyanide in human disease: A review of clinical and laboratory evidence. Fund Appl Toxicol 3:397–399, 1983.

XII. Food Poisoning

54. FOOD POISONING

John Alexis, M.D., and Andrea G. Carlson, M.D.

1. Which agent is responsible for the most reported cases of food-borne illness?

Bacterial contamination has remained the most common etiology of food-borne illness reported to the Centers for Disease Control and Prevention (CDC). Between 1993 and 1997, nearly 75% of bacterial food-borne illnesses were attributed to infection with *Salmonella* species. In 1996, the CDC instituted the Foodborne Diseases Active Surveillance Network (FoodNet) in selected geographic sites to determine more accurately the etiology of food-borne disease outbreaks. Under this new surveillance system, *Campylobacter* emerged as the number one cause of food-borne illness and remained the most common agent until 1999, when it was again outnumbered by *Salmonella* cases.

2. Contamination of which foodstuff results in the greatest number of reported cases of food-borne illness each year?

Despite concerns over meat and dairy products, the majority of cases of food-borne illness reported to the CDC in the last decade has been the result of contaminated fruits and vegetables. Pollution of farm ground water with human and animal sewage, incomplete composting, and inadequate washing of fruits and vegetables prior to consumption likely contribute to this phenomenon.

3. A 31-year-old teacher presents to the emergency department with sudden onset of vomiting, diarrhea, and diffuse abdominal cramps. Four hours before, she was at a picnic with her third-grade students. She denies having any fever or preceding symptoms. What is the likely etiology?

The patient most likely is suffering from a preformed toxin made by bacteria such as *Staphylococcus aureus* or *Bacillus cereus* (type I). Improper food storage is often responsible for poisonings caused by these agents.

S. aureus is associated with rich dairy products and other proteinaceous foods. As food sits at room temperature, the staphylococci grow and produce heat stable enterotoxins. Five enterotoxins (A, B, C, D, and E) have been identified. The foods usually have a normal taste and appearance. Onset of illness is usually < 6 hours after ingestion. Vomiting and diarrhea occur in > 75% of all cases. Fever is uncommon. The disease is usually self-limited, and antibiotics are not indicated.

B. cereus can cause both an emetic (type I) and a diarrheal (type II) syndrome. Onset of the emetic form occurs early, usually within 6 hours, and has been associated with the ingestion of fried rice. Patients suffering from the diarrheal form tend to develop symptoms as late as 12 hours after ingestion of contaminated meats or vegetables. In both cases, improper food storage allows spores to germinate and produce heat-labile toxins. As with *S. aureus*, the illness is generally self-limited and lasts < 24 hours.

4. A 27-year-old senior emergency medicine resident presents with diarrhea and abdominal cramps 12 hours after his last shift. He reports that, having no time to eat at work, he was famished and ate his 2-day-old tuna sandwich at the end of his shift. Which illness is a strong consideration?

Clostridium perfringens or *B. cereus* type II could cause this illness. Unlike *S. aureus*, enterotoxins from these bacteria are produced in the victim. Therefore, the incubation period is longer. Both vomiting and fever are uncommon. Antibiotics are generally not indicated.

5. A 44-year-old man presents to the emergency department complaining of diffuse, painful abdominal cramping, fever, and bloody diarrhea. His last meal was over 24 hours ago, and he currently has no appetite. What bacteria may be responsible for his symptoms?

Several types of enteroinvasive infections can cause this clinical presentation. Timing of symptom onset is a helpful clue. The etiologic agents to be considered are:

Salmonella species
Shigella species
Campylobacter species
Enteroinvasive *Escherichia coli*
Vibrio parahaemolyticus
Yersinia species

Invasion of the abdominal wall by the bacteria can be detected by presence of fecal leukocytes and blood in the stool. The illness typically lasts 2–7 days. The most common laboratory-confirmed bacterial causes of diarrhea are campylobacteriosis and salmonellosis, followed by shigellosis, *Escherichia coli* 0157, yersiniosis, listeriosis, and *Vibrio* species.

6. Outbreaks of *Campylobacter* enteritis are associated with which foods?

Unpasteurized milk and **raw or undercooked poultry** products often are colonized with *campylobacter*. Because the organism is heat labile, sufficient cooking prevents infection. Chlorination of water also helps prevent transmission. The incubation period ranges from 1 to 7 days. Symptoms are often protracted, lasting up to 5–6 days. In 25% of the cases, the infection presents only with vomiting. Antibiotics are often given to decrease the transmission of organisms; however, they do not eradicate the organism completely. Recent studies have shown that the use of ciprofloxacin or azithromycin does shorten the duration of symptoms.

A number of case reports have suggested an association between *Campylobacter* infection and the development of Guillain-Barré syndrome. Investigators speculate that an antibody made in response to the infection may attack peripheral neurons.

7. *Extra credit:* Who was Mary Mallon?

During the beginning of the twentieth century, several small outbreaks of typhoid fever were linked to households in the New York area, all of which employed a cook by the name of Mary Mallon. Although clearly aware that this awful disease followed her from job to job, Mary refused to acknowledge that she could be a carrier of typhoid. She changed employers frequently to evade authorities. In 1915, she was finally found at Sloan Maternity Hospital in New York, where she was working as a cook. A recent outbreak of typhoid at the hospital had led to her discovery.

Typhoid Mary, as the press named her, was placed under permanent quarantine on North Brother Island, where she spent the rest of her life. She died on November 11, 1938, after more than 23 years of isolation. In total, she passed the disease on to at least 51 people, 3 of whom died.

8. Which food item is most commonly associated with *Salmonella enteritidis* infection?

Exposure to *Salmonella enteritidis* most often results from ingestion of **raw or undercooked eggs**. Raw egg is an ingredient in many sauces, dressings, drinks, and desserts. Recent fascination with uncooked cookie dough and the time-honored tradition of "licking the bowl" after dessert preparation have been hampered by fear of exposure to salmonella. Less commonly, outbreaks may result from ingestion of unpasteurized milk.

Salmonella gastroenteritis is extremely common and is usually of the nontyphoidal species. It may present as acute diarrhea or as a systemic infection with central nervous system (CNS), bone, cardiac, or vascular involvement. Patients with sickle cell disease are at increased risk for serious infection.

Treating patients for uncomplicated salmonella enteritis has not proven to be beneficial. Early studies suggest that the carrier state might be prolonged, resulting in higher risk of bacteriologic and symptomatic relapse. There is also increasing resistance to ampicillin and trimethoprim-sulfamethoxazole (TMP-SMX). Immunocompromised individuals may benefit from treatment. Cephalosporins, azithromycin, and the fluoroquinolones are all reasonable treatment options for such patients.

9. The 45-year-old owner of a small neighborhood pet store presents with fever, abdominal cramping, and bloody diarrhea. Stool analysis reveals fecal leukocytes. Which bacteria is the most likely culprit?

Salmonella gastroenteritis has been reported with exposure to various animals, including turtles, iguanas, and chicks.

10. What are the intestinal and extraintestinal manifestations of *Yersinia enterocolitica*?

Yersinia typically affects children and young adults. It is rare in the United States and is more common in Northern Europe and Canada. Fever and diarrhea are common. Mesenteric adenitis secondary to the infection may mimic acute appendicitis. Vomiting is uncommon and occurs in < 40% of the cases. Along with the gastrointestinal effects, many extraintestinal effects occur such as fever, arthritis, pharyngitis, hepatitis, and rash. Transmission is usually from milk, raw pork products, and pets. There is very little evidence to support treating enteritis in the absence of systemic disease. Antibiotics such as the fluoroquinolones or cephalosporins are indicated for systemic disease. The infection may last from 1 day to 4 weeks.

11. Following several days of diarrhea, a young child is brought to the emergency department with fever, rash, lethargy, and anuria. Her parents report that the diarrhea has worsened today and is now bloody. You notice a purpuric rash over the lower extremities. What infection is likely?

The patient's symptoms suggest the development of **hemolytic-uremic syndrome** (HUS). Many types of bacterial gastroenteritis can cause this syndrome, but *E. coli* 0157:H7 is the agent most often implicated. Infected cattle are a common source of this bacterial strain. Incidence of infection peaks during the summer months. The Shiga-like toxin damages vascular endothelial cells of the gut, kidney, and CNS. Purpura, most commonly on the lower extremities, may be present. The illness develops following an 8–10-day incubation period and may last up to 2 weeks.

Laboratory findings include leukocytosis, microangiopathic hemolytic anemia, thrombocytopenia, uremia, renal insufficiency, and fecal leukocytes. Most hospital laboratories do not test for *E. coli* 0157:H7 as part of the stool culture unless specifically directed to do so. Although *E. coli* 0157:H7 is sensitive to a number of antibiotics, there is no clear evidence that treatment will shorten the duration of symptoms. In fact, antibiotic therapy has been shown to increase the risk of developing HUS.

12. Typically, which patients suffer from *Listeria monocytogenes*?

Listeriosis usually occurs in patients who are **immunocompromised**. Patients who are pregnant or have diabetes, malignancy, chronic renal failure, or HIV are at risk. Extraintestinal effects include severe headaches, muscle aches, and pharyngitis. In 1998, a large multistate outbreak of listeriosis was detected by the CDC's FoodNet surveillance system. The source of the outbreak has not been determined. During that year, 88% of reported *Listeria* infections resulted in hospitalization, and 12% of infected patients died. These deaths represented nearly 40% of all deaths from food-borne disease in 1998.

13. A 65-year-old-man presents to the emergency department complaining of a tingling tongue and loose, painful teeth. He adds that although he feels chilled, his skin seems hot, and the warm blanket the nurse provided feels freezing cold to him. He wonders if something was slipped into his food while dining out a few hours ago. Prior to calling psychiatry, you decide to consult the local poison center. What might they ask you?

They will probably want to know what he had for dinner. This patient is describing classic symptoms of ciguatera poisoning, the second most commonly reported fish-borne poisoning.

Ciguatoxin is found primarily in blue-green algae, protozoa, and free algae dinoflagellates. The toxin concentrates as it moves up the food chain from small, herbivorous fish to larger, carnivorous fish. Barracuda, sea bass, red snapper, grouper, amber jack, kingfish, parrotfish, and sturgeon fish are the most common carriers of ciguatoxin.

The toxin is heat stable, lipid soluble, odorless, and tasteless. Symptoms usually occur within 12 hours and involve gastrointestinal as well as neurologic symptoms. Other common symptoms are headaches, myalgias, tremors, ataxia, weakness, visual disturbances, and a metallic taste in the mouth. Seizures and vascular collapse may also occur. These symptoms are thought to result from impairment of the function of the sodium channels on nerve cell receptors.

Treatment is primarily supportive. Intravenous fluids and vasopressors may be necessary. Decontamination is essential. Activated charcoal and a cathartic should be given. Gastric lavage may be considered if ingestion is very recent. IV mannitol has also been reported to be of benefit.

14. Why is scombroid poisoning a misnomer?

Scombroid poisoning most commonly occurs after ingestion of nonscombroid fish such as mahi-mahi and amber jack. Scombroidea fish include large, dark-meat marine tuna, albacore, bonito, mackerel, and skipjack. As fish spoils, the histamine levels increase and approach 100 times normal within 12 hours of improper storage. Histamine is converted to saurine by bacteria that have the histidine decarboxylase enzyme. The agent responsible for symptoms is actually saurine.

Perioral and oral complaints are the most common followed by dysphagia, vomiting, abdominal pain, and diarrhea. The hallmark of scombroid poisoning is the development of facial and upper torso flushing following ingestion of the fish. Allergic-type symptoms are rare but can occur. Treatment includes parenteral antihistamines including both H_1- and H_2-receptor antagonists. Elevated histamine levels in fish can be confirmed if any uncooked fish remains.

15. What is tetrodon poisoning?

Tetrodon poisoning involves tetrodotoxin, which is produced primarily from the puffer-like fish: globefish, balloon fish, blowfish, and toadfish. The toxin is heat stable and concentrated in the skin, liver, intestine, and ovaries. The female fish is, therefore, the most poisonous. Neurotoxicity results from inhibition of the sodium-potassium pump. Symptoms occur within minutes and include headache and facial paresthesias. Dysphagia, dysarthria, and gastroenteritis follow. Ascending paralysis can occur. Mortality approaches 50%. Supportive care including protection of the airway is vital.

16. *Extra credit:* What is a fugu?

A fugu is a Japanese puffer fish that is incredibly toxic. The art of preparing the fugu involves rendering the fish nontoxic without losing the innate euphoric properties of the fish's flesh. Only specially licensed chefs prepare this delicacy.

17. Your friend has just returned from an oyster bar complaining of "floating sensations" and facial paresthesias. He quickly develops ataxia, weakness, and seizures. What has happened?

Your friend most likely has poisoning from saxitoxin. Saxitoxin is made by mollusks (clams, oysters, mussels, and scallops) that live in latitudes between 30° north and 30° south. The mollusks feed on the dinoflagellates *Gonyaulax catenella* and *Gonyaulax tamarensis*, which produce saxitoxin. These dinoflagellates cause the "red tide," and wildlife in the vicinity of a red tide may die. The toxin is heat stable and acts as a depolarizing blocker at the neuromuscular junction. Neurologic, cardiac, and gastrointestinal symptoms can occur. Symptoms usually abate in 24 hours. Gastrointestinal decontamination with gastric lavage and activated charcoal may help to remove the toxin. Less severe symptoms may be caused by *Gymnodinium breve*, which may present symptoms suggesting an allergic reaction.

BIBLIOGRAPHY

1. Altekruse S, Stern NJ, Fields PI, et al: *Campylobacter jejuni*: An emerging foodborne pathogen. Emerg Infect Dis 5:28–35, 1999.
2. Brooks J: The sad and tragic life of Typhoid Mary. Can Med Assoc J 154:915–916, 1996.
3. Centers for Disease Control and Prevention: Incidence of foodborne illnesses—FoodNet, 1997. MMWR 47:782–786, 1998.
4. Centers for Disease Control and Prevention: Incidence of foodborne illnesses: Preliminary data from the Foodborne Diseases Active Surveillance Network (FoodNet)—United States, 1998. MMWR 48:189–194, 1999.
5. Centers for Disease Control and Prevention: Preliminary FoodNet data on the incidence of foodborne illnesses—selected sites, United States, 1999. MMWR 49:201–205, 2000.
6. Chiu CH, Lin TY, Ou JT: A clinical trial comparing oral azithromycin, cefixime, and no antibiotics in the treatment of acute uncomplicated *Salmonella* enteritis in children. J Paediatr Child Health 35:372–374, 1999.
7. Doyle MP: *Escherichia coli* 0157:H7 and its significance in foods. Int J Food Microbiol 12:289–301, 1991.
8. McInerney J, Sahgal P, Vogel M, et al: Scombroid poisoning. Ann Emerg Med 28:235–238, 1996.
9. Mead PS, Slutsker L, Dietz V, et al: Food-related illness and death in the United States. Emerg Infect Dis 5:607–625, 1999.
10. Mines D, Stahmer S, Shepherd SM: Poisonings: Food, fish, shellfish. Emerg Med Clin North Am 15:157–177, 1997.
11. Olsen SJ, MacKinnon LC, Goulding JS, et al: Surveillance for foodborne-disease outbreaks—United States, 1993–1997. MMWR CDC Surveill Summ 49:1–62, 2000.
12. Tauxe RV, David L, James M: Foodborne disease. In Mandell GL, Bennett JE, Dolin R (eds): Principles and Practice of Infectious Disease, 5th ed. Philadelphia, Churchill Livingstone, 2000.

55. BOTULISM

Ilene B. Anderson, Pharm.D., Maerry L. Lee, M.D., and Timothy Erickson, M.D.

1. What is botulism?

Botulism is a paralytic infectious disease caused by a neurotoxin produced from the germination of *Clostridium botulinum* spores. It is characterized by muscle weakness that typically involves the head, neck, and chest muscles initially, commonly described as a descending paralysis. German physicians first recognized botulism in the late 18th century. Their patients developed an often fatal disease after eating spoiled sausage. The term *botulism* is derived from *botulus*, the Latin word for sausage.

2. What conditions favor *C. botulinum* spore germination and toxin production?

C. botulinum is an anaerobic, gram-positive bacterium found in soil, sea water, and air. It is spore-forming and, once ingested, can persist in the human body for a long time. The spores are dormant and highly resistant to damage. They can withstand boiling at 100°C for hours, but 30 minutes of moist heat at 120°C (e.g., pressure cooking) usually destroys them.

The botulinum toxin is produced after the botulinum spore germinates and begins cell growth. The neurotoxin (the causative agent) is released when the mature cell wall lyses. The neurotoxin is not as heat resilient as the spores and can be destroyed by heating to 80°C for 30 minutes or 100°C for 10 minutes.

3. What is the mechanism of action of botulinum toxin?

An enzyme associated with the toxin enables the toxin to cross the cell membrane and enter the presynaptic terminal. Once inside, the toxin prevents acetylcholine release from the presynaptic terminal. Synthesis and storage of acetylcholine is not affected. The result of this activity is flaccid paralysis. Anticholinesterase medications do not modulate the toxic effects of *C. botulinum* because the neurotransmitter is not available for cholinesterase breakdown in the postsynaptic space. The reduction in presynaptic function impairs cholinergic transmission at all acetylcholine-dependent synapses in the peripheral nervous system. Nerve function may be impaired for months until new nerve endings regenerate. There is no effect on the central nervous system or on axonal conduction.

4. What serologic types of *C. botulinum* are responsible for human disease?

There are seven different serologic types of *C. botulinum:* A–G. Types A, B, E, F, and G have been reported to cause illness in humans, whereas types C and D have only been shown to affect birds and nonprimate mammals. Types A, B, and E are the serologic types most frequently responsible for human disease.

5. What are the types of botulism?

1. **Food-borne** (classic). This is caused by ingestion of foods contaminated with the **preformed neurotoxin**.

2. **Infant botulism.** This is the most common type and is caused by ingestion of foods contaminated with the **spores** of *C. botulinum*. Disease occurs when the spores germinate and proliferate in the gastrointestinal (GI) tract, producing the neurotoxin.

3. **Wound botulism.** If wounds become contaminated with the spores of *C. botulinum*, the bacteria germinate and produce toxin that is absorbed systemically.

4. **Adult intestinal colonization.** This classification is undetermined but includes cases of botulism without a food or wound source that occur in patients who are older than 1 year.

6. What is the differential diagnosis for botulism?

Magnesium intoxication, aminoglycoside, and Eaton-Lambert syndrome are highest on the differential. Heavy metals, plants, mushrooms, common bacteria, viral infection, parasitic agents, anticholinergics, buckthorn, carbon monoxide, cerebrovascular accident (CVA), diphtheria, elapid (coral snake) envenomation, encephalitis, bacterial food poisoning, Guillain-Barré syndrome and the Miller-Fisher variant, inflammatory myelopathies, multiple sclerosis, myasthenia gravis, organophosphate, paralytic shellfish poisoning, poliomyelitis, tetanus, and tick bites should also be considered.

Selected Differential Diagnosis for Botulism

ILLNESS	KEY SYMPTOM DIFFERENCES	USEFUL DIAGNOSTIC TESTS
Anticholinergic poisoning	Altered sensorium, absence of paralysis, cranial nerves are intact	Physostigmine will reverse anticholinergic symptoms
Eaton-Lambert syndrome	Intact respiratory function, different EMG findings (post-tetanic facilitation)	EMG
Encephalitis	Altered sensorium, elevated CSF protein	Lumbar puncture
Guillain-Barré syndrome (Miller-Fisher variant)	Normal pupillary response, absent DTR, sensory paresthesias, elevated CSF protein	EMG, lumbar puncture
Guillain-Barré syndrome	Ascending paralysis, normal pupillary response, absent DTR, sensory paresthesias, elevated CSF protein	EMG, lumbar puncture
Myasthenia gravis	Exercise-induced muscle weakness	EMG, pronounced response to edrophonium (Tensilon) test
Paralytic shellfish poisoning	Paresthesias, altered mental status	
Cerebrovascular accident	Focal findings	CT scan or MRI
Tick-related paralysis (*Dermacentor andersoni, D. variabilis, Ixodes holocyclus*)	Ascending muscle paralysis, rigidity, cranial nerve defects are rare	Improvement with tick removal

DTR = deep tendon reflex; CSF = cerebrospinal fluid; EMG = electromyography

7. What laboratory tests should be ordered?

Every patient should have serum, stool, wound, and gastric aspirate specimens submitted for toxin assay and anaerobic culture. However, if these tests are negative, botulism has not been excluded.

8. How is the definitive diagnosis of botulism made?

A patient presents with a neurologic disorder manifested by a descending paralysis and at least one of the following:
- Typical electromyographic findings
- *C. botulinum* in stool or a wound
- Botulinum toxin in serum, stool, or implicated food samples
- A compatible clinical illness in a person who is epidemiologically linked to a laboratory-confirmed case

9. What is the life threat in botulism?

Respiratory compromise. The patient and all individuals suspected of exposure to the possible source should be admitted for airway management. With antitoxin and respiratory support, mortality has decreased from 60% to approximately 10–25%. Recovery is gradual over weeks to months.

10. What are the signs and symptoms of food-borne botulism?

Initial symptoms may occur as soon as 6 hours or up to 8 days later. The most common initial signs are gastrointestinal: nausea, vomiting, diarrhea, and abdominal distention. Patients also may present with neurologic findings caused by the cholinergic blockade, especially visual disturbances, dysarthria, dysphagia, and dry mouth. Progression of the disease leads to oculobulbar signs, descending paralysis, and progressive respiratory weakness, which leads to respiratory failure. Mental status, sensory exam, and reflexes usually remain normal.

11. What is the treatment for food-borne botulism toxicity?

1. Gastric decontamination to remove the spores and toxin from the gut
2. Activated charcoal. Gastric lavage and emesis should be reserved for patients with known ingestion of contaminated foods.
3. Antitoxin can prevent paralysis but does not affect already paralyzed muscles because the antitoxin only binds to free toxin. Antitoxin should be given to patients who are symptomatic and those who were exposed but are currently asymptomatic. The use of antitoxin must be weighed against the risk of serum sickness and anaphylaxis.

12. How can food-borne botulism be prevented?

Prevention of germination is accomplished by acidifying canned or bottled foods to a pH < 4.5. Foods that must have acidifying agents added to them include green beans, corn, beets, asparagus, chili peppers, mushrooms, spinach, figs, olives, and certain nonacidic tomatoes. Jams and jellies can be home-canned safely without a pressure cooker because their high sugar content will not support the growth of *C. botulinum.*

Common home-canning errors include failing to pressure cook and allowing food to putrefy at room temperature. Outbreaks are also associated with specialty foods such as chopped garlic in soy oil, fried lotus rhizome solid mustard, and uneviscerated salted fish.

13. How does infant botulism present?

Infant botulism occurs in children < 1 year (usually 1–3 months old) with normal birth history. Like adult botulism, the symptoms of infant botulism involve a descending muscle paralysis, but the early presentation of symptoms in infants may differ from the classic picture seen in adults. Early characteristics of infant botulism include constipation, hypotonia, listlessness, generalized weakness, and decreased sucking and swallowing reflexes. The cranial nerves can be affected early in the course, resulting in an expressionless face, feeble cry, ptosis, ophthalmoparesis, and poor head control. Infants are commonly described as having a floppy appearance. Some infants develop a sudden onset of symptoms that dramatically worsens over a period of hours; whereas, others decline gradually over several days until the illness becomes more clinically manifest.

14. What is differential diagnosis of infant botulism?

Dehydration
Failure to thrive
Hypotonia of unknown etiology
Sepsis
Viral syndrome

15. Describe the pathophysiology of infant botulism.

Infant botulism is due to the in vivo germination of botulism spores with subsequent toxin production, as opposed to food-borne variety where the preformed toxin is ingested. The infant

GI tract is a more hospitable location for proliferation because it is more alkaline, has a paucity of normal flora, and lacks mature mucosal immunologic defenses including lysozyme, complement, and secretory IgA.

16. How is infant botulism treated?

The bivalent and trivalent horse serum–derived antitoxin is not recommended for infants. It has no effect on the toxin-producing organisms in the gut, and it does not stop the progression of the syndrome. In addition, only very low levels of circulating toxin are found in the serum. However, a recent double-blind, clinical trial of botulism immune globulin (BIG) has shown promising results in the treatment of infant botulism. BIG is a human tissue–derived botulism immune globulin. It is currently available for use in cases of infant botulism and is pending U.S. Food and Drug Administration (FDA) approval. The role of antibiotics is unclear. Survival rate is high, but there is a risk of respiratory and feeding problems during the acute and recovery phases.

17. How does infant botulism differ from food-borne botulism?

Illness results from the ingestion of botulism spores, not toxin. The spores germinate in the GI tract and produce toxin in vivo that is absorbed systemically. The protective normal bacterial flora found in adults has not yet been established in the GI tract of this young population. In addition, these infants lack the bile acids found in adults that inhibit the growth of *C. botulinum* spores.

18. How can infant botulism be prevented?

Raw honey should never be given to infants. Objects and foods should be washed thoroughly before they are placed in an infants mouth.

19. What is the treatment for wound botulism?

Surgical debridement of the wound and intensive respiratory care. Penicillin has excellent in vitro efficacy against *C. botulinum*, but there is no evidence that antibiotics affect the disease course or outcome. Coincidental tetanus prophylaxis is essential. The benefit of botulism antitoxin has not been established. Mortality is approximately 10%.

20. How does wound botulism differ from both adult and infant food-borne botulism?

Wound botulism occurs when botulinum spores contaminate a wound site, germinate, and produce toxin in vivo. The toxin is then absorbed systemically, resulting in illness. Wound botulism has been reported with open fractures, dental abscesses, lacerations, puncture wounds, gunshot wounds, sinusitis, and, most commonly, following illicit injection of drugs of abuse. At the time of presentation, the wound itself may not be very impressive. The routes most commonly associated with this illness among injection drug users are intramuscular and subcutaneous ("skin popping") with a rare report following intranasal abuse.

GI symptoms of nausea and vomiting are usually absent in patients suffering from wound botulism. Fever may be present. The incubation period is generally longer (1–3 weeks) than in food-borne botulism because the toxin is being formed in vivo at the wound site rather than from ingestion of the preformed toxin.

21. Why is adult intestinal colonization botulism so unusual?

Intestinal colonization botulism is the rarest form of botulism reported. Like infant botulism, ingested spores germinate in the GI tract producing toxin in vivo. The toxin is absorbed systemically, causing illness. By definition, it occurs in persons who have no other documented wound or food source of botulism and are older than 1 year of age. This condition is unusual because the ingestion of spores is normally considered harmless in adults. However, in this population, spores have been shown to produce toxin in vivo that results in illness.

All reported cases of this disorder have had predisposing factors that altered the protective conditions normally present in the adult GI tract. Predisposing conditions include a history of GI surgery, decreased presence of gastric or bile acids, decreased gut motility, and alteration of GI bacterial flora following prolonged antimicrobial therapy. These conditions are presumed to allow spore germination and toxin production.

22. What is the role of the health department?

The local or state health departments or the Centers for Disease Control and Prevention (CDC) should be contacted immediately whenever the clinical diagnosis of botulism is suspected. Public health agencies can aid in the diagnosis, treatment, microbiological testing, and prevention of further cases of botulism. Typically, state health departments store and control the release of all available forms of botulism antitoxin (including BIG). Their laboratories conduct testing of all biological samples and all suspected food items. In addition, these agencies conduct an on-site investigation to collect potential food sources for testing and interview individuals who may have been exposed, referring any at-risk cases to medical care.

Regional poison control centers are important resources to contact when the clinical diagnosis of botulism is suspected. They can be instrumental in diagnosis, management of patients, and notification of public health agencies when indicated.

23. *Extra credit:* Emperor Leo VI of Byzantium (A.D. 886–911) forbade the eating of this food because of its potential harm to the people's health. Name this food.

Blood sausage, a notable source of botulism.

24. *Extra credit:* In 1990, the Food and Drug Administration approved the use of Oculinum (an injectable form of type A botulinum toxin) for the treatment of what medical conditions?

The eye muscle disorders strabismus and blepharospasm.

BIBLIOGRAPHY

1. Burningham MD, Walter FG, Mechem C, et al: Wound botulism. Ann Emerg Med 24:1184–1187, 1994.
2. California Department of Health Services: Botulism from fresh foods—California. MMWR 34:157, 1985.
3. Cherington M: Clinical spectrum of botulism. Muscle Nerve 21:701–710, 1998.
4. Li LY, Kelkar P, Exconde RE, et al: Adult-onset "infant" botulism: An unusual cause of weakness in the intensive care unit. Neurology 53:891, 1999.
5. Midura TF: Update: Infant botulism. Clin Microbiol Rev 9:119–125, 1996.
6. Mills DC, Arnon SS: The large intestine as the site of *Clostridium botulinum* colonization in human infant botulism. J Infect Dis 156:997–998, 1987.
7. Passaro DJ, Werner SB, McGee J, et al: Wound botulism associated with black tar heroin among injecting drug users. JAMA 279:859–863, 1998.
8. Schmidt RD, Schmidt TW: Infant botulism: A case series and review of the literature. J Emerg Med 10:713–718, 1992.
9. Shapiro RL, Hatheway C, Swerdlow DL: Botulism in the United States: A clinical and epidemiologic review. Ann Intern Med 129:221–228, 1998.

56. AIR AND WATER POLLUTION

*Richard J. Geller, M.D., M.P.H., Samuel Dorevitch, M.D.,
and David D. Gummin, M.D.*

1. What environmental interactions are responsible for air pollution?

Environmental air quality depends on a balance between production of pollutants and dispersion (the ability of the air to carry pollutants away). Production of pollution is both anthropogenic (human-caused) and natural, including biogenic and geogenic causes. Anthropogenic air pollution comes from transportation vehicles (approximately 56% by weight), stationary source fuel combustion (23%), industrial processes (12%), solid waste disposal (3%), and other causes (6%).

Factors that influence dispersion include topography, wind, air turbulence and atmospheric stability. Flat topography contains no barriers to wind and benefits from wind dispersion. Localities surrounded by mountain ranges, such as the Los Angeles basin and California's San Joaquin Valley, suffer from less-effective wind dispersion. Three-dimensional movement of air, called turbulence, is a positive influence on dispersion. Mechanical turbulence is produced by air moving past a fixed obstruction, such as a building or a varied landscape. Thermal turbulence results from air moving in response to atmospheric heating.

2. What are the constituents of polluted air?

Pollutants are classified as **gaseous** (90% of pollution by weight) or **particulate** (10%). Another classification important from a regulatory perspective is the distinction between **stationary** and **mobile** (vehicular) sources. Major categories of air pollutants are:

1. **Particulate matter**. Examples include smoke, fly ash, metallurgic dust and fumes, coal dust, cement dust, soil, pollen, and sea dust.

2. **Ozone**. Ozone at high altitudes (stratospheric ozone) absorbs harmful ultraviolet rays and infrared radiation. Depletion of the stratospheric ozone layer is thus a human health concern. Ozone at ground level (tropospheric ozone) can lead to adverse human health effects. It is produced in the atmosphere by a photochemical reaction between oxygen, hydrocarbons, oxides of nitrogen, and sunlight.

3. **Carbon oxides** (CO and CO_2)

4. **Hydrocarbons**. Multiple hydrocarbons are discharged into the atmosphere in the refining and use of petroleum products.

5. **Nitrogen oxides**. Oxides of nitrogen are formed when the heat generated in combustion processes combines N_2 and O_2. Nitrous oxide (N_2O) is a relatively nontoxic gas with anesthetic properties, but it can destroy stratospheric ozone and thus is a possible contributor to global warming. Nitric oxide (NO) is another relatively nontoxic gas that can destroy ozone. Nitrogen dioxide (NO_2) is an irritating gas and a potent oxidizer. It imparts a yellow-orange to brown color to air depending on concentration and is a major contributor to the appearance of "dirty air."

6. **Sulfur oxides** (SO_2 and SO_3; also referred to as SO_x). These are produced naturally from volcanoes and anthropogenically from burning of sulfur-containing fuel such as coal and petroleum. The combination of sulfur dioxide and water forms sulfuric acid ($SO_2 + H_2O = H_2SO_3$), a major cause of acid rain.

3. What does an ozone alert have to do with ozone depletion?

Nothing. These are two separate ozone issues. Ozone depletion refers to **stratospheric ozone** miles above the earth's surface. The depletion is due to chlorofluorocarbons (CFCs), which have been used in cooling systems and as aerosol spray propellants. Depletion of the stratospheric ozone layer has been documented by sampling and satellite imaging, and its depletion has resulted in increased ultraviolet-B exposure. Consequently, increased incidences of skin cancer and cataracts are expected.

An ozone alert warns of contaminated tropospheric ozone, the result of a photochemical reaction involving nitrogen oxides, hydrocarbon vapors, and sunlight. Primary sources of nitrogen oxides include motor vehicle exhaust and electrical power generation. Ozone causes respiratory tract irritation and bronchospasm and may cause respiratory tract malignancies.

4. What properties of air does one examine with respect to air pollution?

1. **pH**. In the United States, hydrogen ion atmospheric precipitation increases as one travels from west to east. Water has a pH of approximately 7.0 upon evaporation. Interacting with CO_2 in the air, cloud water has a natural pH of about 5.7. In the western U.S., rainfall pH is in the range of 5.0–6.0. As one travels east, rain pH drops below 5, with values of approximately 4.2 seen in the Ohio Valley and Pennsylvania. Acids are formed in the atmosphere from oxides of sulfur and nitrogen, with sulfuric acid accounting for approximately 65% of the acid and nitric acid 30%.

2. **Ozone level**. Ozone chemistry is a complicated interplay between sunlight, oxygen, oxides of nitrogen, and hydrocarbons, both halogenated and nonhalogenated.

3. **Temperature**. Temperature affects air quality of cities because the air over cities is warmer than surrounding rural air. The city air rises and is replaced by lower, colder air from surrounding locales. As a result, a dirty air mass tends to accumulate in the center of the heat island over the city, and is referred to as a "dust dome."

4. **Visibility**. Visibility refers to how far through the prevailing air objects can be clearly seen. Visibility is decreased by air pollution because light rays are absorbed or scattered by pollutants in various ways.

5. **Turbidity**. Whereas visibility is a function of horizontal light scattering, vertical light interference is referred to as turbidity.

5. How is air pollution measured?

Particle size is the critical consideration in the assessment of particulate pollution on health. In general, particles > 10 μm are eliminated by the upper respiratory tract. Particles < 10 μm are called **inhalable** because they can enter and be deposited in the respiratory system. Particles < 2.5 μm are called **respirable** because they can be deposited in lower respiratory tract tissue. The most common measure of air quality is called PM_{10}. PM_{10} is the weight of particles that are ≤ 10 μm collected from a standard volume of air passed through a filter over a 24-hour period. Particles > 10 μm are excluded from the collection process. Values are expressed in micrograms per cubic meter ($\mu g/m^3$).

Concentrations of gases such as CO, ozone, NO_x, SO_x, and hydrocarbons are measured using a variety of technologies and are reported in parts per million by volume (ppmv).

6. What air pollutants are most harmful to human health?

Not surprisingly, most of the clinical effects seen from polluted air are pulmonary in nature, with asthmatics especially effected. Of the hundreds of substances that contaminate air, only a few are present in sufficient quantity in ambient air to be established as definite concerns to human health. Thus, classical closed-space toxicological concerns about the gases that pollute air have limited applicability when assessing toxicologic risk to outdoor air exposure. The substances for which the U.S. Environmental Protection Agency (EPA) has promulgated National Ambient Air Quality Standards (NAAQS) include:

Carbon monoxide (CO). Most cases of acute CO poisoning result from closed-space inhalational exposures such as those in homes, campers, or buildings. However, epidemiologists report an increase in population deaths from coronary artery disease (CAD) during periods of increased outdoor ambient CO levels. Outdoor ambient air levels of CO vary in a range from 1 to approximately 140 ppm, with the high concentrations found in urban areas with heavy automobile density. The Occupational Safety and Health Administration (OSHA) permissible exposure limit (PEL) for carbon monoxide, as an 8-hour time-weighted average (TWA) is 50 ppm. The NAAQS is 35 ppm as a 1-hour average. Exposures above this are uncommon, and clinical acute CO poisoning occurring from outdoor air exposure would be unusual.

Lead. During the era of leaded gasoline, air was a significant source of environmental lead exposure, because lead is absorbed inhalationally as well as by ingestion. Since leaded gasoline was phased out beginning in the 1970s, the average population blood lead levels have declined substantially. The OSHA PEL as an 8-hour TWA is 50 $\mu g/m^3$. The NAAQS is 1.5 $\mu g/m^3$ as a 3-month average. Average levels in vehicle-laden California are now approximately 0.06 $\mu g/m^3$.

NO_2. NO_2 facilitates the formation of ozone, and this is probably its major health effect outdoors. NO_2 is unique as an air pollutant in that it is usually present in higher concentrations inside buildings than outdoors. Pulmonary edema occurring in an ice hockey player has been attributed to accumulation of CO and NO_2 from an ice-surfacing machine. Acute occupational illness from NO_2 is seen in people who work around grain storage silos, welding, and industries involving processing or combustion of certain nitrogen compounds. Delayed onset of cough, dyspnea, and pulmonary edema are characteristic of acute NO_2 exposure. The NAAQS is 0.053 ppm as a yearly average.

Nonmethane hydrocarbons (NMHCs). Although NMHCs produce no clearly defined human disease from ambient outdoor air, they are implicated in the photochemical processes that produce ozone, so an air quality standard has been established for them. In addition, derivatives of hydrocarbons, such as formaldehyde and acrolein, contribute to mucous membrane irritation.

Ozone. Exposure to ambient outdoor levels of ozone has produced increased airway reactivity in healthy patients, decreased exercise capability in athletes, and increased hospitalizations in asthmatics and others with respiratory illnesses. Symptoms of acute ozone exposure include cough, dyspnea, wheezing, chest tightness, headache, malaise, and nausea. The OSHA PEL as an 8-hour TWA is 0.10 ppm. The NAAQS is 0.12 ppm as a 1-hour average.

Particulate matter and **SO_2**. Increases in particulate matter often are accompanied by increases in SO_2. Health effects of particulate matter exposure include an increase in respiratory symptoms in healthy populations and increased mortality in populations with underlying asthma or other chronic lung disease. The NAAQS for particulate matter and SO_2 are computed on an annual basis, with values of 50 $\mu g/m^3$ and 0.03 ppm, respectively.

7. What are the U.S. National (Primary) Ambient Air Quality Standards (NAAQS)?

The EPA defined a group of six common air pollutants that are detrimental to human health and the environment. These pollutants are those to which most people are routinely exposed in their daily lives. For each of these agents, a scientifically-based EPA manuscript called a *Criteria Document* forms the basis for setting permissible limits. For each of the six **criteria air pollutants**, two sets of permissible levels were defined: one set (the primary standard) is designed to protect human health; the other set (the secondary standard) is to protect the environment. Geographic regions in compliance with the primary standard are called **attainment areas**. Those not meeting the primary standard are called **nonattainment areas**. The criteria pollutants and their permissible limits form the NAAQS-set and are monitored by the EPA. The six criteria pollutants are sulfur dioxide, carbon monoxide, ozone, nitrogen dioxide, inhalable particulate matter, and lead.

8. What are HAPs?

The EPA also designated hazardous air pollutants (HAPs; also called air toxics), natural or man-made air pollutants that are measurable in the air in specific areas. HAPs typically present a risk of carcinogensis or other significant risk to human health. The criteria pollutants are explicitly excluded from this designation. The agents are usually specific to certain industries, and regulation is directed toward limiting airborne emissions from those industries. More than 100 HAPs have been identified, and over 30 are specifically regulated in urban areas. HAPS encompass a variety of chemical species, including hydrazine, acetaldehyde, acrylonitrile, benzene, styrene, carbon tetrachloride, acrolein, asbestos, heavy metal compounds, and pesticides.

9. How does air pollution harm the environment?

Air contaminants that damage the plant kingdom are referred to as **phytotoxic pollutants**. Chemicals that cause widespread injury to plants include ozone, peroxyacylnitrate (PAN), SO_2 (via acid rain), fluorides, and ethylene. Leaves are the primary target for damage by air pollutants, because they are the organs of gas exchange for plants.

Livestock are adversely effected by fluorosis, which is caused by discharge of fluorides into the atmosphere in various manufacturing processes. Lead poisoning resulting from atmospheric lead has also affected animals.

The natural corrosion process of metals used in man-made structures is accelerated by acid, largely by sulfuric acid produced from atmospheric SO_2. Stone exteriors, paint, paper, leather, and textiles are other man-made items destroyed by air pollution.

10. A group of people who work in the same office building have all developed nonspecific neurologic and respiratory tract symptoms. What may be the cause?

Because this is an office building, industrial chemicals are unlikely. Carbon monoxide poisoning must be considered, but simple ambient air or blood measurements could rule this out. **Building-related illness** is a medical condition with known causes that are triggered by indoor air. Examples include hypersensitivity pneumonitis, building-related asthma, Legionnaire's disease, and inhalation fevers. These can be caused by animal, plant, or microbial allergens, workplace chemicals, or, in the case of Legionnaire's disease, infectious agents.

The **sick building syndrome** refers to an outbreak of symptoms in a number of building occupants in the absence of a clear medical explanation. Symptoms include headache, concentration difficulties, mucous membrane and respiratory irritation, and dry skin. Many theories have been proposed to explain this syndrome including poor ventilation, indoor volatile organic compounds (from carpeting, furniture, photocopiers, computer printers), and fungal toxins. There is some evidence to support each of these theories, as well as data that point to psychosocial factors.

11. What lung cancer-causing compound is found in the basements of millions of Americans?

Cigarette smoke would be an acceptable answer here, but a better response is radon. Radon itself does not cause cancer but rather decays into other radioactive compounds. These radon progeny emit alpha particles that can be inhaled and then damage DNA in lung tissue. This results in lung cancer. After cigarette smoking, radon may be the number 2 cause of lung cancer. Uranium miners are exposed to radon occupationally, but radon gas is an environmental threat in homes as well. The gas is odorless and colorless. It enters homes through defects in the foundation, drains, and sumps. The EPA recommends that indoor levels be < 4 pCu/L of air. About 6% of homes exceed this level. A lifetime of exposure to 4 6Cu/L is associated with a 1 in 500 chance of developing lung cancer in a nonsmoker. This compares with a less than 1 in 1000 risk for a nonsmoker with a lifetime exposure to 1.3 pCu/L, the average indoor radon level. Cigarette smoking increases the risk of lung cancer due to radon by a factor of about 15.

12. What are the general sources of water pollution?

In the U.S., half the population gets its drinking water from groundwater (wells that draw from underground reservoirs or aquifers), and the other half drinks surface water (from lakes, rivers, above-ground reservoirs). Pollution of surface water occurs from point (stationary) and nonpoint (diffuse or mobile) sources. Point-source pollution includes sewage, industrial plants, oil tanks, and mining operations. Nonpoint sources include natural sources (e.g., forest fires, giardia amplification by beavers) and man-made sources (e.g., pesticides, petroleum products on roads, acid rain). Groundwater is contaminated by septic and storage tanks, uncapped wells, municipal solid waste tanks, illegal dumps, and agricultural chemicals.

13. What are the constituents of polluted water?

Water is polluted primarily by biological and chemical entities. Algae, bacteria, viruses, helminths, and protozoa make up the majority of biological health hazards. Standards for the chemical quality of drinking water have been defined as primary and secondary. Primary standards are approved limits for health, and have been defined for organic and inorganic chemicals, radionuclides and for turbidity. Secondary standards address not necessarily health hazards but aesthetics and have been set for water color, odor, corrosivity, inorganic chemicals, and dissolved salts. Secondary standards are not enforceable by the EPA. Waste water is assessed by biochemical oxygen demand, ammonia nitrogen, chlorine residual, fecal coliforms, grease, oil, phosphorus, and suspended solids.

Certain substances that create harm and environmental persistence are referred to as **toxic water pollutants** by the EPA. Compounds include ethers, halogenated aliphatic compounds, heavy metals, monocyclic aromatics, nitrosamines, pesticides, phthalate esters, polycyclic aromatic hydrocarbons, and polychlorinated biphenyls.

14. How are water pollutants measured?

The EPA has established numerical limits on the content of water through the following measurements:

1. **Biochemical oxygen demand** (BOD) refers to the amount of oxygen usable by microorganisms in polluted water as they pursue aerobic metabolism. It is thus an indirect measure of organic pollution. BOD is measured over a standard 5-day period and is used to estimate the amount of pollution in waste water.

2. **Fecal coliform measurements** are performed as "indicator organisms." Testing for a broad range of organisms is technically difficult and expensive. Therefore, only the presence or absence of fecal coliform bacteria is used as presumptive evidence of the presence or absence of microbiologic contamination.

3. **Chlorine** is toxic to fish, and the EPA has established a total chlorine residual limit of 2.0 μg/L for salmonid fish and 10.0 μg/L for other fish. **Unionized ammonia** is also toxic to fish, and limits have been set at varying levels of pH.

4. **Oil and grease** standards are set not to exceed 0.01 of the LC_{50} for a particular species over a 96-hour exposure. The LC_{50} is the concentration found to be lethal to 50% of an exposed cohort.

5. **Phosphorus**

6. **Suspended solids**

15. What water pollutants are hazardous to human health?

1. Multiple **biologic hazards** exist in water in the form of infectious diseases. Human and animal feces are significant contaminants of water, with sewage being the largest public health concern. Cross-contamination of drinking water by sewage was common in the U.S. until the mid-nineteenth century and is still a significant problem in third-world countries.

- **Bacterial pathogens** in water include *Salmonella* (typhoid and paratyphoid fevers) species, *Shigella* (bacillary dysentery) species, *Vibrio* (cholera), and *Yersinia*. Infection with these organisms causes various gastrointestinal and systemic illnesses, usually with diarrhea.
- **Viral pathogens** include adenoviruses (respiratory infections), enteroviruses (aseptic meningitis and polio), coxsackie viruses (aseptic meningitis), and hepatitis A (infectious hepatitis).
- **Protozoal pathogens** include *Giardia lamblia* and *Entamoeba histolytica*. *Giardia* species are found in mountain streams and are a hazard to campers. Beavers are a biologic amplifier of *Giardia* and can excrete up to 1 million fecal cysts per orally ingested cyst.
- Multiple types of **helminths** (worms) can be found in sewage.

2. **Chemical contamination** of water can be caused by a broad range of substances. The EPA regulates the safety of water by promulgating enforceable primary standards known as maximum contaminant levels (MCLs), generally expressed in milligrams per liter. MCLs are established for:

- **Inorganic chemicals**—asbestos, arsenic, barium, cadmium, chromium, copper, fluoride, lead, mercury, nitrate, nitrite, and selenium
- **Volatile organic chemicals**—solvents, pesticides, and industrial chemicals. Trihalomethanes are regulated as a group at a 0.10 mg/L level.
- **Other organic chemicals**
- **Radionuclides**
- **Turbidity**

16. What is TCE?

Trichloroethylene is a chlorinated hydrocarbon commonly used as a degreaser—meaning it is used to remove oils and impurities from the surfaces of many materials. Historically, TCE was also used as an anesthetic agent. Recently, TCE was made infamous in Jonathan Harr's book *A Civil Action* and the movie based on it. Like other organic solvents, acute exposure can cause drowsiness, confusion, headache, and ataxia. Chronic exposure may cause trigeminal neuropathy, cancer, and immune dysfunction. Specifically, leukemia and bladder cancer risk is increased in people exposed to TCE from contaminated drinking water. Exposure to TCE can be assessed by measuring trichloroacetic acid in urine or blood.

TCE has been identified in over one third of all of the EPA's "superfund" sites (hazardous waste sites in need of large scale clean-up assistance. In over 90% of these sites, TCE contaminated the groundwater.[2] Even where there are no superfund sites, TCE contaminates well water in many areas of the U.S.

17. What are PCBs? How do people unknowingly ingest them?

Polychlorinated biphenyls (PCBs) belong to a family of chemicals that derive from chlorination of carbon atoms within two linked benzene rings (biphenyls). They were used widely in electrical transformers and capacitors because of their physical and chemical stability. Like other organochlorines, they are toxic persistent organic pollutants (POPs) that both bioaccumulate and biomagnify up the food chain. While their concentrations may be relatively low in the sediments of lakes and rivers, PCBs become progressively more concentrated in the fat of animals. People are exposed by eating contaminated fish. Occupational exposure to PCBs cause liver disease, biliary tract, and skin rashes, including the classic (but rare) chloracne.

18. What are POPs?

Persistent organic pollutants are a threat both to human health and to ecosystems worldwide. These organic toxicants are not degraded by known biotic (biodegradation) or abiotic (e.g., photolysis or hydrolysis) mechanisms. These synthetic compounds include PCBs, dioxins, and organochlorine pesticides such as DDT. Because POPs persist in ecosystems for decades, they have ample opportunity to be taken up by species within those ecosystems. In particular, POPs are ingested by fish, where they can remain in fatty tissue permanently. As larger fish eat smaller fish, the POP concentration increases up the food chain in a process known as **biomagnification**. It was through this process that DDT caused eggshell thinning in birds that ate contaminated fish. Humans are, of course, at risk for ingesting POPs in this way as well. Human health hazards associated with POPs include abnormal child development.

19. How can a bottle of formula make an infant turn blue?

About 40% of the nitrates in fertilizer leach from soil to groundwater. About 2% of wells exceed the U.S. Environmental Protection Agency's (EPA) limit of 10 parts per million (ppm) of nitrates. Infant formula mixed with water from such a source can contain significant quantities of nitrates. Once ingested these nitrates can cause methemoglobinemia directly or after conversion to nitrites by bowel flora. Infants are at particular risk for methemoglobinemia because of the immaturity of the enzyme nicotinamide adenine dinucleotide (NADH) methemoglobin reductase, which protects against oxidative stresses. Nitrates in well water either may be a marker for bacterial contamination (which leads to gastroenteritis and increased endogenous nitric oxide production) or may increase the nitrate load in those already producing excess nitrites.

20. *Extra credit:* **In the 1970s, 53,000 kg of what insecticidal compound was discharged into the James River through the Hopewell, Virginia, city sewage system?**
Kepone.

21. What laws and regulatory agencies govern the quality of air and water in the U.S.?

Regulatory Agencies that Govern Air and Water Quality

AGENCY	RESPONSIBILITIES
Environmental Protection Agency (EPA)	Established to protect human health and to safeguard the natural environment
	Conducts risk assessments of the dangers of substances in the air and water
	Issues standards and regulations
	Cleans up hazardous waste sites
Occupational Safety and Health Administration (OSHA)	As part of the Department of Labor, creates and enforces standards for workplace safety
	Sets PELs for many industrial toxins (e.g., benzene, silica, lead)
Agency for Toxic Substance and Disease Registry (ATSDR)	Studies the hazards of chemicals
	Works with the EPA at toxic waste sites
	Assists health care providers and local governments with hazardous exposures

Significant Federal Legislation Governing Air Quality

LAW	YEAR	FEATURES
Clean Air Act	1963	Developed air quality criteria
		Gave federal government the authority to act on interstate air pollution abatement
National Environmental Policy Act (NEPA)	1970	EPA was created to enforce the provisions of this act
Clean Air Act of 1970	1970	Mandated NAAQS
		Instituted the state implementation plans (SIPs) for pollution reduction
		Set national standards for automobile and stationary source emissions
		Authorized federal authority in air pollution emergencies
Resource Conservation and Recovery Act (RCRA)	1976	Mandates "cradle-to-grave" management of hazardous chemicals
Clean Air Amendment of 1977	1977	Regulated ozone-causing pollutants
Comprehensive Environmental Response, Compensation, and Liability Act (CERCLA)	1980	Authorized tax on chemical and petroleum industries to defray cost of hazardous waste clean up
		Gave federal government control over hazardous sites
		Commonly known as Superfund
Various toxic-specific laws	varies	Ban or regulate individual toxins (e.g., DDT, chlorofluorocarbons)

Significant Federal Legislation Governing Water Quality

LAW	YEAR	FEATURES
Water Quality Act	1965	Mandated quality standards for interstate waters only
Clean Rivers Restoration Act	1966	Funded waste-water treatment plants
Wild and Scenic Rivers Act	1968	Protects notable free-flowing rivers
Clean Water Act	1972 (revised 1977)	Established national standards for polluted water
Safe Drinking Water Act	1974 (revised 1986)	Established national standards for drinking water in all public water systems

22. Why are children more susceptible to the effects of air and water pollutants?
- Children have a smaller ratio of body mass to body surface area, leaving them relatively more exposed to the environment.
- Children have higher ventilatory and metabolic rates than do adults, thus they eat more food, drink more water, and breathe more air (on a per kilogram basis) than adults.
- Children typically spend more time outdoors, are engaged in physical activity more, and spend more time close to the floor or ground.
- Young children exhibit more hand-to-mouth activity and are in contact with objects from the environment more frequently than the typical adult.
- Children may not attend to personal hygiene as well as adults and may forget to wash substances off their hands before eating.
- Children handle xenobiotic compounds differently than do adults. Significant differences in absorption of exogenous compounds have been documented by inhalational, transcutaneous, and gastrointestinal routes for children. This appears related to differences in membrane composition, perfusion, and surface area. A good example is lead, which is absorbed more extensively both by inhalation and by ingestion in youngsters.
- Children have a longer anticipated life span, giving toxicants with long latency periods more time to express themselves.
- Children are more vulnerable than adults to the cumulative effects of multiple exposures.
- Toxicants may alter the process of organ (particularly neurologic) growth and development in children.

BIBLIOGRAPHY

1. Bascom R, Bromberg PA, Dosta DL, et al: Health effects of outdoor air pollution. Part I. Am J Respir Crit Care Med 153:3–50, 1996.
2. Bascom R, Bromberg PA, Dosta DL, et al: Health effects of outdoor air pollution. Part II. Am J Respir Crit Care Med 153:477–498, 1996.
3. Dunnick JK, Melnick RL: Assessment of the carcinogenic potential of chlorinated water: Experimental studies of chlorine, chloramine and trihalomethanes. J Natl Cancer Inst 85:817–822, 1993.
4. Godish T: Air Quality, 3rd ed. New York, Lewis Publishers, 1997.
5. Goldfrank L, Flomenbaum N, Lewin N, et al (eds): Goldfrank's Toxicologic Emergencies, 6th ed. Stamford, CT, Appleton & Lange, 1998.
6. Kindschy JW, Kraft M, Carpenter M: Guide to Hazardous Materials and Waste. Point Arena, CA, Solano Press Books, 1997.
7. Sullivan JB, Krieger GR: Hazardous Materials Toxicology. Baltimore, Williams & Wilkins, 1992.
8. Viessman W, Hammer MJ: Water Supply and Pollution Control, 5th ed. New York, Harper Collins, 1993.

XIII. Botanicals

57. MUSHROOM POISONING

Binh T. Ly, M.D.

1. What is the frequency of mushroom poisoning in the United States?

Serious poisoning from mushroom ingestion in North America is rare. Of the 1.6 million poisoning exposures reported to the American Association of Poison Control Centers in 1998, only 9839 cases (0.3%) were attributed to mushrooms. Extrapolation of these data along with those from the North American Mycological Association suggests an incidence of 5 mushroom exposures per 100,000 population per year. Of the 9839 cases of mushroom exposure, the species was identified in only 1183 (12%). One death was reported from mushrooms in 1998 from an unknown species. The majority of mushroom exposures (56%) had no clinical effect.

2. Match the following mushroom structures to the appropriate letters in the figure: annulus (ring); (lamellae (gills); mycelium; pileus (cap); stem (stipe); and volva (cup).

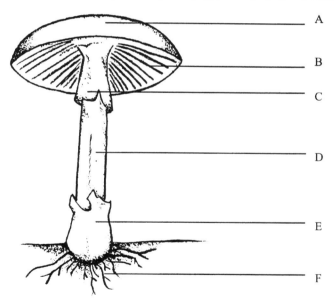

A

B

C

D

E

F

A. pileus
B. lamellae
C. annulus
D. stem
E. volva
F. mycelium

3. How should mushroom poisonings be approached?

Although most mushroom exposures are benign, some can be life threatening. Efforts must be concentrated on good supportive care, as with any poisoning. Assessment of airway patency and respiratory and circulatory adequacy (ABCs) takes precedence, followed by appropriate resuscitation measures as indicated. After immediate life-threatening conditions have been addressed, a detailed history of the exposure can be determined. Factors in the exposure history that are important include time of ingestion, time of symptom onset, how many types of mushrooms ingested, how the mushrooms were prepared, and symptoms of others who ingested the mushroom meal. Most patients will present with symptoms of gastrointestinal (GI) irritation. In these cases, the latency period of symptom onset must be established. An attempt should be made to characterize the constellation of symptoms into one of the specific toxin categories. Identifying mushrooms by their physical characteristics is challenging. Any mushrooms, spores, or fragments remaining from the meal or recovered from emesis should be collected and sent to a mycologist, if possible, for identification. Because GI symptoms predominate and can be severe, specific attention should be given to intravascular volume status and electrolyte balance. Activated charcoal may be of benefit and should be administered even in cases of delayed presentation because certain toxins (amatoxin) may be enterohepatically recirculated. Some toxins may be identified by using sophisticated laboratory techniques such as radioimmunoassay, mass spectrometry, spectrophotometry, and thin-layer, gas, or high-performance liquid chromatography. However, these tests are not widely available, and their reliability is unproved. Mushroom or toxin identification, albeit important, should never take priority over caring for the patient and addressing symptomatology.

4. What are the eight generally recognized toxic groups of mushrooms?

1. Cyclopeptide
2. Gyromitrin
3. Orellanine
4. Muscarine
5. Coprine
6. Ibotenic acid/muscimol
7. Psilocybin
8. GI toxins

5. What is the clinical presentation or syndrome associated with each group?

TOXIN	GENUS AND SPECIES	SYMPTOM ONSET	SYMPTOMS
Cyclopeptides Amatoxin Phallotoxin Virotoxin	*Amanita phalloides* ("death cap") *A. verna* ("death angel") *A. virosa* ("destroying angel")	6–12 hrs	*Stage 1:* gastroenteritis, profuse diarrhea, abdominal cramping
	A. ocreata *Galerina autumnalis* *G. marginata*	12–24 hrs	*Stage 2:* apparent resolution of GI symptoms, ↑ hepatic enzymes
	Lepiota helveola *L. josserandii*	24–72 hrs	*Stage 3:* hepatic and renal failure, encephalopathy, death in 10–30% of cases
Gyromitrin Monomethyl- hydrazine	*Gyromitra esculenta* ("false morel") *G. gigas* *G. infula*	6–12 hrs	Gastroenteritis, dizziness, headache, intractable seizures
Orellanine Orelline	*Cortinarius orellanus* *C. speciosissimus*	24–36 hrs	Gastroenteritis, oliguria
	C. gentilus	Days to weeks	Acute renal failure, tubulo-interstitial nephritis and fibrosis

(Table continued on next page.)

TOXIN	GENUS AND SPECIES	SYMPTOM ONSET	SYMPTOMS
Muscarine	*Clitocybe cerrusata* *C. dealbata* *Inocybe fasigiata* *I. geophylla* *Boletus calopus* *B. luridus*	0.5–3 hrs	Bronchorreha, broncho-spasms, vomiting, diarrhea, salivation, urination, lacrimation
Coprine 1-Aminocyclo-propanone	*Coprinus atramentarius* ("inky cap") *C. quadrificus* *C. variegatus* *Clitocybe claviceps*	0.5–3 hrs after in-gestion of ethanol	Facial and truncal flushing, palpitations, nausea, vomit-ing, dyspnea, possible hypotension
Ibotenic acid Muscimol	*Amanita muscaria* ("fly agaric") *A. pantherina* *A. gemata*	0.5–3 hrs 10–15 hrs	Excitatory-hyperactivity, hallucinations, euphoria, tremors, myoclonus, con-vulsions, delirium Inhibitory-hypersomnolence, exhaustion, coma
Psilocybin	*Psilocybe cubensis* *P. cyanescens*	0.5–2 hrs	Euphoria, hallucinations, agitation, hyperthermia, possible convulsions
GI toxins	*Agaricus hordensus* *Chlorophyllum molybdites* *C. esculentum* *Clitocybe nebularis* *Omphalates illudens* "Little brown mushrooms" and various other genera	0.5–3 hrs	Nausea, vomiting, diarrhea

6. How do amatoxins cause cellular injury?

Cellular injury in cyclopeptide mushroom poisoning is primarily due to amatoxins. These toxins are heat stable and water insoluble; therefore, cooking is not likely to eliminate toxic ef-fects. Amatoxin has been shown in vitro to produce cellular damage by binding to and inhibiting RNA polymerase II, thus preventing mRNA synthesis and DNA transcription. The organs most adversely affected are those with high cellular turnover rates. The liver is the primary site of tox-icity, but the kidneys and GI tract are also damaged.

7. What therapies have been reported to be beneficial in cyclopeptide poisoning?

Because of the lethality of cyclopeptide mushroom poisoning, there has been an extensive search for a remedy. The use of thiotic acid was beneficial in a small series of poisonings. Although its mechanism of action is unclear, thiotic acid has been postulated to be a free radical scavenger. Some authors have advocated the use of penicillin G alone or in combination with sili-binin, an extract from the thistle *Silybum marianum*. Both agents are thought to inhibit amatoxin uptake by hepatocytes. Silibinin stimulates DNA-dependent RNA polymerases and may also scav-enge free radicals. Because amatoxins have been reported to undergo enterohepatic recirculation, the administration of multiple doses of activated charcoal (MDAC) has also been advocated. Other unproved interventions include cimetidine, corticosteroids, ascorbic acid, cytochrome C, hyper-baric oxygen, forced diuresis, hemodialysis, hemoperfusion, and plasmapheresis. Although many regimens have been tried and anecdotally reported to be beneficial, none have been prospectively validated in controlled trials. For this reason, the cornerstone of therapy remains supportive care and perhaps MDAC. Silibinin has no apparent major side effects and can be used if available. Many amatoxin-poisoned patients will recover with conservative management alone.

Although liver transplantation may be necessary in some cases of cyclopeptide-induced hepatic failure, no clearly defined indications have been established. In addition, no laboratory tests provide reliable prognostic values. Individuals presenting with significant hepatic injury following cyclopeptide-containing mushroom ingestion should be referred to a regional liver transplantation center for evaluation.

8. What is a spore print and how is one made?

A spore print is an impression of mushroom spores used by mycologists to assist in the identification of mushroom species. One can be made by cutting the stem from the cap, placing the cap onto a white sheet of paper, and allowing the spores to fall from the cap onto the paper. Because this process may take several hours, care should be taken to prevent air currents from blowing the spores away by covering the mushroom cap with a glass or bowl. The spore color is, for the most part, species specific.

9. Why is it important to determine the time delay from mushroom ingestion to the onset of symptoms?

This can be useful in cases of unidentified mushroom ingestion to assess the likelihood that a cyclopeptide-containing mushroom is responsible for the symptoms. A delay of 6–8 hours in the onset of GI symptoms after a mushroom meal is highly suggestive of cyclopeptide poisoning. Because 95% of all mushroom fatalities involve the cyclopeptide-containing species, it is imperative to identify these exposures and initiate appropriate therapy. Monomethylhydrazine and orellanine poisonings also have long latency periods (> 6 hours) prior to the onset of their characteristic symptoms. All other species have shorter latency periods (< 6 hours).

10. Do *Amanita* species that contain ibotenic acid and muscimol cause hepatotoxicity?

No. Ibotenic acid is an isoxazole derivative that is structurally similar to the excitatory neurotransmitter glutamic acid. Ibotenic acid is decarboxylated in vivo to form muscimol, which happens to have structural similarity to the inhibitory neurotransmitter gamma aminobutyric acid (GABA). In addition to their structural relationship, ibotenic acid and muscimol have neuropharmacologic effects similar to glutamic acid and GABA. Intoxication usually occurs about 30 minutes after ingesting these mushrooms and is marked by hyperactivity, ataxia, euphoria, hallucinations, anxiety, agitation, and tremors. Delirium, psychosis, coma, myoclonic movements, and convulsions may be seen with severe poisonings. This excitatory period, typically lasting about 3 hours, is followed by a 10–15-hour period of exhaustion and somnolence. Because of the low concentrations of psychoactive substances in these mushrooms, large amounts must be ingested to achieve the psychedelic effect. Accidental poisoning with ibotenic acid–containing mushrooms is rare. Treatment is supportive, with the administration of benzodiazepines as needed for the excitatory effects. Administration of activated charcoal can also be considered.

11. What non-*Amanita* mushrooms have been reported to cause hepatic failure?

Although cyclopeptide-containing *Amanita* species are notorious for causing hepatic damage, some species of *Galerina* and *Lepiota* have also been implicated. These mushrooms contain hepatotoxic cyclopeptides. *L. helveola* contains more cyclopeptides than *A. phalloides* and can result in similar devastating hepatic failure. The *Galerina* species are much smaller, brown mushrooms with lower amatoxin content. It is estimated that one *A. phalloides* contains as much amatoxin as 15–20 *Galerina* mushrooms, the approximate amount needed for hepatotoxicity.

12. What is paxillus syndrome?

Paxillus syndrome is a rare condition characterized by immune-mediated hemolytic anemia occurring in some individuals after the consumption of *Paxillus involutus* mushrooms. Most people only experience symptoms of GI irritation, typically 1–2 hours after ingestion. If syncope, oliguria, anuria, and hemoglobinuria are present, hemolysis should be suspected, and a diagnosis of paxillus syndrome should be considered. The antigen or toxin responsible for initiating this immune-mediated hemolysis has not yet been identified. Treatment is primarily aggressive intravascular volume resuscitation. Plasmapheresis has been tried in a severe case, but no conclusive evidence exists to show that this intervention is beneficial.

13. Describe the Meixner test.

The Meixner test is a simple, rapid assay used to screen for the presence of amatoxins. Although more sensitive methods such as radioimmunoassay and high-performance liquid chromatography exist, they are not routinely available. The Meixner assay, which can be done at the beside, is performed by expressing fluid from the fresh mushroom onto wood pulp paper, such as newspaper, and allowing it to dry. Several drops of 10–12 N hydrochloric acid are applied to the paper. If only dried mushroom samples are available, fluid can be extracted from the mushroom with methanol. A positive result is characterized by the development of a blue coloration in 1–2 minutes, although results may take longer if amatoxin concentration is low. Because false-positive results do occur, this test should not be regarded as conclusive, and further testing should be performed to confirm the presence of amatoxin. Psilocybin, along with other terpenes, has been reported to give a false-positive Meixner test.

14. Which mushroom poisoning has clinical features similar to disulfiram's reaction with ethanol?

Coprine is a toxin contained in *Coprinus* mushrooms. It is likely that its metabolite, 1-aminocyclopropanol, is responsible for the inhibition of acetaldehyde dehydrogenase, the same enzyme involved in the metabolism of ethanol and inhibited by disulfiram. Because of this inhibition, acetaldehyde accumulation occurs within 30 minutes to 2 hours after the ingestion of ethanol in each case, resulting in truncal and facial flushing (vasodilation), palpitations, dyspnea, nausea, vomiting, and diaphoresis. Hypotension has been reported and is probably due to peripheral vasodilation. Symptoms gradually improve over several hours. There are no specific antidotes available to treat this syndrome, and therapy consists of symptomatic and supportive measures. Symptoms will only develop if ethanol is coingested or subsequently consumed in the 48–72 hours after *Coprinus* mushroom ingestion.

15. How is gyromitrin (monomethylhydrazine) poisoning related to poisoning by isoniazid?

Gyromitra species mushroom poisoning can have presenting symptoms and signs similar to that of isoniazid toxicity. These mushrooms are typically found in the spring and contain N-formyl-monomethyl hydrazones, most notably gyromitrin, that are hydrolized to monomethylhydrazine (MMH). Gyromitrin is a volatile, heat-labile, and water-soluble toxin; therefore, toxicity may be prevented by cooking or boiling the mushrooms, but because of the volatility of the toxin, inhaling the fumes during cooking can also lead to poisoning. The clinical presentation of MMH poisoning is similar to that of isoniazid because both compounds inhibit the formation of GABA in the brain by inducing pyridoxine (vitamin B_6) depletion. Pyridoxine is a cofactor in the synthesis of GABA. As can be expected, a deficiency of an inhibitory neurotransmitter will leave the brain in a relatively excited state. Unregulated neuroexcitation in these cases manifests as seizures that can be resistant to routine anticonvulsant therapy with GABA receptor agonist such as benzodiazepines and barbiturates because these agents require the presence of endogenous GABA for their anticonvulsant action. For this reason, pyridoxine should be coadministered with anticonvulsants to aid in GABA synthesis. A generally accepted dose of pyridoxine for these patients is 25 mg/kg up to 5 gm.

16. Which type of mushrooms are referred to as "magic mushrooms"?

Psilocybin-containing mushrooms have psychotropic properties similar to lysergic acid diethylamide (LSD). Psilocybin mushrooms have been used for centuries by North American Indians in their religious ceremonies. Not surprisingly, the chemical structure of psilocybin is similar to LSD and serotonin. Serotonin activity has been implicated in the mechanisms of other hallucinogenic compounds. Symptoms of intoxication are usually present 30–60 minutes after mushroom ingestion and include euphoria, disorientation, vertigo, hallucinations, agitation, hyperthermia, headache, bradycardia, and possibly hypotension or convulsions. Therapy is emotional support because the symptoms are self-limited. Benzodiazepines may be helpful with uncontrolled or unpleasant hallucinations ("bad trips").

17. What are some pitfalls in the treatment of mushroom poisoning?
- Concentrating on identification of the mushroom instead of providing supportive care
- Allowing mushroom appearances, which may be misleading, to direct therapy instead of the patient's symptomatology
- Failing to recognize that symptoms may be due to pesticides or other chemicals (including drugs) placed on the mushrooms
- Forgetting that other medical or surgical conditions can present similar to mushroom poisonings (i.e., coprine-ethanol reaction, allergic reaction)
- Dismissing toxic mushroom ingestion as benign if symptoms occur prior to 6 hours in cases of mixed mushroom ingestion (i.e., GI toxins coingested with *Amanita phalloides*)
- Not recognizing that symptoms from some toxic species can be delayed
- Forgetting that not all persons ingesting the same mushroom meal will be symptomatic because poisoning is sometimes dependent on the quantity ingested, bioavailability, variability in toxin content, and susceptibility of certain individuals

18. *Extra credit:* **The mushroom** *Galerina sulcipes*, **thought to be the world's most toxic, is responsible for the deaths of 31 people, on two separate occasions, in 1934 and 1937. On what Asian island did these disastrous deaths occur?**
Java, Indonesia.

19. *Extra credit:* **What do rockets and mushrooms have in common?**
The chemical MMH is a rocket guidance propellant as well as a toxic compound found in certain species of *Gyromitra* mushrooms.

BIBLIOGRAPHY

1. Brent J, Kulig K: Mushrooms. In Haddad LM, Shannon MW, Winchester JF (eds): Clinical Management of Poisoning and Drug Overdose, 3rd ed. Philadelphia, W.B. Saunders, 1998, pp 365–374.
2. Goldfrank LR: Mushrooms: Toxic and hallucinogenic. In Goldfrank LR, Flomenbaum NE, Lewin NA, et al (eds): Goldfrank's Toxicologic Emergencies, 6th ed. Stamford, CT, Appleton & Lange, 1998, pp 1207–1219.
3. Köppel C: Clinical symptomatology and management of mushroom poisoning. Toxicon 31:1513–1540, 1993.
4. Lampe KF, McCann MA: Differential diagnosis of poisoning by North American mushrooms, with particular emphasis on *Amanita phalloides*–like intoxication. Ann Emerg Med 16:956–963, 1987.
5. Trestrail JH: Mushroom poisoning in the United States: An analysis of 1989 United States Poison Center data. Clin Toxicol 29:459–465, 1991.

58. HERBAL PREPARATIONS

Christine Haller, M.D.

1. What is the current prevalence of herbal preparation use in the United States?

Approximately 1 in 3 Americans uses herbal remedies for health purposes. Annual sales of herbal preparations exceed $3 billion.

2. What are the most commonly used herbal preparations?

The ten top-selling herbs of 1997 (in the U.S.) were:

1. Ginseng
2. Garlic
3. Ginkgo biloba
4. Echinacea
5. St. John's wort
6. Saw palmetto
7. Echinacea-goldenseal
8. Grapeseed
9. Goldenseal
10. Evening primrose

3. How are herbal medicines different from conventional drugs?

Federal regulation of these compounds is totally different. In 1994, Congress passed the Dietary Supplement Health and Education Act (DSHEA), which defined herbs, vitamins, minerals, amino acids, and organ extracts as dietary supplements, thereby classifying them as foods, not drugs. Any product sold as a supplement prior to passage of DSHEA was "grandfathered" in as a dietary supplement. In contrast to drugs, Food and Drug Administration (FDA) approval is not required prior to marketing of dietary supplements. Premarket testing for safety and efficacy is not mandated, and adherence to good manufacturing practice and quality control standards is not enforced. Dietary supplements are only restricted from making claims of preventing or treating disease but are allowed to claim effects on body structure or function. For example, a label on glucosamine can claim to improve joint mobility but cannot claim to treat arthritis.

4. Aren't herbal preparations fairly innocuous unless contaminated with a toxin?

It is true that a number of poisonings related to herbal preparations were caused by contaminants such as cadmium, lead, arsenic, mercury, and undeclared pharmaceutical adulterants such as diazepam, acetaminophen, phenylbutazone, and prednisone. However, some herbs are intrinsically toxic, and poisoning results from misidentification, mislabeling, and improper purification of plant parts. For instance, more that 48 cases of renal failure resulted from an herbal weight-loss preparation sold in Belgium that was supposed to contain fang-ji (*Stephania tetrandra*) but which actually contained the nephrotoxic herb guang-fang-ji (*Aristolochia fangchi*). The confusion arose from the similar Chinese names of the herbs.

5. What herbal preparations are considered unsafe for consumption?

The table lists common herbs that are considered unsafe for general use. Other herbs such as chamomile, echinacea, and ginkgo may be harmful to individuals with a history of hypersensitivity to similar plants. Bee pollen and royal jelly can cause anaphylaxis in persons allergic to hymenoptera stings. Topical herbal remedies such as tea tree oil (*Melaleuca alternifolia*) and aloe vera may cause clinical toxicity if orally ingested.

Potentially Harmful Herbs and Their Toxic Effects

COMMON NAME	BOTANICAL NAME	POTENTIAL TOXIC EFFECT
Aconite (monkshood, wolfsbane)	*Aconitum* species	Cardiac and neurologic toxicity
Blue cohosh (squaw root)	*Caulophyllum thalictroides*	Nicotinic toxicity
Broom	*Cytisus scoparius*	Nicotinic toxicity
Calamus	*Acorus calamus*	Carcinogenic
Chaparral	*Larrea tridentata*	Hepatotoxic
Coltsfoot	*Tussilago farfara*	Hepatotoxic, carcinogenic
Comfrey	*Symphytum officinale*	Hepatotoxic, carcinogenic
Dong quai	*Angelica sinensis*	Photosensitization, anticoagulation, abortifacient (?)
Germander	*Teucrium chamaedrys*	Hepatotoxic
Jin bu huan	*Lycopodium serratum* *Stephania, Corydalis* species	Hepatotoxic
Licorice	*Glycyrrhiza glabra*	Hypokalemia, sodium and water retention, hypertension
Life root	*Senecio aureus*	Hepatotoxic, carcinogenic
Ma huang	*Ephedra sinica*	Insomnia, nervousness, headache, palpitations, hypertension, stroke, psychosis, myocardial infarction
Pennyroyal	*Mentha pulegium* *Hedeoma pulegoides*	Hepatotoxic
Sassafras	*Sassafras albidum*	Carcinogenic
Wormwood (absinthe)	*Artemisia absinthium*	Psychosis, hallucinations
Yohimbe	*Pausinystalia yohimbe*	Hypertension, headache, anxiety, insomnia, nausea, vomiting

6. Which herbal preparations have demonstrated therapeutic benefits?

St. John's wort (*Hypericum perforatum*) is effective in the treatment of mild to moderate depression.

Ginkgo biloba has been shown in clinical trials to reduce symptoms associated with circulatory impairment including vertigo, tinnitus, and intermittent claudication. Ginkgo may also improve cognitive and social functioning in adults with Alzheimer's disease and multi-infarct dementia.

Saw palmetto (*Serenoa repens*) appears to be an effective agent for treating symptoms associated with benign prostatic hypertrophy.

Ginger (*Zingiber officinale*) taken in 1-gm doses may relieve postoperative nausea and vomiting as well as seasickness and motion sickness.

Valerian (*Valeriana officinalis*) is a mild anxiolytic and sedative that may be useful for disturbances of sleep.

Feverfew (*Tanacetum parthenium*) has been shown to be effective in migraine prophylaxis, reducing both the frequency and intensity of headaches.

7. Do herbal preparations interact with prescription or over-the-counter (OTC) drugs?

Yes. The herbal sedatives valerian and kava kava should not be coingested with opioids, ethanol, or any sedative-hypnotic drug including barbiturates and benzodiazepines. St. John's wort and yohimbe inhibit monoamine oxidase in vitro and should not be taken with tricyclic anti-depressants, OTC diet aids, or decongestants containing phenylpropanolamine or pseudo-ephedrine. St. John's wort has been demonstrated to inhibit the uptake of serotonin and has been associated with serotonin syndrome when used in combination with selective serotonin reuptake inhibitors. Furthermore, St. John's wort has been recognized as a potent inducer of the cy-tochrome P450 metabolic enzyme system and may lead to significant reductions in blood levels and effectiveness of drugs such as cyclosporine and oral contraceptives. Ginkgo biloba, ginseng, garlic, and dong quai are reported to have anticoagulant effects and should be avoided by patients on heparin or warfarin (Coumadin). Stimulant-laxative herbs such as senna (*Cassia angustifolia*) and cascara (*Cascara sagrada*) can decrease the intestinal absorption of drugs. Licorice may po-tentiate the action of corticosteroids.

8. What advice should be given to pregnant and breast-feeding patients regarding herbal preparations?

As with all drugs, herbal preparations may cross the placenta and be secreted in breast milk. In general, herbal preparations should not be taken during pregnancy or lactation. However, many herbalists advocate the therapeutic use of ginger for nausea associated with pregnancy. In Chinese medicine and throughout the world, millions of pregnant women have consumed ginger without documented adverse effects. In controlled clinical trials, ginger was found effective for hyperemesis gravidarum. However, high doses of ginger have demonstrated mutagenicity in vitro.

Herbs that promote menstruation (emmenagogues), such as blue cohosh, tansy, rue, mother-wort, and goldenseal, may also induce abortion. Confusion over the use of pennyroyal as an em-menagogue has led to several cases of severe poisoning. The essential oil of pennyroyal is highly concentrated and toxic and can cause massive hepatic damage. However, herbalists sometimes advocate small quantities of pennyroyal tea for menstrual irregularities. Pennyroyal use should be suspected in any pregnant patient with liver failure.

9. What should I do if I suspect herbal medicine poisoning in my patient?
- Have the patient stop taking all herbal preparations immediately and bring them in the orig-inal packaging.
- Determine if the product was imported or manufactured domestically.
- Write down a history of all medications and herbal medicines taken, including method of preparation and dose consumed.
- Call a regional poison control center for advice on management of the poisoning.
- Collect and freeze urine and blood samples for possible diagnostic testing.
- Consider having the herbal product evaluated by a qualified botanist or tested for chemical contaminants or toxins.
- Report the adverse event to the FDA's MedWatch program (1-800-FDA-1088).

10. What recommendations are suggested for people who want to use herbal preparations?

Warn patients not to believe unsubstantiated claims for benefits that seem too good to be true. Explain the difference between research and regulation of drug formulations and anecdotal information on herbal therapies. Recommend that herbs be purchased from a reputable source and be manufactured in the U.S.

Encourage patients to bring in herbal preparations so you can familiarize yourself with what they are taking. Carefully check the labels for ingredient lists and source of herbs. In summary, ask about herbs, listen to reasons for use, and learn.

11. *Extra credit:* If you sailed to an island and joined in a native ceremony where partici-pants used the powdered roots of the kava kava (*Piper methysticum*) to prepare a hypnotic herbal drink, in which area of the world's oceans would you be sailing?

The South Pacific, mainly the islands of Fiji, Tonga, and Samoa.

12. *Extra credit:* **This herbal substance, which is flown into the U.S. daily from Yemen and Turkey, was of some concern to soldiers who, in 1992, were assigned to the military operations in Somalia, where it is chewed by the residents for its stimulant effects. What is it?**

Khat (*Catha edulis*).

BIBLIOGRAPHY

1. Almeida JC, Grimsley EW: Coma from the health food store: Interaction between kava and alprazolam. Ann Intern Med 125:940–941, 1996.
2. Anderson IB, Mullen WH, Meeker JE, et al: Pennyroyal toxicity: Measurement of toxic metabolite levels in two cases and review of the literature. Ann Intern Med 124:726–734, 1996.
3. Barrett B, Kiefer D, Rabago D: Assessing the risks and benefits of herbal medicine: An overview of scientific evidence. Altern Ther Health Med 5:40–49, 1999.
4. Blumenthal M (ed): The Complete German Commission E Monographs: Therapeutic Guide to Herbal Medicines. Austin, TX, American Botanical Council and Integrated Medicine Communications, 1998.
5. Borins M: The dangers of using herbs. What your patients need to know. Postgrad Med 104:91–95, 99–100, 1998.
6. Cupp MJ: Herbal remedies: Adverse effects and drug interactions. Am Fam Physician 59:1239–1245, 1999.
7. Eisenberg DM, Davis RB, Ettner SL, et al: Trends in alternative medicine use in the United States, 1990–97. JAMA 280:1569–1575, 1998.
8. Ernst E. Harmless herbs? A review of the recent literature. Am J Med 104:170–178, 1998.
9. Fugh-Berman A: Herb-drug interactions. Lancet 355:134–138, 2000.
10. Hung OL, Lewin NA, Howland MA: Herbal preparations. In Goldfrank LR, Flomenbaum NE, Lewin NA, et al (eds): Goldfrank's Toxicologic Emergencies, 6th ed. Stamford, CT, Appleton & Lange, 1998, pp 1221–1241.
11. Huxtable RJ: The myth of beneficent nature: The risks of herbal preparations. Ann Intern Med 117:165–166, 1992.
12. Klepser TB, Klepser ME: Unsafe and potentially safe herbal therapies. Am J Health System Pharm 56:125–138, 1999.
13. Ko RJ: Causes, epidemiology, and clinical evaluation of suspected herbal poisoning. J Toxicol Clin Toxicol 37:697–708, 1999.
14. McIntyre M: A review of the benefits, adverse events, drug interactions, and safety of St. John's wort (*Hypericum perforatum*): The implications with regard to the regulation of herbal medicines. J Altern Complement Med 6:115–124, 2000.
15. O'Hara MA, Kiefer D, Farrell K, Kemper K: A review of 12 commonly used medicinal herbs. Arch Fam Med 7:523–536, 1998.
16. Shannon M: Alternative medicines toxicology: A review of selected agents. J Toxicol Clin Toxicol 37:709–713, 1999.

59. PLANTS

Anne-Michelle Ruha, M.D.

1. How common are plant exposures?

Plants ranked as the fourth largest category of exposures reported to the American Association of Poison Control Centers (AAPCC) in 1998. Of the 122,578 plant exposures reported, over 2100 were considered to have moderate or major outcomes, and 4 resulted in death.

2. What populations are most at risk

Children younger than 6 years of age account for the greatest number of plant exposures because of their attraction to bright flowers and berries and their tendency to put accessible objects in their mouths. Most of these exposures are benign because of the low toxicity and small amount of plant ingested.

More serious exposures tend to involve adults who deliberately ingest plants. The populations at greatest risk for adverse effects include suicidal patients, foragers and herbalists who mistake poisonous plants for edible ones, and recreational plant users in search of psychotropic effects.

3. How should a patient with an unknown plant ingestion be managed?

As with all toxic exposures, immediate attention should be given to the airway, breathing, and circulation (ABCs). If dermal exposure has occurred, the patient should be decontaminated with soap and water. Patients who present early after a plant ingestion with an intact airway should receive activated charcoal.

Attempts should be made to identify the plant involved. Poison centers, local botanists, and even the Internet may aid in this task. In general, treatment is symptomatic and supportive. Intravenous fluids, vasopressors, and antiarrhythmic agents should be used for hypotension and dysrhythmias. Seizures may be controlled with benzodiazepines and barbiturates. If rhabdomyolysis develops, urinary alkalization may be achieved using intravenous sodium bicarbonate. With most plants, if symptoms have not developed within 6 hours of ingestion, toxicity is unlikely to occur.

4. Why is *Dieffenbachia* referred to as "dumbcane"?

Dieffenbachia, a common houseplant, has large green leaves with ivory splotches in their centers. The leaves contain needle-like calcium oxalate crystals that are bundled in raphides. The raphides are packaged together with proteolytic enzymes into idioblasts. When a dieffenbachia leaf is damaged, as with mastication, the idioblasts fire, releasing the sharp crystals and proteases. This may produce severe pain and swelling of the tongue, lips, and oral mucosa, rendering the victim mute, or "dumb."

5. Which houseplants are the most toxic?

A review of AAPCC data from 1985–1994 found dieffenbachia and philodendron, another calcium oxalate-containing houseplant, to be the most commonly reported plant exposures. Despite the many exposures reported, serious toxicity was rare, and most patients developed only minor mucous membrane irritation. Severe swelling, pain, and salivation may occur, with the potential for airway compromise. The majority of exposures respond to cool liquids or ice cream.

6. What plant ingestions are most likely to result in cardiac glycoside toxicity?

Although foxglove (*Digitalis purpurea, D. lanata*), from which digitoxin and digoxin are derived, is the most well known of the cardiac glycoside–containing plants, those most likely to cause toxicity following ingestion include common oleander (*Nerium oleander*), yellow oleander

(*Thevetia peruviana*), and lily of the valley (*Convallaria majalis*). Other plants containing cardiac glycosides include *Urginea maritima* (squill), *Helleborus niger* (Christmas rose), and *Strophanthus gratus* (ouabain). Common oleander is responsible for most of the exposures reported in the United States each year.

Oleander contains several cardiac glycosides, including oleandrin and digitoxigenin. These act similarly to digoxin by inhibiting the membrane-bound sodium-potassium-adenosine triphosphatase (Na-K-ATPase). Intracellular sodium and calcium concentrations rise, and, in severe poisonings, hyperkalemia may develop. The increased sodium and calcium levels lead to late afterdepolarizations and increased automaticity. Similar depolarization of baroreceptors innervated by the ninth cranial nerve produces increased vagal tone.

7. How does plant-derived cardiac glycoside toxicity present? How is it treated?

Clinical presentation of poisoning with plant-derived cardiac glycosides is similar to that seen with digoxin toxicity. Symptoms include nausea, vomiting, visual changes, mental status changes, and cardiac arrhythmias. The dysrhythmias experienced are varied and may include premature ventricular contractions, bradycardia, atrioventricular block, and ventricular tachycardia and fibrillation.

Plant-derived cardiac glycosides may cross-react with immunoassays for digoxin, aiding diagnosis. However, the levels obtained do not correlate with toxicity and cannot be used to guide treatment. Patients with life-threatening dysrhythmias or hyperkalemia may benefit from administration of digoxin-specific antibody fragments (Digibind). The dose required should be based on the patient's clinical response. If Digibind is unavailable, dysrhythmias may respond to lidocaine or phenytoin. Management of cardiac glycoside toxicity is otherwise supportive. Calcium should never be given to patients poisoned with cardiac glycosides, because the intracellular calcium concentration is already elevated, and exogenous calcium may result in a sustained contraction ("stone heart").

8. Which plants exert cardiotoxic effects that are clinically difficult to distinguish from cardiac glycoside toxicity?

1. **Aconitine** is derived from *Aconitum* species (monkshood, wolfsbane), and its use in herbal preparations has resulted in many poisonings.

2. **Veratrum alkaloids** are found in the *Veratrum* species (white hellebore, false hellebore) and *Zigadenus* species. Toxicity has resulted from ingestion of sneezing powders made from pulverized roots of *Veratrum* species and from ingestion of *Zigadenus* species when mistaken for wild onions.

3. **Grayanotoxins** are resins present in rhododendrons, mountain laurels, and azaleas. Most grayanotoxin poisonings are the result of consumption of honey made by bees that collected nectar from these plants.

These toxins act by increasing the permeability of voltage-sensitive sodium channels, resulting in increased automaticity and enhanced vagal tone. Bradycardia, supraventricular tachycardia, atrioventricular blocks, and ventricular dysrhythmias may develop. Aconitine has also been associated with torsades de pointes. Other effects include nausea, vomiting, and central nervous system (CNS) changes. There are no antidotes for these toxins. Management is supportive and includes activated charcoal, intravenous fluids, atropine, vasopressors, and aggressive treatment of dysrhythmias.

9. What toxicity has been associated with the ingestion of apricot kernels?

Ingestion of the kernels of the *Prunus* species (cherries, peaches, plums, apricots) and the seeds of the *Malus* species (apples) may produce fatal cyanide poisoning. The cyanogenic glycoside, amygdalin, is present in these plants and yields hydrocyanic acid upon hydrolysis. The degree of toxicity is determined by the amount of amygdalin ingested and hydrocyanic acid released. (See Chapter 53, Cyanide and Hydrogen Sulfide, for treatment of cyanide poisoning.)

10. An adolescent develops confusion, mydriasis, dry axilla, and tachycardia following the recreational use of a plant. What plants may cause this syndrome?

The patient's symptoms are characteristic of an anticholinergic toxidrome, which is often described by the mnemonic blind as a bat, hot as a hare, red as a beet, dry as a bone, and mad as a hatter. Anticholinergic plants contain tropane, or belladonna, alkaloids including atropine, hyoscyamine, and scopolamine. These act through competitive inhibition of acetylcholine at central and peripheral postsynaptic muscarinic receptors.

Common Anticholinergic Plants

COMMON NAME	TAXONOMIC CLASSIFICATION
Deadly nightshade	*Atropa belladonna*
Jimsonweed	*Datura* species
Angel trumpet	*Brugmansia* species
Henbane	*Hyoscyamus niger*
Mandrake	*Mandragora officinarum*

The most likely cause of this patient's symptoms is jimsonweed (*Datura* species), which is popular among teenagers who have learned of its hallucinogenic effects. The plant grows abundantly along roadsides and in fields and is distinguished by its spiny round fruit, which contains 50–100 seeds. The seeds are the most toxic part of the plant, and ingestion of the contents of a single fruit may provide the equivalent of 6 mg of atropine.

11. How is jimsonweed toxicity treated?

Toxicity develops as early as 30 minutes after ingestion and can last up to 48 hours. Symptoms include tachycardia, mydriasis, dry flushed skin, decreased bowel sounds, urinary retention, sedation, and hallucinations. Hyperthermia, seizures, and coma may occur with severe toxicity, and rhabdomyolysis is not unusual.

Treatment of these patients is supportive. Some authors recommend physostigmine to treat patients with CNS effects (coma, hallucinations). Physostigmine inhibits cholinesterase, reversing the anticholinergic effects by increasing the amount of acetylcholine available at muscarinic receptors. The risks of this therapy may outweigh the benefits, however, because intravenous physostigmine administration has resulted in convulsions, bradycardia, heart blocks, and asystole. If physostigmine is used, consultation with a toxicologist or poison control center is recommended.

12. What toxin is found in water hemlock?

Cicutoxin is a resin that is present in all parts of water hemlock (*Cicuta* species) and is responsible for the plant's toxic effects. Water hemlock grows along lakes, streams, and marshes. Its roots, tuberous structures with air-filled chambers, contain the highest concentration of toxin. The stems are hollow, and both the stems and roots have a strong carrot-like odor. Poisoning most often occurs when the plant is ingested after being mistaken for a wild carrot, parsnips, or a nontoxic member of the Umbelliferae family, such as Queen Anne's lace (*Daucus carota*).

Just a few bites from the root of water hemlock can result in fatal cicutoxin poisoning. Nausea, vomiting, abdominal pain, and diaphoresis occur within 60 minutes of ingestion, followed by seizures. Death occurs secondary to status epilepticus and cardiac arrest. Treatment is supportive and includes airway protection, administration of activated charcoal, and seizure control with benzodiazepines and barbiturates.

13. Which plant was reportedly used to execute Socrates?

Poison hemlock (*Conium maculatum*) was used in ancient times for capital punishment and murder and was likely responsible for the death of the Greek philosopher. Poison hemlock grows throughout the United States along roadways and railroads. It is very similar in appearance to *D. carota* (Queen Anne's lace) and *Cicuta* species (water hemlock) and is sometimes mistaken for edible plants. Purple spots on the hollow stems aid in identification of this plant. Although all parts of the plant are toxic, the roots are the most poisonous.

Poison hemlock contains the nicotine alkaloid coniine. Coniine acts through activation and then blockade of nicotinic acetylcholine receptors. Initial effects of stimulation include salivation, nausea, vomiting, diarrhea, and tachycardia and are followed by effects of blockade including bradycardia, paralysis, and coma. Treatment should be initiated with activated charcoal and supportive care, with intravenous fluids, benzodiazepines for seizures, and mechanical ventilation as needed.

14. What toxin was implicated in the death of Georgi Markov, an exiled Bulgarian broadcaster?

In London in 1978, Markov was injected with **ricin** in the posterior thigh with a small spherical capsule from the tip of an umbrella. He died 3 days later from severe gastroenteritis and multiorgan failure. Though no toxin was identified on autopsy, it was determined that only ricin was capable of producing such effects in the small quantity injected.

15. What is ricin?

Ricin, a toxalbumin, is found in the seeds of the castor bean (*Ricinus communis*). Despite its reputation as the most potent of plant toxins, ricin is unlikely to cause toxicity if the whole seeds are ingested. The toxin is protected by a hard shell and is released only if this shell is disrupted, as with mastication. Surprisingly, ingestion of chewed castor beans rarely results in significant morbidity. Ricin is much more toxic when administered parenterally.

Ricin acts by binding to the 60s ribosomal subunit in cells and interfering with protein synthesis. With severe poisoning, gastroenteritis with shock, dehydration, and hepatorenal dysfunction can develop. Mental status changes, seizures, and hyperthermia may also occur. Management includes gastric decontamination and supportive care.

16. What plants are responsible for the majority of plant dermatitis?

Rhus species (also called *Toxicodendron*), which include poison ivy (*R. radicans*), poison oak (*R. diversiloba*), and poison sumac (*R. vernix*), are responsible for a significant amount of allergic contact dermatitis in North America. An estimated 50–70% of the adult population is sensitive to the antigenic sap material, urushiol contained within these plants.

17. How is plant dermatitis treated?

Many people have learned to identify and avoid poison ivy and poison oak with the saying "leaves of three, leave them be." If exposure does occur, antigen from an injured leaf enters the skin rapidly and, if not completely removed within 10–30 minutes, will cause dermatitis in susceptible individuals within 8 hours to 10 days. Any resin remaining under the fingernails may continue to spread antigen to other parts of the body, so fingernails should be scrubbed with soap and water.

Dermatitis is characterized by redness, papules, vesicles, bullae, and linear streaking. Fluid from ruptured vesicles is not antigenic and does not cause spread of the dermatitis. Mild dermatitis may be treated with steroid creams and oral antihistamines. More severe cases may require oral corticosteroids, which should be tapered over a 2–3-week period to avoid rebound of the dermatitis. Hydrocarbon-type products now sold in some outdoor recreation stores can be applied to the exposed areas to limit the chance of skin reaction to the antigen.

18. What findings are expected in a patient who has ingested improperly prepared pokeweed?

Pokeweed (*Phytolacca americana*) contains the saponin glycosides phytolaccatoxin and phytolaccagenin, which may produce severe gastrointestinal toxicity if ingested. Pokeweed grows in the eastern U.S. and has red stems and stalks and dark purple berries that grow in groups of twenty to thirty. Consumption of this plant in poke salads is not uncommon and is usually harmless if the toxins are removed by parboiling. The leaves should be boiled twice, and the contaminated water should be discarded after the first boiling. Ingestion of various poke-weed recipes, including pokeberry tea and pokeberry wine, may lead to vomiting and diarrhea that can be foamy in appearance if toxin remains. Symptoms can progress to severe dehydration and hypovolemia.

Pokeweed also contains a mitogenic protein that may be ingested or absorbed through broken skin. Effects from this mitogen can produce a plasmacytosis seen on peripheral smear for up to 2 weeks following exposure. Eosinophilia and thrombocytopenia may also occur. A final clue to a diagnosis of pokeweed toxicity may be purple staining of the skin from handling the berries. Treatment is supportive, with activated charcoal and fluid resuscitation.

19. A child presents with vomiting and hypoglycemia after eating fruit that has been imported from Jamaica. What is the likely toxin responsible?

Hypoglycin A, found in unripe akee fruit from the *Blighia sapida* tree, is a potent hypoglycemic agent. Unripe, damaged, or decayed akee fruit may contain 100 times the amount of hypoglycin A that is in ripe fruit. Ingestion of this toxin results in inhibition of beta-oxidation of fatty acids, leading to microvesicular steatosis of the liver, hyperammonemia, metabolic acidosis, and hypoglycemia.

The akee fruit tree is native to West Africa but also grows in the Caribbean and southern Florida. It is a regular part of the Jamaican diet, with poisonings commonly referred to as "Jamaican vomiting sickness." Fatal toxicity occurs more often in children than in adults. In West Africa in 1998, an outbreak of encephalopathy, in which 29 children between the ages of 2 and 6 died, was attributed to ingestion of unripe akee fruit.

Toxicity is characterized by nausea and vomiting with severe hypoglycemia. Hypotonia, convulsions, and coma may ensue. Treatment should include administration of activated charcoal, glucose, intravenous fluids, and benzodiazepines and barbiturates for seizure control. Carnitine may offer some therapeutic value.

20. What is khat?

Khat (*Catha edulis*) is a plant that is popular among populations of East Africa and southwestern Arabia for its stimulant effect. In recent years, khat has been imported to the United States and Europe. The active constituent of this plant is cathinone, a potent amphetamine-like substance found in highest concentrations in fresh young leaves. Chewing these leaves produces euphoria and excitation. In large amounts, agitation and psychosis may occur. Effects last for about 3 hours and are followed by a depressive phase. Dependence is mainly psychological, although minor withdrawal symptoms may develop after discontinuation of prolonged use.

21. How does betel nut toxicity present?

Betel nut (*Areca catechu*) is used by 600 million people worldwide and is an integral part of the culture in Far East Asia, East Africa, India, and the South Pacific. It is an addictive drug with effects similar to nicotine. Cholinergic effects may occur in first-time users or following excessive use. The toxin, arecoline, is a cholinergic alkaloid that stimulates both nicotinic and muscarinic receptors. Effects may include nausea and vomiting, salivation, diaphoresis, bronchospasm, bronchorrhea, bradycardia or tachycardia, dysrhythmias, hypertension, hallucinations, seizures, paralysis, and coma. Betel-nut users can be identified by the deep red oral mucosa, red saliva, and dark-stained teeth that is caused by coloring contained in the preparation.

22. Name some plants that have a reputation of being poisonous but are in fact of low toxicity.

The most common are the popular Christmas plants, poinsettia and holly. The poinsettia (*Euphorbia pulcherrima*) is most undeserving of its reputation, which is based on a solitary case report from 1919. Ingestion of this plant rarely causes symptoms but may occasionally result in minor gastrointestinal irritation. Similarly, holly (*Ilex* species) has bright red berries that are frequently ingested but are rarely of consequence. When symptoms do occur from holly berry ingestion, they are also gastrointestinal.

23. *Extra credit:* **At Christmastime, this plant part is used in a popular drink, but in the prison population, it has been abused as a hallucinogenic substance. What is the common name of this plant material?**

Nutmeg, the fruit of the tree *Myristica fragrans.*

24. *Extra credit:* **American colonists called this fruit, which is often mistaken for a vegetable, the "love apple" but avoided it because they believed it was poisonous. Name this fruit.**

The tomato, *Lycopersicon esculentum.*

BIBLIOGRAPHY

 1. Chapel TA, Chapel J: Toxicodendron dermatitis. In Tintinalli JE, et al (eds): Emergency Medicine: A Comprehensive Study Guide, 4th ed. New York, McGraw-Hill, 1996, pp 1111–1112.
 2. Furbee B, Wermuth M: Life-threatening plant poisoning. Crit Care Clin 13:849–887, 1997.
 3. Graeme DA, Braitberg G, Kunkel DB, et al: Toxic plant ingestions. In Auerbach PS (ed): Wilderness Medicine, 4th ed. St. Louis, Mosby, 2000.
 4. Kalix P: *Catha edulis,* a plant that has amphetamine effects. Pharm World Sci 18:69–73, 1996.
 5. Krenzelok EP, Jacobsen TD: Plant exposures: A national profile of the most common plant genera. Vet Human Toxicol 39:248–249, 1997.
 6. Litovitz TL, Klein-Schwartz W, Dyer KS, et al: 1998 Annual report of the American Association of Poison Control Centers Toxic Exposure Surveillance System. Am J Emerg Med 17:435–487, 1999.
 7. Meda HA, Diallo B, Buchet JP, et al: Epidemic of fatal encephalopathy in preschool children in Burkina Faso and consumption of unripe akee (Blighia sapida) fruit. Lancet 353:536–540, 1999.
 8. Mrvos R, Dean BS, Krenzelok EP: Philodendron/dieffenbachia ingestions: Are they a problem? J Toxicol Clin Toxicol 29:485–491, 1991.
 9. Nelson BS, Heischober BH: Betel nut: A common drug used by naturalized citizens from India, Far East Asia, and the South Pacific Islands. Ann Emerg Med 34:238–243, 1999.
10. Shih RD, Goldfrank LR: Plants. In Goldfrank LR, Flomenbaum NE, Lewin NA, et al (eds): Goldfrank's Toxicologic Emergencies, 6th ed. Stamford, CT, Appleton & Lange, 1998, pp 1243–1255.

XIV. Envenomation

60. SNAKES AND OTHER REPTILES

Marianne Ingels, M.D.

1. What impact do snakebites have on the world's human population?

Snakebites do not represent a major public health problem in North America. The World Health Organization (WHO) estimates that, although 10,000 people per year in the United States and Canada are bitten by venomous snakes, only 15 die as a result. The American Association of Poison Control Centers reports an average of one snakebite death per year. Worldwide, WHO statistics are more grim. WHO estimates that there are 5,400,000 snakebites annually, over 2,500,000 of which cause symptoms and more than 125,000 deaths. Most of the deaths occur in Asia (100,000), Africa (20,000), and Central and South America (5000).

2. What are the main families of venomous snakes?

This is not as easy to answer as one might think. Classification schemes, from family to subspecies, are debated and revised continuously. Crotalids and sea snakes have been considered distinct families by many sources, but recent reviews instead classify them as members of the Viperidae and Elapidae families, respectively. The burrowing asps were thought to be members of the Viperidae, but they have been reclassified as their own family. With this disclaimer in mind, the venomous snake families are:

Atractaspididae (burrowing asps). These small snakes are found in Africa and parts of the Middle East. They have large maxillary fangs that they use one at a time to bite with backward stabbing motions. The bites are rarely fatal.

Colubridae. This is a large and poorly defined family, in which most of the species are either nonvenomous or lack a venom delivery apparatus capable of causing significant human envenomation. Colubrids are found throughout the world except for the Arctic, Antarctic, southern Australia, and some islands. Most of the nonvenomous snakes in the U.S. belong to this family. At least 50 species of colubrids have caused human envenomation, and, although the symptoms are usually mild, some species have caused fatalities. Important venomous colubrids include the African boomslang (*Dispholidus typus*), bird or twig snake (*Thelotornis kirtlandii*), Japanese garter snake or yamakagashi (*Rhabdophis trigrinus*), and red-necked keelback (*R. subminiatus*). African colubrids are considered the most dangerous members of this family.

Elapidae. Elapids have short fangs located at the anterior end of the maxilla. The predominant characteristic of envenomation by most of these snakes is neurotoxicity. This family includes coral snakes (*Micrurus* and *Micruroides* spp.) found in the Americas, the African and Asian cobras (*Naja, Ophiophagus, Hemachatus, Boulengerina,* and *Pseudohaje* spp.), African mambas (*Dendroaspis* spp.), and Asian kraits (*Bungarus* spp.). It also includes all of the major venomous snakes of Australia, including the taipan (*Oxyuranus scutellatus*), death adder (*Acanthophis*), tiger snake (*Notechis* spp.), brown snake (*Pseudonaja*), red-bellied black snake (*Pseudechis porphyriacus*), and king brown snake (*P. australis*).

- **Hydrophiidae** (sea snakes). These snakes are very similar to the Australian land-based elapids. They are found mostly in the coastal waters off Australia and Southeast Asia. An exception is the pelagic sea snake (*Pelamis platurus*), which also lives in the eastern Pacific Ocean from Baja California to Ecuador. Although sea snakes are now considered members of the Elapidae family, their taxonomy continues to evolve.

Viperidae. This family of snakes has highly specialized fangs. The large fangs. which are either tubular or deeply grooved, are mobile and attached to a relatively small maxillary bone. Viperid envenomation is characterized by tissue necrosis and hematologic disturbances.

- Subfamily Viperinae (Old World vipers). Species of this subfamily are located in Africa, Asia, and Europe, and many are extremely dangerous. Examples include:
    Asia: Russell's viper (*Vipera russelli*)
    Near and Middle East: Levantine viper (*V. labetina*) and Palestine viper (*V. palaestinae*)
    Africa, Asia, and Middle East: saw-scaled viper (*Echis* spp.)
    North Africa and Middle East: desert horned viper (*Cerastes* spp.)
    Africa: puff adder (*Bitis arietans*) and Gaboon viper (*B. gabonica*)
    Europe: European viper (*V. berus*).
- Subfamily Crotalinae (pit vipers). This subfamily includes the rattlesnakes (*Crotalus* and *Sistrurus* spp.), *Agkistrodon* species (copperheads, cottonmouths, and others in the Americas and Asia), *Bothrops* species (fer-de-lance and other snakes in Mexico, Central America, and South America), and *Trimeresurus* species (habu, white-lipped tree viper, and others found in Asia).

3. Which venomous snakes are found in the U.S.?

All of the snakes native to the U.S. that are capable of causing significant human envenomation are either crotalids or coral snakes. The crotalids include rattlesnakes (*Crotalus* spp.), pygmy rattlesnakes (*Sistrurus* spp.), cottonmouths or water moccasins (*Agkistrodon piscivorus*), and copperheads (*A. contortrix*). Rattlesnake bites are typically more severe than cottonmouth or copperhead bites. Native coral snakes include the eastern coral snake (*Micrurus fulvius fulvius*), the Texas coral snake (*M. fulvius tenere*), and the Sonoran coral snake (*Micruroides euryxanthus*). The Sonoran coral snake is much smaller than the other species, with a maximum length of 20 inches. It is considered much less dangerous, with no reported fatalities from envenomation. The vast majority of venomous snakebites in the United States are inflicted by crotalids. Coral snakes account for less than 0.5% of envenomations.

4. Are there states that don't have poisonous snakes?

Alaska, Hawaii, and Maine do not have native poisonous snakes. However, North American and exotic venomous snakes are located throughout the United States in zoos and in private collections. Although the pelagic sea snake is sometimes found in Hawaiian waters, it is not considered native.

5. What time of year do most snakebites occur? Who is most likely to be bitten?

In the U.S., most snakebites occur in the spring and summer, with approximately 90% occurring between April and October. Fifty percent of snakebite victims are between the ages of 18 and 28, and there is a male-to-female ratio of 9:1. Most bites are on the extremities, with 80% involving the fingers or hand and 15% involving the foot or ankle.

6. What is an "illegitimate bite"?

Illegitimate bites are those that are sustained when the victim intentionally handles the snake. At least 40% of rattlesnake bites are thought to be illegitimate, a statistic reflected in the predominance of bites to the hand. There have been several cases in which patients were bitten on the face while attempting to kiss a pet rattlesnake. Alcohol intoxication, not surprisingly, is frequently a factor in illegitimate bites.

7. Define dry bite.

A snakebite is considered "dry" when the snake bites but does not inject any venom. This occurs in up to 25% of rattlesnake bites and up to 60% of coral snake bites. If rattlesnake bite-patients are observed for at least 8 hours and have no signs of local tissue toxicity (bruising, blistering), edema, hematologic abnormalities, evidence of neurotoxicity, or vital sign abnormalities at any point in that time period, the bite is considered a dry bite. This rule cannot be applied to snakes other than crotalids. Neurotoxicity from coral snakes may develop up to 13 hours after envenomation and is not as often associated with significant local damage or hematologic abnormalities.

8. What are some identifying characteristics of pit vipers?
Triangular head
Vertical, elliptical pupils
Heat-sensing pit between the eye and nostril
Single row of ventral scales leading to the anal plate
Rattles on tail (rattlesnakes only)

9. Are there any rattleless rattlesnakes?
Yes. The Santa Catalina Island rattlesnake, *Crotalus catalinensis*, has only a vestigial rattle. This snake is found only on the Santa Catalina Island in the Gulf of California.

10. *Extra credit:* The habitat of the rattlesnake *Crotalus viridis abyssus* is restricted to what popular American tourist attraction?
The Grand Canyon.

11. *Extra credit:* When a rattlesnake makes a noise with its rattle, what is the musical pitch of the sound that is produced?
Between C and $C^\#$ (128–135 vibrations/second).

12. Do rattlesnakes always rattle before they strike?
No. Rattlesnakes may strike without warning. Another misconception is that rattlesnakes must be coiled to strike. In fact, they can strike from almost any position. Although the peak traveling speed of a rattlesnake is only about 3 miles per hour, the strike speed is very rapid, approximately 8 feet per second. The striking range of a snake is estimated as half the length of the snake. It may be longer, however, particularly if the snake is traveling down hill.

13. Is it true that baby rattlesnakes are more dangerous because they can't control the amount of venom they inject?
Definitive data are not available to answer this question despite the considerable amount of discussion and folklore surrounding this issue. Nonetheless, baby rattlesnakes clearly are capable of causing very serious and potentially lethal envenomation. Children have been bitten after mistaking baby rattlesnakes for toys. It is not the size of the snake but the clinical manifestations of the bite that determine severity.

14. Describe the signs and symptoms of crotalid envenomation.
General complaints. Patients may experience anxiety, nausea, vomiting, and a metallic taste.
Cardiovascular. Patients may become hypotensive, usually from volume depletion. Hypotension may be exacerbated by coagulopathy and by venom-induced release of vasoactive amines.
Local injury. The following are usually seen at the bite site:
• Fang marks. Fang marks may not appear as two well-defined puncture wounds. There may be only one puncture mark or even just scratches, and fang marks from baby snakes may not be easy to find. Commonly, a small amount of blood will ooze from the puncture site even in the absence of systemic coagulopathy. The presence of fang marks is indicative of a snakebite, but not necessarily of envenomation.
• Discoloration, swelling, and pain. With significant envenomation, ecchymosis develops from bleeding into the local tissues; this is usually not significant enough to cause anemia. The exception may occur in small children, because the extravasated blood represents a

larger proportion of their blood volume. The swelling, with or without ecchymosis, typically spreads from the bite site to surrounding tissues over the course of several hours and may extend from an extremity into the trunk. Bites to the face are particularly dangerous because swelling can obstruct the airway.

• Local tissue destruction. Rattlesnake venom contains many enzymes (proteases, hyaluronidase, phospholipase A_2, L-amino acid oxidase, and several others) to help digest their prey and which may cause significant tissue destruction at the human bite site. Patients may suffer necrosis of a bitten fingertip or require skin grafting.

Neurotoxicity. Neurotoxicity is not usually an important factor in crotalid envenomation. However, Mojave rattlesnakes, particularly those that live in California, Utah, and southwestern Arizona, have been known to cause respiratory paralysis in the absence of significant local injury and hematologic abnormalities. Several other species, including the southern Pacific rattlesnake, are also known for their milder neurotoxic properties. Patients may develop fasciculations, commonly noted in the face. The available crotalid antivenin does not treat neurotoxicity very well.

Hematologic abnormalities. Envenomated patients frequently develop thrombocytopenia, hypofibrinogenemia, and prolonged coagulation times. Disseminated intravascular coagulation (DIC)–like syndrome is common, but true DIC is rare.

15. Explain the DIC-like syndrome associated with crotalid envenomation.

During the normal clotting process, thrombin cleaves fibrinopeptides A and B from fibrinogen to form fibrin monomers, which then aggregate in chains. Thrombin also activates factor XIII, which stabilizes the fibrin clot. Crotalid venom, by contrast, contains a thrombin-like enzyme that incompletely cleaves fibrinopeptide A or B from fibrinogen. This enzyme does not activate factor XIII. The net results of this thrombin-like enzyme's activity are the depletion of fibrinogen with formation of fibrin split products and the development of ineffective and easily lysed clots. Therefore, true intravascular clotting with platelet consumption, red cell fragmentation, tissue infarction, and significant bleeding do not occur. The thrombocytopenia seen in rattlesnake-envenomated patients is thought to occur by a different mechanism, most likely sequestration by the venom at the bite site.

16. When, if ever, does rattlesnake envenomation cause true DIC?

Although rattlesnake bites can cause true DIC, this is rare. It is thought to be due to rapid systemic absorption of a large volume of venom, perhaps from an intravascular injection of venom. True DIC is a sign of severe envenomation.

17. What is appropriate first aid for crotalid bites?

This question has caused a great deal of argument and anxiety. The general consensus is:

• Keep the patient (and the bystanders) calm. The victim should be at rest as much as possible.
• Immobilize the bitten extremity.
• Transport the victim to an appropriate health care facility as soon as possible.

18. Which first aid measures are potentially (or definitely) dangerous, of questionable efficacy, and therefore *not* recommended?

• Tourniquets. They should not be used in the treatment of any snakebite. They cause tissue ischemia and complicate the injury that the patient has already sustained. Some authors recommend the use of constriction bands, which are circumferential wraps intended to occlude lymph vessels and superficial veins only. A constriction band should be loose enough so that two fingers fit easily underneath it. Because efficacy data are limited, this treatment is not widely recommended.
• Ice. Patients have suffered serious frostbite from the application of ice to snakebite wounds.
• Excision of the bite site
• Electric shock to the bite site

- Cutting on the wound to extract venom. Cutting on the bite site is not effective in removing venom and risks damage to nerves, vessels, tendons, and other important structures.
- Sucking on the wound. This is not an effective way to remove significant amounts of venom and serves to introduce mouth flora into the wound, which increases the risk of infection.

19. What about negative-pressure venom extraction devices?

Commercial negative-pressure venom extractors have been shown in animal studies to remove some venom when applied immediately after the injection of venom. These devices do not require cutting the skin. Although there is little evidence that outcome is changed by these devices, little harm is done by using one as long as it does not delay getting the patient to a hospital for further treatment. However, some data suggest that the negative pressure that is generated may itself cause tissue injury.

20. Does the snake need to be identified in order to treat the patient appropriately?

No. Although it is helpful to know the exact identity of the snake, it is not necessary, particularly in the U.S. where there are only a few venomous native species. Many people have been envenomated while handling or attempting to catch or kill snakes for identification. People have even been envenomated by rattlesnakes that were dead or nearly dead. Do not risk being bitten to identify a snake.

21. What do you do if you are all alone in the wilderness and a rattlesnake bites you?

Most experts suggest that you splint the involved extremity and then slowly hike out to get help, taking plenty of breaks to rest. If you are bitten in the leg, use a makeshift crutch. Drink plenty of fluids to prevent hypotension from third-spacing of fluid into tissues.

22. What should be done for a patient who comes to the hospital with a tourniquet in place?

Some authors advocate that the tourniquet should remain in place until the victim has received antivenin, because there have been reports of sudden deterioration in patient condition following tourniquet release. However, these cases are rare, and, if blood flow to the distal extremity is occluded (the job of a tourniquet, after all), tissue ischemia is a much more definite risk to the patient. The tourniquet should be removed, or at least converted to a constriction band, preferably with antivenin available nearby. Be prepared for sudden deterioration in the patient's condition, not only from release of venom but also from sudden return of blood from an ischemic extremity to the central circulation. The exception to consider in the immediate removal of a tourniquet is a patient who has signs of severe systemic toxicity with cardiovascular instability or frank DIC. In such a case, administer antivenin as soon as possible and then release the tourniquet.

23. Can people be poisoned by sucking out rattlesnake venom?

Rattlesnake venom is absorbed poorly through the gastrointestinal tract, and therefore it is unlikely that significant poisoning would occur by this route. Nevertheless, people who choose to suck on snakebite wounds should spit and then rinse out their mouths.

24. What laboratory tests should be ordered for crotalid-bite patients?

A complete blood count including platelets, fibrinogen, fibrin split products, prothrombin time, and partial thromboplastin time should be drawn. A peripheral blood smear, urinalysis, and creatine phosphokinase are also helpful.

25. If the patient has no swelling after 6–8 hours, are lab tests necessary?

Yes. Some patients show little sign of swelling and yet have significant defibrination and thrombocytopenia. Anecdotal reports indicate this occurs more often after envenomation by baby rattlesnakes.

26. When is skin testing done? What can be determined by the results?

Skin testing with horse serum should be done only when the conclusion has been reached that antivenin therapy is needed. The skin test itself can cause anaphylaxis and can sensitize patients to horse serum. Skin test results are not reliable in predicting a patient's response to antivenin. Patients with a negative skin test may still develop anaphylaxis with antivenin therapy, and patients with a positive skin test may tolerate antivenin without a reaction. Skin tests are usually still performed to comply with package insert instructions for use of the product.

27. When should you *not* do skin testing?

Patients who should not receive the skin test are those with a known allergy to horses or horse serum and those who have received horse-derived antivenin before. These patients should be presumed to be allergic. The skin test should not be administered to patients who may not need antivenin.

28. Can patients with a positive skin test or horse serum allergy still get antivenin?

Yes. In cases of life-threatening envenomation, allergic patients may still receive antivenin in a critical care setting under close and direct physician supervision. The patient should be pretreated with antihistamines and possibly steroids, and an epinephrine drip should be infusing or immediately available. The antivenin must be administered extremely slowly. At any sign of anaphylaxis, the antivenin must be stopped, and the epinephrine infusion rate should be increased. By titrating the epinephrine infusion to the patient's symptoms, physicians are usually able to administer the needed antivenin.

29. What about pregnant patients?

Insufficient data are available on the proper management of pregnant patients with crotalid envenomation. There is some evidence that envenomation may be harmful to the fetus, but this must be balanced against the risk of anaphylaxis to both the mother and fetus with antivenin therapy. Most sources advocate treating pregnant patients as you would any other patient, with the exception that epinephrine should be avoided if possible. Epinephrine decreases blood flow to the placenta. Ephedrine and terbutaline have been suggested as alternatives.

30. How should the dose of antivenin be adjusted for pediatric patients?

It shouldn't. Antivenin neutralizes the venom in the patient's body, and this is independent of the patient's size.

31. How is antivenin administered?

The patient must be in a critical care setting such as the emergency department or intensive care unit. There must be close physician supervision, and drugs and equipment should be available if needed to treat anaphylaxis. Antivenin is administered intravenously, usually in 10-vial increments. There is no benefit to local injection of antivenin. A seriously ill patient may require 50 vials, and the adequacy of the hospital supply should be established.

32. What are the complications of antivenin therapy?

Because the antivenin contains a large amount of foreign protein, patients are at risk for hypersensitivity reactions. In the short term, this manifests as anaphylaxis and in the longer term as serum sickness. Serum sickness usually occurs 1–2 weeks after antivenin administration and is characterized by fever, joint aches, and an urticarial rash. It is usually treatable with steroids and antihistamines.

33. When should blood products be used in the treatment of crotalid envenomation?

Blood products are not routinely needed for crotalid envenomation. Thrombocytopenia, hypofibrinogenemia, and elevated coagulation times are treated with antivenin. Blood products should be considered for those patients with active bleeding. Although adults do not generally become anemic from crotalid envenomation, it is possible for very small children to lose significant amounts of their blood volume into the soft tissues surrounding the bite, and they may require transfusion.

34. When is fasciotomy indicated?

Fasciotomy should be considered only when a compartment syndrome is clearly present, preferably confirmed by objective measurement of increased compartment pressures. True compartment syndrome can occur following deeper penetrating crotalid bites but is rare because most bites do not penetrate the fascia. There are cases in the literature of elevated compartment pressures that have resolved with antivenin therapy alone.

35. Should patients envenomated by rattlesnakes be given antibiotics?

Some authors recommend prophylactic antibiotics because the appearance of rattlesnake envenomation can be difficult to distinguish from infection. Others argue against the routine use of these drugs, citing a low incidence of bite infections and evidence that rattlesnake venom may have intrinsic antimicrobial properties. Higher risk patients include those who have made cuts on their wounds, particularly if they introduced mouth flora to the area by sucking on it. If the patient is not given antibiotics, very clear wound care instructions must be given to the patient at discharge, with cautions to return for signs of infection. Tetanus prophylaxis should be addressed.

36. What are the physical characteristics of coral snakes?

These snakes are elapids and have round pupils, short and fixed anterior fangs, and a double row of subcaudal scales. The coral snakes found in the U.S. have black snouts and a red, black, and yellow or white banding pattern. Coral snakes are shy and generally do not bite unless provoked. When they do bite, they tend to chew rather than strike and release. Their small mouths make it difficult for them to bite anywhere other than digits, web spaces, or other skin folds.

37. What is the mnemonic for identifying coral snakes? How reliable is it?

"Red on yellow, kill a fellow. Red on black, venom lack." This refers to the banding pattern on the snake. Although it is reliable in the U.S. for native species, it not reliable from Mexico City southward.

38. Describe the signs and symptoms of coral snake envenomation.

Patients initially may be asymptomatic, with minimal local trauma. There is generally little edema and no necrosis, and the bite marks may be difficult to see. Patients may develop fasciculations and paresthesias near or at the bite site and in severe cases may develop flaccid paralysis and respiratory failure. Patients may also experience vomiting, dizziness, tremors, diplopia, diaphoresis, myalgias, dyspnea, hypersalivation, and confusion. Death is rare.

39. What is the treatment for coral snake envenomation?

Prolonged observation is required for these patients because local signs are minimal and neurotoxicity can be delayed. In patients with suspected eastern or Texas coral snake bites, early treatment with antivenin is recommended, even if the patient is asymptomatic. If treatment is delayed, paralysis is difficult or impossible to reverse. The antivenin is a horse-derived product and carries with it the same risks of anaphylaxis as crotalid antivenin. Supportive care with intubation and mechanical ventilation may be needed in patients with serious envenomation. No antivenin is available specifically for the Sonoran coral snake, but symptoms are generally mild.

40. What about exotic snakes?

Non-native snakes are imported into the U.S. and are frequently bought by snake enthusiasts for their private collections. An estimated 75,000 snakes are legally imported each year, and about 6800 are venomous. Among the commonly collected venomous species are cobras (*Naja naja*), Gaboon vipers (*Bitis gabonica*), African puff adders (*B. arietans*), kraits (*Bungarus* spp.),

European vipers (*Vipera* spp.), European asps (*V. aspis*), and mambas (*Dendroaspis* spp.). Four percent to 13% of snake envenomation patients in the U.S. attribute their bites to exotic species. The most commonly involved snakes are cobras.

41. What is the treatment for a patients who has been bitten by an exotic snake?

Fortunately, the bitten snake collector is often able to provide the identity of the responsible snake. Unfortunately, specific antivenin can be difficult to locate and may not be available at all. Zoo workers may bring the appropriate antivenin with them to the hospital, but private collectors are rarely as prepared. A regional poison center should be contacted for assistance in locating antivenin and for help with management. Good supportive care often is all that can be provided.

42. What about compression-immobilization?

Compression-immobilization is a technique that has been shown to slow the systemic absorption of elapid venom and is used primarily in Australia. The entire bitten extremity is wrapped with an elastic or crepe bandage with the same tension that is used in wrapping a sprain. The extremity is then splinted. Although this has been proven effective in treating Australian neurotoxic snakebites, it is not recommended for treatment of envenomation by snakes with local tissue toxicity.

43. What should be done for patients who are attacked by spitting cobras?

The most important initial first aid is copious irrigation of the eyes. Spitting cobras (*Naja nigricollis, N. mossambica,* and *Hemachatus*) are African snakes that can eject venom accurately at targets up to 3 meters away. Eye exposure to the venom does not cause significant systemic absorption but can cause corneal ulceration and permanent blindness. Bites from these animals generally cause severe local damage with hemorrhage and necrosis but not neurotoxicity.

44. How many venomous lizards are there in the world?

So far only two are known, the Gila monster (*Heloderma suspectum*) and the Mexican beaded lizard (*H. horridum*), and both are native to North America. They live primarily in the desert and are found in Arizona, California, Nevada, New Mexico, Utah, and Mexico.

45. What is the treatment for venomous lizard bites?

The treatment is general supportive care and local wound care. There is no antivenin available. In animal studies, heloderma venom causes hypotension and respiratory arrest, but these symptoms are rare in humans. Envenomated patients usually report severe, burning pain and may develop edema and cyanosis at the bite site. Tissue necrosis is rare, but pain may persist at the bite site for several weeks. Systemic signs of envenomation are weakness, light-headedness, and diaphoresis. Gila monsters are known for their tendency to hang onto their victims, and they can be quite difficult to remove. Measures involving significant force (e.g., crowbars, flames) have been reported by some authors. In any event, lizard teeth may break off into the wound during the bite or removal of the lizard and should be sought when evaluating the wound. Tetanus immunization status should be addressed, and the wound should be watched for the development of secondary infection.

BIBLIOGRAPHY

1. Bush SP, Hegewald KG, Green SM, et al: Effects of a negative pressure venom extraction device (Extractor) on local tissue injury after artificial rattlesnake envenomation in a porcine model [abstract]. Acad Emerg Med 7:495, 2000.
2. Chippaux J-P: Snake-bites: Appraisal of the global situation. Bull World Health Org 76:515–524, 1998.
3. Dunnihoo DR, Rush BM, Wise RB, et al: Snake bite poisoning in pregnancy: A review of the literature. J Reprod Med 37:653–658, 1992.
4. Holstege CP, Miller MB, Wermuth M, et al: Crotalid snake envenomation. Crit Care Clin 13:889–921, 1997.
5. Integrated Taxonomic Information System: www.itis.usda.gov/plantproj/itis/index.html.

6. Minton SA, Norris RL: Non–North American venomous reptile bites. In Auerbach PS (ed): Wilderness Medicine: Management of Wilderness and Environmental Emergencies, 3rd ed. St. Louis, Mosby, 1995, pp 710–730.

7. Roberts JR, Otten EJ: Snakes and other reptiles. In Goldfrank LR, Flomenbaum NE, Lewin NA, et al (eds): Goldfrank's Toxicologic Emergencies, 6th ed. Stamford, CT, Appleton & Lange, 1998, pp 1603–1619.

8. Stewart RM, Page CP, Schwesinger WH, et al: Antivenin and fasciotomy/debridement in the treatment of severe rattlesnake bite. Am J Surg 158:543–547, 1989.

9. Sullivan JB, Wingert WA, Norris RL: North American venomous reptile bites. In Auerbach PS (ed): Wilderness Medicine: Management of Wilderness and Environmental Emergencies, 3rd ed. St. Louis, Mosby, 1995, pp 680–709.

10. U.S. Department of the Navy: Poisonous Snakes of the World. New York, Dover Publications, 1991.

61. ARTHROPOD ENVENOMATION

Sean Patrick Nordt, PharmD, and Richard F. Clark, M.D.

1. What are arachnids?

Arachnids are any member of the class Arachnida, phylum of Arthropoda, and include spiders, scorpions, ticks, and mites. The latter two are rarely involved a toxicologic concern because although they are significant vectors of infectious diseases, they are not venomous.

2. Are all spiders venomous?

Virtually all spiders are venomous because they require venom to kill and digest their prey. However, of the 20,000 species of spiders found in the United States, only a few (e.g., *Latrodectus, Loxosceles*) are thought to be poisonous or of medical importance to humans. The main difference in the poisonous group of spiders is that they possess fangs large enough to penetrate human skin.

3. What is latrodectism?

Latrodectism is the clinical syndrome resulting from an envenomation of a spider in the genus *Latrodectus*. In the U.S., the most common *Latrodectus* species are the black widow *L. mactans*), red widow (*L. geometricus*), and brown widow (*L. variolus*). At least one *Latrodectus* species inhabits each of the fifty states.

4. What are the clinical signs and symptoms of latrodectism?

The signs and symptoms are largely neurologic, resulting from the neurotoxic venom. The patient often feels the bite, described as a "pin prick," which is a positive identification of a black widow in many cases. Initially, only local pain near the puncture marks from the spider's fangs may be present. An irregularly circular area of erythema with central blanching, often referred to as a "target lesion," may be seen around the site accompanied by local diaphoresis. Systemic symptoms generally begin within 30 minutes but may be delayed for several hours. The absence of systemic symptoms suggests either mild or no envenomation. Pain following a black widow bite can be severe and out of proportion to the patient's other physical examination findings. The victim is often agitated and restless and can be seen writhing on the gurney.

Muscle cramping or tightness is one of the hallmark signs of latrodectism and frequently involves the abdomen. Peritonitis is sometimes misdiagnosed, resulting in unnecessary laparoscopy. Pain from latrodectism is often intermittent; this sometimes gives the erroneous impression that the patient is improving and needs no analgesics when in fact he or she is still significantly envenomated. The natural waxing and waning course of this illness likely explains the proposed efficacy of unproven treatments such as calcium and muscle relaxants.

Autonomic nervous system activation is common in latrodectism, with diaphoresis, nausea, diarrhea, tachycardia, and hypertension. If untreated, symptoms generally peak by 12 hours and may persist for 48–72 hours after envenomation.

5. Is a male black widow dangerous?

Although both male and female *Latrodectus* spiders are venomous, only the female is large enough to pierce human skin and deliver enough venom to cause severe symptoms. The severity of envenomation depends a number of factors including the amount of venom delivered to the patient, the location and number of bites (i.e., a well-vascularized region of the body such as male genitalia would be deemed severe), the age and size of the victim, and the victim's physical condition and underlying disease state.

6. What physical characteristics identify a black widow spider?

Both the immature male and female spiders are light-brown, but the female grows to be much larger (8–10 mm) and changes color to a shiny black with a red hourglass on its abdomen. The hourglass may or may not be present, and its absence does not rule out the possibility of a black widow envenomation. In addition, because the hourglass is on the ventral surface, it may not be seen from the superior view of the victim onto the dorsum of the spider.

7. Are any spiders commonly mistaken for a widow?

A species of spider called *Phidippus* (jumping spider) can have red markings on its dorsal surface. Unlike the black widow, which is docile and nonthreatening, *Phidippus* species can be aggressive. *Phidippus*, however, does not deliver neurotoxic venom to humans, although there may be local pain at the site of envenomation from fang penetration.

8. Where are black widows generally found?

Black widows are nocturnal and prefer woodpiles, crevices, garages, storage spaces, and rock fences. Favorite habitats are portable chemical toilets (e.g., Port-o-sans, Port-a-potty) and out-houses, resulting in male genitalia and the buttocks of both sexes as common sites of envenomation.

The black widow's web is strong but not sticky. Therefore, the spider is alerted to something in its web before the victim is aware of the spider's bite.

9. What is the mechanism of action of black widow spider venom?

Latrodectus venom is one of the most potent neurotoxins discovered. The venom binds to nerve membranes and forms ion channels that allow an influx of calcium ions. In addition, the venom produces a nonspecific spontaneous release of neurotransmitters including gamma aminobutyric acid (GABA), norepinephrine, and acetylcholine by facilitating exocytosis of synaptic vesicles.

10. Is an antivenin available for black widow spider bites?

There is a commercially available antivenin prepared from *L. mactans* that is an IgG horse-serum derived product. Although its clinical efficacy is not disputed, its indication often is. Envenomation from a black widow often is excruciatingly painful but rarely life threatening. Because of the risk of an anaphylactic reaction with horse serum products, the antivenin should be reserved for patients who are refractory to standard supportive measures or who demonstrate more serious effects of envenomation (e.g., dyspnea, severe hypertension, cardiac dysrhythmias). The usual dose is 1 vial (2.5 ml) diluted in 50 ml of normal saline infused intravenously over 30 minutes.

11. What supportive care can be given for black widow spider bites?

Muscle relaxants such as methocarbamol have been suggested. However, clinical experience has demonstrated that benzodiazepines are often more effective than methocarbamol in relieving rigidity and cramping. In addition, benzodiazepines appear to have a favorable effect on lowering blood pressure and tachycardia while providing the patient with some anxiolytic and amnestic effects. The use of an opioid analgesic such as morphine sulfate is also recommended. These patients may require high doses of morphine to achieve significant pain relief. Standard precautions such as monitoring respiratory and mental status and having naloxone readily available are recommended.

12. Where in the U.S. is the brown recluse spider (*Loxosceles reclusa*) predominantly found?

The midwestern and south central parts of this country.

13. Can any other spider bites or lesions be mistaken for the brown recluse?

Because the brown recluse's bite initially is painless, positive identification is almost never possible. As a result, many skin lesions of an unknown etiology are often attributed to the brown recluse. Two spiders that have become more widely known in recent years for producing similar necrotic lesions are *Agelenopsis aperta* (grass spider) and *Tegenaria agrestis* (hobo spider). Both of these are now believed to be responsible for many bites previously attributed to brown recluse spiders.

The grass spider is found throughout the western U.S. from California to Texas and north to Colorado and Wyoming. There are no brown recluse spiders in southern California, although other *Loxosceles* species have been identified. Similarly, brown recluse spiders have never been collected in the Pacific Northwest, where the hobo spider is now thought to be responsible for numerous necrotic lesions in humans.

Other *Loxosceles* species found in the U.S. include *L. deserta* (in western deserts), *L. arizonica* (in Arizona), and *L. refescens* (in the eastern United States). These species are not believed to be as venomous as the brown recluse. One dangerous variety, *L. laeta*, emigrated from South America to the Los Angeles area in the late 1960s, although no severe envenomations by this spider have been reported in the U.S.

14. Why is the brown recluse spider also known as the violin spider?

The brown recluse is also known as the violin spider or fiddleback spider because of a distinctive upside-down violin-shaped marking on its cephalothorax.

15. What components does *Loxosceles* venom contain?

The venom contains a considerable number of enzymes, including sphingomyelinase D, phospholipase, protease, esterase, collagenase, hyaluronidase, and dermanecrosis factors 33 and 37, which are most likely responsible for the classic necrotic lesions.

16. Describe the clinical presentation of a brown recluse spider bite.

Typically, patients present with a skin lesion of unclear etiology. Bites can vary from a minimal wound with local pain and erythema to serious full-thickness skin necrosis. A local burning sensation may develop around the injury shortly after the bite and last for 30–60 minutes. Pruritis around the area may accompany the pain. A small bleb or vesicle may develop at the lesion. This can rupture and form pustules. Central necrosis of varying depths can develop over several days and can measure up to 8–10 cm in diameter with severe necrosis invading underlying muscle tissue. Most cases, however, heal with minimal or no necrosis.

Systemic effects also may be seen with brown recluse envenomations, and the severity of skin lesion does not appear to correlate with the degree of severity of the systemic symptoms. The symptoms of systemic toxicity include fever, chills, malaise, nausea, vomiting, hemolysis, disseminated intravascular coagulation, renal failure, and, rarely, death.

17. What is the treatment of a brown recluse spider bite?

There is no commercially available antivenin for brown recluse spider envenomations. As a result, many therapies have been proposed including corticosteroids, hyperbaric oxygen, colchicine, dapsone, and surgical excision with skin grafting. Scientific data regarding efficacy of any of these therapies are lacking, and there have not been any randomized, controlled studies in humans. Animal studies show no benefit of any of these therapies over routine wound management.

Brown recluse venom causes selective damage to vascular endothelium. Neutrophils adhere to capillary walls with sequestration and activation of these cells. Neutrophil migration into the site of the lesion suggests a possible benefit from dapsone. However, in animal studies and clinical trials, dapsone failed to demonstrate definitive benefit. Dapsone also has an extensive adverse effect profile, including hemolysis, methemoglobinemia, hypersensitivity reactions, and agranulocytosis.

18. What is *Atrax robustus*?

Atrax robustus is the Sydney funnel-web spider that is only found in a 160-km area around Sydney, Australia. This spider is aggressive and rears up when approached. The male is more venomous than the female. The funnel-web spider's venom is neurotoxic, containing atratoxin.

Atratoxin causes the release of acetylcholine, norepinephrine, and epinephrine. Clinical signs of envenomation include muscle fasciculations, tachycardia, dysrhythmias, hypertension, cholinergic crisis, and, rarely, pulmonary edema.

Although 13 deaths have been recorded following *A. robustus* envenomations since 1927, no deaths have been reported since the advent of an antivenin in 1984. In addition, review of the previously reported deaths suggests many may have resulted from a lack of supportive care.

19. Are tarantulas venomous to humans?

Despite popular belief, no. In the 17th century, the European wolf spider (*Lycosa tarantula*) was wrongly implicated as a major cause of morbidity in humans because of its distinctive large size and appearance. A dance called the "tarantella" was actually developed to ward off this imposing spider. It is now believed a *Latrodectus* species was responsible for many spider envenomations during this time period.

In North America, common tarantulas are not usually poisonous to humans, although they may produce a bite that causes local pain and swelling. In addition to biting, the tarantulas' other defensive maneuver is to flick body hairs from their abdomen; the hairs can become embedded in the skin or eyes, resulting in pain or an urticarial reaction.

20. What is the most venomous scorpion in the United States?

The scorpion considered most venomous in the United States is *Centruroides exilicauda*, formerly known as *C. sculpturatus*. Its common name is the **bark scorpion**. *C. sculpturatus* mostly inhabits Arizona, although some may be found in Texas, New Mexico, Nevada, and the very eastern parts of the Californian desert.

Scorpion stings from other less toxic species are much more common in most of the U.S. The clinical effects of these stings are similar to that of Hymenoptera and only require treatment for local pain.

21. Describe the mechanism of *C. sculpturatus* venom.

C. sculpturatus venom causes repetitive firing of neurons by binding to sodium channels and impeding neuronal channel inactivation. This results in a prolongation of neuron action potentials and spontaneous depolarization of both sympathetic and parasympathetic nervous systems.

22. What is the clinical presentation of *Centruroides* envenomation?

Clinical symptoms vary from mild pain at the site of envenomation to severe cranial nerve dysfunction. Typically, patients have pain and paresthesias around the site of envenomation. This may progress to perioral numbness. Skeletal muscle dysfunction may be seen with agitation, restlessness, and myoclonic jerks. Autonomic nervous system effects such as tachycardia, hypertension, and hypersalivation can occur. In severe envenomations, patients may develop ptosis, blurred vision, tongue fasciculations, slurred speech, dysphagia, and dyspnea. Severe respiratory dysfunction may require mechanical ventilation, particularly in patients younger than 6 years of age. Convulsions are not found with *C. exilicauda* stings.

23. What is the tap test?

Often, the site of the scorpion sting cannot be seen because there is no swelling, ecchymosis, or erythema. Tapping the area around the suspected envenomation site with a finger determines the site of a scorpion envenomation. The tap test is positive when pain increases over or around the envenomation site with percussion.

24. Is there an antivenin available for *Centruroides* envenomation in the U.S.?

Although there is no commercially available antivenin, a goat-derived antivenin has been produced by Arizona State University. The usual dose is 1 vial (10 ml) diluted in 50 ml of D_5W or normal saline and infused over 30 minutes after a skin test. This antivenin is only available for use in the state of Arizona by a special action of the Arizona State Board of Pharmacy because of the high incidence of hypersensitivity reactions and serum sickness associated with it. In a series of 116 patients treated with *Centruroides* antivenin, 4 had immediate hypersensitivity reactions and 60 patients developed serum sickness.

25. What is the treatment of non-*Centruroides* scorpion envenomation?

The treatment is primarily supportive, using analgesics for local pain (e.g., acetaminophen, ibuprofen). Although rare, acute hypersensitivity reaction to scorpion stings is possible.

26. What is tick paralysis?

Tick paralysis is an ascending flaccid paralysis affiliated with the bites from several different types of ticks in this country, including *Dermatocentor* species, *Amblyomma* species, and *Ixodes* species. Symptoms are related to a toxin that is released after the bite. Signs and symptoms include lethargy, muscle weakness, incoordination, and nystagmus; respiratory paralysis may develop. Treatment involves locating the tick, which is often well hidden in the hair or embedded in the scalp, and removing it. Symptoms generally resolve within several hours of tick removal.

27. Which ticks have Lyme disease?

Ixodes ticks in some parts of the country contain the spirochete that causes Lyme disease. These ticks must be attached for > 48 hours for the illness to occur. Signs and symptoms include fever, myalgias, and rashes. Although prophylaxis is not recommended, macrolide antibiotics can be used to treat Lyme disease when laboratory tests confirm the suspected diagnosis.

28. *Extra credit:* When the French were testing nuclear weapons in the Sahara Desert, what type of venomous animal was able to withstand the most radiation?

Scorpions.

29. *Extra credit:* All centipedes are poisonous, and they possess an unusual means of administering their venom. What is it?

They do not bite but use specialized claws on their front feet.

BIBLIOGRAPHY

1. Clark RF, Wethern-Kestner S, Vance MV, et al: Clinical presentation and treatment of black widow spider envenomation: A review of 163 cases. Ann Emerg Med 21:782–787, 1992.
2. Goldfrank LR, Flomenbaum NE, Lewin NA, et al (eds): Goldfrank's Toxicologic Emergencies, 6th ed. Stamford, CT, Appleton & Lange, 1998.
3. Klassen CD: Casarett and Doull's Toxicology: The Basic Science of Poisons, 5th ed. New York, McGraw-Hill, 1996.
4. LoVecchio F, Welch S, Klemmens J, et al: Incidence of immediate and delayed hypersensitivity to *Centruroides* antivenin. Ann Emerg Med 34:615–619, 1999.
5. Miller TA: Latrodectism: Bite of the black widow spider. Am Fam Physician 45:181–187, 1992.
6. Vetter RS: Envenomation by a spider, *Agelenopsis aperta* (family: Agelenidae) previously considered harmless. Ann Emerg Med 32:739–741, 1998.
7. Wright SW, Wrenn KD, Murray L, et al: Clinical presentation and outcome of brown recluse spider bite. Ann Emerg Med 30:28–32, 1997.

62. MARINE ENVENOMATIONS

Cyrus Rangan, M.D.

1. What is a sponge?

Considered plants until the mid-1800s, sponges are multicellular animals of varying size that can injure victims through numerous spicules made of silica and calcium carbonate. Contact produces an immediate localized dermatitis, similar to poison ivy. Burning and erythema may accompany the exposure. Crinotoxin, the primary component of sponge venom, can cause systemic reactions such as erythema multiforme and anaphylactoid reactions, particularly from the poison bun sponge (*Fubula nolitangere*). Adhesive tape can be used to remove spicules. Acetic acid may assist removal.

2. What is the *maladie des plongeurs*?

Sponge fisherman's disease. This illness actually comes from sea anemones that grow on the sponge. This disease was first identified in French fishermen who used to locate sponges by feeling for them with their hands on the ocean bottom. They would clean the sponges and package them into a mesh sack, which they would carry by a strap suspended from their necks. Because these fishermen worked au naturel, there was ample opportunity for stings.

3. How do you pronounce Cnidaria?

Ask ten toxicologists, and you will get ten different answers. Ask a marine biologist, and you will get the appropriate answer: ni-DAR-ee-uh.

4. More importantly, what *is* Cnidaria?

Cnidaria is an animal phylum, also known as Coelenterata. It comprises the classes Hydrozoa (e.g., Portuguese man-of-war), Scyphozoa (most other jellyfish), and Anthozoa (sea anemones and corals). The common bond they share is the presence of numerous tiny weapons known as cnidoblasts.

5. What is the most poisonous sea creature?

The majority of marine envenomations are not fatal. However, a sting from the dreaded **box jellyfish**, or Australian sea wasp (*Chironex fleckeri*), can lead to immediate wheals and blisters, followed by hypotension, respiratory paralysis, cardiovascular collapse, and death within minutes. Death rates have been recorded at 15–20%. The box jellyfish is camouflaged by its translucent light-blue color, and its tentacles can extend for several meters. Lucky victims may benefit from ovine-derived *Chironex* antivenin, which is available in Australia. One ampule is administered over 5 minutes every 2 hours until progression of symptoms has stopped. A newer, more available treatment is called Stingose, a topical aluminum sulfate-surfactant preparation. Evidence is still being gathered regarding its efficacy.

6. Are other jellyfish lethal?

Death has been attributed to the West Indies sea wasp (*Chiropsalmus quadrigatus*), which closely resembles the box jellyfish, but reports are much less common. Envenomations from more common jellyfish such as the moon jelly (*Aurelia aurita*), the stinging hydroid (*Aglaophenia cupressina*), and the sea nettle (*Chrysaora quinquecirrha*) cause nonfatal but potentially painful stings.

7. What about the Portuguese man-of-war?

Severe envenomations can result from the Portuguese man-of-war (*Physalia physalis*). Stings are extremely painful and are capable of inducing respiratory depression and death if not treated. It is found close to the shores of Florida between July and September. The bell of the man-of-war is about a foot long with tentacles that can stretch 10 feet. Cnidoblasts cover the entire surface of the tentacles.

8. How do cnidoblasts work?

Numerous cnidoblasts are spread along the surfaces of all jellyfish tentacles, on the surfaces of fire coral, and on the finger-like projections of sea anemones. On the outer surface of the cnidoblast is the cnidocil, a bayonet-shaped trigger mechanism. Inside a large vacuole of each cnidoblast is a nematocyst. Each nematocyst is a tightly coiled, ejectable, thread-like package with a sharp barb on the tip that is bathed in viscous venom. Both mechanical stimulation of the cnidocil and electrochemical stimulation (pH changes in particular) can stimulate cnidoblasts to open up and release thousands of nematocysts onto human skin. A spring-loaded mechanism ejects the thread-like substance with great velocity, and the barbs pierce the skin to allow venom injection. Curiously, a lack of surrounding chloride anions will allow nematocyst extrusion but will prevent ejection of the stinging thread.

9. What are the symptoms after nematocyst discharge?

Remember immediate symptoms by the 4 P's: *p*ain, *p*aresthesia, *p*aralysis, and *p*ruritic rash. All, some, or none of these effects might be reported by a patient. The exact mechanism of pain induction is not well understood. Initially, it was thought to be mediated by the direct effect of 5-hydroxytryptamine (5-HT) on dermal pain receptors, because a significant amount of this neurotransmitter is found in jellyfish tentacles. However, very little 5-HT is actually present in nematocysts. The neurotoxicity seems to result from the action of two chemicals: tetramethyl ammonium (tetramine) and *N*-methyl betaine (homarine), which possess curare-like properties. The rash results from various histamine-releasing substances present in the venom. Rare systemic symptoms include anaphylactoid reactions, hypotension, and hemolysis. Possible long-term effects include keloid formation, paresthesias, and peripheral neuritis.

10. What are tentacle tracks?

Characteristic lines of inflammation along the site of exposure to jellyfish tentacles.

11. What is the Irukandji syndrome?

The Irukandji were an aboriginal tribe who inhabited the coast of Cairns, Queensland, Australia. The coast was rich in Carybdeid jellyfish (*Carukia barnesi*). Dr. Hugo Flecker, of *Chironex fleckeri* fame, an Australian radiologist with a strong interest in natural history and marine science, described this constellation of symptoms as a relatively insignificant sting on any part of the body, followed by local erythema. Early pain spreads and becomes exponentially worse over the first hour. Backache, headache, and arthralgias follow. Nausea is present throughout and may be accompanied by vomiting. Profuse sweating is universal, and accompanying symptoms may also include restlessness, pyrexia, tachycardia, cough, hemoptysis, hematemesis, and chest tightness. Patients recover gradually over 1–2 days. Although many types of jellyfish stings *can* result in this described clinical syndrome, the majority of stings are not that serious.

12. Can a floating, detached jellyfish tentacle be harmful?

Yes! Detached tentacles are just as dangerous as attached tentacles. Jellyfish with particularly long tentacles, such as the Portuguese man-of-war, continually lose tentacles, which contain thousands of fully functional nematocysts. A dead jellyfish is just as harmful. Stray tentacles may reside on sponges and other marine creatures.

13. Can jellyfish larvae hurt you *before* they become jellyfish?

Yes! Some jellyfish larvae (*Linuche unguiculata*) can cause atopic dermatitis, especially when they collect in the fibers or waistbands of swimsuits. Also known as sea lice, this malady responds well to topical corticosteroids and antihistamines.

14. What are the "dos" of jellyfish sting management?

- Do wash with salt water or 5% acetic acid (vinegar) for 30 minutes to incapacitate nematocysts. Meat tenderizer (papain) also has been shown to deactivate nematocysts.
- Do carefully remove tentacle fragments with double-gloved hands or forceps. The ejected threads of nematocysts can penetrate surgical gloves!
- Do treat pain. It is the most forgotten aspect of jellyfish sting management.

15. What are the "don'ts" of jellyfish sting management?

- Don't rub or scrape the injured area. Intact nematocysts may discharge.
- Don't use fresh water to wash affected areas. Nematocysts discharge in hypotonic solutions.
- Don't use isopropyl alcohol. It does not deactivate nematocysts and may actually cause them to fire.
- Don't use acidic solutions on stings from the American sea nettle, the little mauve stinger jellyfish (*Pelagia noctiluca*), or the hair jellyfish (*Cyanea capillata*) because their nematocysts may fire under acidic conditions. Instead, an aqueous solution of baking soda applied for 10 minutes is recommended.

16. What's the bottom line?

When in doubt, just wash jellyfish stings with good ol' pH-neutral normal saline and treat the pain with appropriate analgesics. The pain always feels worse than the wound looks!

17. What other creatures have nematocysts?

The phylum Echinodermata contains corals, sea urchins, starfish, and sea cucumbers, many of which have species that contain nematocysts or modified forms of them. Victims are usually skin divers, snorklers, and tide-pool waders. One species of mention is the fire coral (*Millepora alcicornis*). Taxonomically speaking, it is not a true coral—it is a coelenterate in the same class as the Portuguese man-of-war. It contains numerous nematocysts capable of inflicting severe burning pain and urticaria that can persist for weeks. Treatment should include seawater rinse or acetic acid. Some clinicians have used systemic corticosteroids for persistent rash.

18. What was the first recorded toxicity from sea urchins?

Hippocrates first reported on the propensity of sea urchins to cause diarrhea after ingestion. Several early 20th-century studies documented the similarity of gastrointestinal poisoning between ingestion of sea urchin ova and the ingestion of puffer fish.

19. How do sea urchins envenomate?

Sea urchins (*Diadema* spp.) have relatively flat bodies with numerous spines. Some spines are solid and can inflict deep punctures and lacerations, sometimes with retained spine fragments. However, some spines are hollow and communicate with a venom sac. Venom is also administered via triple-fanged jaws called pedicellariae, which are flexible stalk-like appendages used for gathering food. The venom contains histamine-like and kinin-like mediators. Dye within the spines can stain the wounds a dark blue or purple color. The Pacific sea urchin (*Tripneustes gratilla*) secretes a neurotoxin that affects the facial and cranial nerves. Treatment of stings involves immersion in hot water (> 104°F) and careful removal of spines. Spines are radiopaque. Careful inspection of injuries to joints is imperative. Analgesics and prophylactic antibiotics are useful for several days after the injury. Sea urchin venom is unique in that it can cause delayed inflammatory reactions, such as granulomas and nodules. These nodules are painless, sterile, and nonsuppurative and generally need excision only when located on the sole of the foot.

20. My children handled starfish all day at the amusement park tide pool last week. Should I have taken them to the Ferris wheel instead?

Most starfish are not poisonous to humans. However, a few possess venom that is coated along several small spines encountered on the arms. Venom enters the victim passively through puncture wounds. Some stars, such as the Australian crown-of-thorns sea star (*Acanthaster planci*), contain high levels of neurotoxic venom capable of inflicting severe pain, with accompanying erythema and paresthesias. Hot water immersion is recommended to relieve pain.

21. Are sea cucumbers edible?

Sea cucumber ingestion has resulted in significant gastrointestinal distress and even death. However, more sea cucumbers are consumed by humans than by fish. The animal is first boiled and then dried in the sun or smoked. Thus prepared, it is known as trepang or bêche-de-mer in the Indo-Pacific region, where it is sold as a flavoring agent for soups and stews.

22. What is the mechanism of envenomation by sea cucumbers?

These elongated, sausage-shaped creatures have no rigid appendages like starfish and sea urchins. Instead, they have a concentric series of tentacles around the mouth. The venom is contained in the organs of Cuvier. The chief ingredient is holothurin, which causes a rather intense dermatitis. Skin care includes acetic acid or isopropanol along with hot water immersion and pain control.

23. What are the organs of Cuvier?

These sticky tubules are attached to the stem of the respiratory tree of sea cucumbers. Also called Cuvierian tubules, they are emitted through the anus when the animal is irritated or provoked. Because they are filled with a hypertonic solution, they swell and elongate when they come into contact with sea water. Potential predators get tangled in the tubules, the tubules break off, and the venom is released. Eventually, these tubules are replenished within the organism.

24. Why might it be good *not* to "keep an eye out" for sea cucumbers?

Holothurin contact with the eye can cause severe keratoconjunctivitis and even blindness. Areas of water heavily populated with sea cucumbers may contain significant ambient water concentrations of holothurin, which can irritate the eyes of unmasked (and unsuspecting) swimmers. Eye involvement requires copious irrigation, inspection, and prompt ophthalmologic consultation.

25. What do sea cucumbers have in common with red squill, foxglove, oleander, lily of the valley, and *Bufo* species toad venom?

Holothurin is a cardiac glycoside and can cause significant digitalis-like symptoms when ingested.

26. What is a whelk?

An aggressive family of carnivorous snails found throughout Europe and Japan. Japanese whelks have been the source of several poisonings. Venom is concentrated in the salivary glands and contains tetramine. Symptoms of envenomation include headache, dizziness, nausea, and vomiting. Treatment is symptomatic.

27. Are other marine snails venomous?

Cone shells, also called cone snails, are nocturnal mollusks that immobilize their prey with a neurotoxin similar to the basic peptides found in hymenoptera venom. The venom apparatus is part of their feeding mechanism. The proboscis of the snail is launched into the victim, and venom is injected through a detachable, harpoon-like tooth. Two specific toxins mediate the majority of the paralytic effects: (1) ω-conotoxin acts presynaptically and prevents the release of acetylcholine at the neuromuscular junction by deactivating voltage-gated calcium channels, and (2) μ-conotoxin acts on muscle cells to prevent the propagation of action potentials by blocking voltage-gated sodium channels. Hot water immersion can inactivate the toxins. Mechanical ventilation may be necessary in cases of severe respiratory muscle involvement. Most symptoms resolve over 6–8 hours.

28. How dangerous is the octopus?

Next to the great white shark, no marine creature has received more fictional misrepresentation than the octopus. Most octopi are extraordinarily shy and nonpoisonous animals. In fact, the larger the octopus, the more likely it is to avoid human contact. The blue-ringed octopus (*Hapalochlaena maculosus*) is the most common poisonous species, found in shallow waters off the coast of Australia. It has a dull, light-brown color when dormant, but when provoked or threatened, it develops bright-blue rings. Adult poisonous octopi are generally quite small (around 5–6 inches long). The blue-ringed octopus venom contains maculotoxin and cephalotoxin. These toxins are almost identical in structure to tetrodotoxin and prevent the propagation of action potentials by blocking sodium channels. All other marine tetrodotoxin exposures occur through the ingestion of tetrodotoxin-containing fish. Initially, the sting of an octopus can be quite numbing, resulting in an innocuous or even painless injury. A slightly delayed but intense pain follows. Other symptoms of envenomation include paresthesias, rash, numbness, aphonia, dysphagia, and cardiorespiratory collapse secondary to autonomic ganglionic blockade. Death has been reported. Treatment is generally supportive.

29. Why is it important to watch your step in shallow waters?

Stingrays (*Urolophus* spp.) are bottom dwellers and usually lie partially covered in mud or sand. Their venom apparatus is located in the tail. Shy creatures, stingrays reflexively whip their tails upward when stepped on or provoked. Therefore, most injuries are to the lower extremity. The tail barb can even penetrate a thick fisherman's boot! The venom contains phosphodiesterases, nucleotidases, and serotonin, which inflict severe pain and burning out of proportion to the visible wound. Rarely, symptoms include cardiac dysrhythmias, seizures, and coma. Like other marine venom, stingray venom is heat labile. Continuous soaking in hot water (running tap water, as opposed to immersions, is preferred by many patients for comfort) is recommended to deactivate the neurotoxin. The major morbidity associated with the injury is the deep, jagged laceration commonly left by the serrated spines on the dorsum of the tail. An analgesic regimen plus a third-generation cephalosporin or quinolone antibiotic to cover for *Vibrio* species (especially *Vibrio vulnificus*) should be considered.

30. What other dangers lurk among the algae and coral?

Weeverfish (*Trachinus* spp.) are mostly sedentary animals that bury in the sand of shallow Atlantic waters with their heads peeking out. They can survive for long periods of time out of water and can envenomate after death if the fish are improperly handled. Venom contains ichthyoacanthotoxin that is administered by a forward dorsal fin. Symptoms include pain, paresthesias, nausea, vomiting, fever, chills, hypotension, and, in some reported cases, cardiac dysrhythmias and respiratory paralysis. The pain can spread quickly through a limb. The venom is partially heat labile and may be inactivated by hot water immersion.

31. Can your next step in the ocean be your last?

Yes! The Scorpaenidae family contains about 300 species of fish, many of which have envenomated fishermen, scuba divers, and waders. The most notorious is the **stonefish** (*Synanceja horrida*). The dorsal, anal, and pectoral fins of this fish are extremely sharp and have been known to penetrate scuba suits and rubber flippers. The stonefish, a sedentary, well-camouflaged creature, is found in shallow, tropical waters. The venom is poorly characterized but extremely potent.

The Australian stonefish delivers the most venom of all the members of the Scorpaenidae family. Envenomation results in excruciating pain and may lead to hypotension, tachycardia, cardiac dysrhythmias, and cardiovascular collapse. Generalized muscular spasticity is common, and mechanical ventilation may be necessary secondary to respiratory muscle paralysis. Affected areas should be immersed in hot water. Antivenin is available and is stored at various marine research facilities. A regional poison control center can locate antivenin if needed.

Scorpaenidae in the genus *Pterois*, such as the lionfish, turkeyfish, zebrafish, tigerfish, and scorpionfish, all have spines that can deliver venom, but their stings are not known to be life threatening like those of the stonefish. Their prostaglandin-containing venom can cause severe pain. Hot water immersion is usually effective treatment. Analgesics should be administered if needed, and pain can last for up to 2 weeks. Large blisters should be excised. High prostaglandin levels can be found in the blister fluid.

32. What about the moray eel?

Much folklore has been passed through generations regarding the "venomous" moray eel. Research has shown a lack of venom or venom glands in these creatures. Although these creatures can pack quite a bite with their powerful jaws and can be difficult to remove from a bitten extremity, the venomous nature of the moray eel has not been proven.

33. *Extra credit:* Endotoxins found in the dinoflagellates *Ptychodiscus breves* cause "red tides" in the Gulf of Mexico that adversely affect fish, shore animals, and humans. As a group, what are these toxins called?

Brevetoxins.

34. What are the take-home points?
- The majority of marine envenomations can be treated with proper irrigation or immersion and supportive care as dictated by symptoms.
- Tetanus prophylaxis and antibiotics should be administered in all penetrating marine wounds.
- Pain management is important and should be administered early.
- The majority of marine envenomations activate at least one arm of the immune system; as such, systemic oral and parenteral corticosteroids have been prescribed for many patients. However, there is no controlled evidence to indicate the use of nontopical steroids in any of these cases, and they are generally not recommended.

BIBLIOGRAPHY

1. Auerbach PS: Hazardous marine animals. Emerg Med Clin North Am 2:531–542, 1984.
2. Baden DG, Burnett JW: Injuries from sea urchins. South Med J 70:459–460, 1977.
3. Burnett JW, Calton GJ: Venomous pelagic coelenterates: Chemistry, toxicology, immunology, and treatment of their stings. Toxicon 25:581–607, 1987.
4. Fenner PJ, Williamson JA, Burnett JW, et al: The "Irukandji syndrome" and acute pulmonary edema. Med J Aust 149:150–156, 1988.
5. Halstead BW: Dangerous Aquatic Animals of the World. Princeton, Darwin Press, 1992.
6. Halstead BW: Current status of marine biotoxicology—an overview. Clin Toxicol 186:1–24, 1981.
7. Kizer KW, McKinney HE, Auerbach PS: Scorpaenidae envenomation: A five-year poison center experience. JAMA 253:807–810, 1985.
8. Lumley J, Williamson JA, Fenner PJ, et al: Fatal envenomation by *Chironex fleckeri*, the north Australian box jellyfish: The continuing search for lethal mechanisms. Med J Aust 148:527–534, 1988.
9. Olivera BM, Gray WR, Zeikus R, et al: Peptide neurotoxins from fish-hunting cone snails. Science 230:1338–1343, 1985.
10. Tu AT: Biotoxicology of sea snake venoms. Ann Emerg Med 16:1023–1028, 1987.

63. HYMENOPTERA STINGS

Anthony S. Manoguerra, PharmD

1. What are hymenoptera?

The order Hymenoptera contains venomous insects that have the ability to sting through a modified ovipositor on the terminal end of their abdomen. The three groups that are of medical importance are Apoidea (bees), Vespoidea (wasps, hornets, and yellow jackets), and Formicidae (ants). Hymenoptera are social insects that live in large colonies and vigorously defend their colonies when threatened. Single stings may occur when one insect feels threatened, and multiple stinging incidents may occur when the colony perceives a threat to the hive. Hymenoptera are thought to cause between 50 and 100 deaths in the United States each year, primarily from allergic reactions to their venom.

2. Is there a difference among stings of the different members of this order of arthropods?

Each member of the order Hymenoptera has a venom sac attached to the stinging apparatus. All species with the exception of the honeybee have the ability to sting multiple times and, with each sting, inject a portion of the contents of the venom sac. Honeybees are only capable of a single sting because the stinger is barbed and remains in the skin of the victim. When the honeybee attempts to fly away, the stinger and venom sac are ripped from the bee's abdomen, resulting in the death of the bee.

The components of the venom may vary widely among different members of the order. This results in different clinical effects from stings. For example, fire ant stings produce a distinctly different syndrome than do stings of honeybees, wasps, or yellow jackets.

3. How do the venoms differ in their chemical components?

Apoidea	Vespoidea	Formicidae (specifically, fire ants)
Biogenic amines	Biogenic amines	Biogenic amines
Phospholipases	Phospholipases	Phospholipases
Hyaluronidases	Hyaluronidases	Hyaluronidase
Acid phosphatases	Antigen 5	Unidentified others
Minimine	Acid phosphatases	Piperidines
Mellitin	Mast cell degranulating	
Apamin	peptide	
Mast cell degranulating	Kinins	
peptide		

The enzymatic components are thought to be the major allergens in the venoms and are common to all three groups. The biogenic amines are responsible for the local pain, swelling, and erythema seen immediately after the sting. These, along with the other ingredients, are responsible for many of the systemic symptoms seen in massive stinging incidents. Mellitin is thought to contribute the most to the systemic toxicity seen in massive honeybee stings.

4. What are Africanized honeybees (AHBs)?

AHBs, the so-called killer bees, are a hybrid that was developed between the common European honeybee, which is the normal honeybee of commerce in Europe and the Western Hemisphere, and an African honeybee that was brought to Brazil in the 1950s as an experiment to increase honey production and parasite resistance. Several African queen bees and their swarms escaped from the apiary in 1957 and have slowly hybridized with local bees. They have now spread through South and Central America and Mexico and into the United States. As of spring 2000, they had colonized Texas, New Mexico, Arizona, southern Nevada, and southern

281

California. Because these bees have difficulty surviving prolonged spells of below-freezing temperatures, their migration will be limited to those areas where temperatures remain above freezing most of the winter.

5. How do AHBs differ from European honeybees?

AHBs are slightly smaller than their European cousins but contain venom that is practically identical in composition and toxicity. The major difference between the two varieties of bees is their behavior when threatened. AHBs evolved in an environment where there was a great deal of competition for resources and frequent attacks on their hives by marauding animals, including humans. As a result, they developed a highly exaggerated response mechanism when the hive is perceived to be threatened. They respond more quickly and send out a larger proportion of workers in response to a threat to the hive, sting in large numbers, and pursue the threat for up to 1 km from the hive. The net result is that more people will experience multiple stinging incidents as the migration of AHBs expands. It had initially been hoped that hybridization of the Africanized bees with local European bees would decrease the African bees' aggressiveness. This has not been the case, and bees that have migrated into the U.S. have maintained aggressiveness similar to the bees that originally were released in Brazil.

6. What are the effects of a single sting by a honeybee? How should they be managed?

Bee, wasp, and yellow jacket stings produce a sharp, stabbing pain followed by a burning sensation that gradually subsides over 15–30 minutes. The wound develops a wheal and flare, with erythema and edema that may persist for several hours. In nonallergic individuals, this is the usual extent of the injury. The stinger, if present, should be removed and the area washed with soap and water and then treated symptomatically with superficial cooling. Occasionally, there may be exaggerated local effects with extended swelling that may involve an entire extremity. This should be managed with over-the-counter analgesics and topical corticosteroids. The most significant risk to health occurs in patients who are allergic to hymenopteron venom. This IgE-mediated anaphylactic reaction results in a local wheal and flare, generalized urticaria, throat and chest tightness, stridor, wheezing, and cardiovascular collapse. The onset is typically rapid, and death may occur within minutes. Management includes rapid airway and cardiovascular support, fluid resuscitation to maintain blood pressure, and the administration of epinephrine to produce airway dilation and peripheral vasoconstriction. Intravenous (IV) administration of epinephrine is preferred, but if IV access is not readily available, the subcutaneous or intratracheal route should be used. Additional medications such as H1 antihistamines and corticosteroids may be helpful, but these are secondary in importance to administering epinephrine and maintaining airway patency and respiratory and cardiovascular support. Delayed hypersensitivity reactions, such as Arthus reactions and serum sickness, following an acute reaction may require corticosteroid therapy.

7. Will people who are allergic to European honeybee venom also be allergic to AHB venom?

Yes. The venom of the two bees is practically identical not only in the components but also in the percentage of each component. Allergic cross-reactivity is to be expected.

8. What are the effects of a multiple stinging incident involving AHBs?

AHBs will produce massive stinging incidents ranging from a few hundred stings to thousands of stings depending on the size of the hive and the ability of the victim to run from the swarm. Unlike the allergic reaction, which is not dose related and occurs following a single sting, the severity of a multiple stinging incident is directly related to the number of stings inflicted. Depending on the health of the victim and the availability of emergency medical care, as few as 100–300 stings have been fatal, but survival has occurred following more than 2200 stings. In general, the LD_{50} in humans has been estimated at 20 stings/kg. The main toxic ingredient in bee venom is mellitin, which is approximately 50–60% of the venom by weight. Phospholipase A

(12% by weight) also contributes significantly to the toxicity. The other ingredients are in smaller amounts, and their significance to the overall reaction is unclear. The net result of a massive stinging incident is intravascular hemolysis, increased capillary permeability, and hypertension from catecholamine release followed by hypotension from vasodilation, bronchospasm, histamine release, central nervous system excitability, vomiting, diarrhea, rhabdomyolysis, and acute renal failure. Death is usually from acute respiratory and cardiovascular failure. Myocardial ischemia has been reported. Skin surfaces involved in massive stinging incidents may become necrotic. Acute hepatic necrosis has also been observed, but it is unclear if this is a direct toxic effect or the result of hypotension and shock.

9. Who is most at risk from a massive stinging incident?

Children and the elderly. Both age groups may have difficulty fleeing the area of the attack and will therefore sustain a greater number of stings. In addition, children may receive a large dose of venom in proportion to their body weight. The elderly may have preexisting health conditions, such as hypertension and coronary artery disease, which will predispose them to the damaging effects of the venom. Young, healthy adults are more likely to outrun the bees and receive fewer stings and are able to withstand the effects of the venom.

10. How should a massive bee sting injury be managed?

Maintaining a patent airway is of utmost importance. AHBs tend to sting heavily in the head and face area, and early endotracheal intubation should be performed. Administration of inhaled beta agonists may be helpful, but most patients will require IV epinephrine to produce bronchodilation. Hypotension may be managed with epinephrine, norepinephrine, dopamine, or phenylephrine or a combination of these drugs. Because histamine release may play a significant role in the symptoms, antihistamines such as diphenhydramine or hydroxyzine may be helpful either alone or in combination with an H_2-receptor blocker such as cimetidine or ranitidine. While the patient is being stabilized, efforts should be made to remove as many stingers and venom sacs from the skin as possible. They can be removed with a gentle scraping or by adhering tape to them and then removing the tape. It was once thought that squeezing the venom sacs with tweezers would introduce more venom, but a recent study of the anatomy of the stinging apparatus has shown that this is not the case. Nonetheless, removing one stinger at a time with tweezers is a slow and tedious process, and it is likely that all of the venom will be introduced before this process can be completed. Severe hemolysis may require blood transfusions, whereas rhabdomyolysis may require urinary alkalization to minimize deposition of myoglobin in the renal tubules. Acute renal failure may require short-term hemodialysis.

11. Is there a difference in a multiple stinging incident caused by AHBs versus yellow jackets or wasps?

Although the chemicals in the venom sacs differ between the vespids and the honeybees, for all practical purposes the clinical syndromes observed are nearly identical and the management of a multiple stinging incident is the same.

12. What are fire ants?

Fire ant is the common name for *Solenopsis richteri* and *invicta*, two ant families that were introduced in the U.S. from South America in the 1920s, most likely from a ship docked in Mobile, Alabama. They have spread throughout the southern U.S. from Florida to southern California. All members of the ant family can sting, but the fire ant is the most vicious and has the most damaging venom of any of the ants in the U.S. The ant is bright red in appearance and inhabits a loose dirt mound that typically is about 30 cm across and 5–10 cm in height. Thousands of colonies may inhabit a single acre. When their nest is disturbed, the ants exhibit intense ferocity and can inflict thousands of stings in a matter of seconds. They will attach their mandibles to the skin and then pivot their bodies and sting repeatedly until they are removed.

13. Describe the clinical effects seen following a fire ant attack.

Fire ant venom produces an intense, immediate burning pain. A wheal forms quickly followed by clear vesicles and then pustules that break, leading to necrosis and scarring. The venom is composed primarily of substituted piperidines that have hemolytic, cytotoxic, insecticidal, and bacteriostatic activity. Other components such as hyaluronidases and phospholipases may account for some degree of allergic cross-reactivity with other hymenoptera venoms. Massive fire ant attacks have caused the death of grazing animals and pets and are suspected of causing human deaths in infants and nursing home patients who could not protect themselves from the attack.

14. What is the management of fire ant envenomation?

Treatment is supportive in nature. Local wound care should be implemented with thorough cleansing and cold compresses to relieve pain and minimize infection. Antihistamines, topical and systemic corticosteroids, analgesics, and antibiotics should be administered as needed.

15. *Extra credit:* What is unusual about the royal Mayan bee?

It doesn't sting; it bites.

16. *Extra credit:* What is unusual about the velvet ant (*Dasymutilla* spp)?

It is really a wasp.

BIBLIOGRAPHY

1. Clark RF: Hymenoptera. In Olson KR (ed): Poisoning and Drug Overdose, 3rd ed. Stamford, CT, Appleton & Lange, 1999, pp 189–190.
2. Franca FO, Benvenuti LA, Fan HW, et al: Severe and fatal mass attacks by "killer" bees (Africanized honey bees—*Apis mellifera scutellata*) in Brazil: Clinicopathological studies with measurement of serum venom concentrations. Q J Med 87:269–282, 1994.
3. Jones E, Joy M: Acute myocardial infarction after a wasp sting. Br Heart J 59:506–508, 1988.
4. Kim KT, Oguro J: Update on the status of Africanized honey bees in the Western states. West J Med 170:220–222, 1999.
5. Lewin NA: Arthropods. In Goldfrank LR, Flomenbaum NE, Lewin NA, et al (eds): Goldfrank's Toxicologic Emergencies, 6th ed. Stamford, CT, Appleton & Lange, 1998, pp 1625–1634.
6. Lockey RF, Turkeltaub PC, Baird-Warren IA, et al: The hymenoptera venom study 1: 1979–1982: Demographics and history-sting data. J Allerg Clin Immunol 82:370–381, 1988.
7. Mejia G, Arbelaez M, Henao J, et al: Acute renal failure due to multiple stings by Africanized bees. Ann Intern Med 104:210–211, 1986.
8. Nelson DR, Collins AM, Hellmich R, et al: Biochemical and immunological comparison of Africanized and European honeybee venoms. J Allerg Clin Immunol 85:80–85, 1990.
9. Reisman RE, Livingston A: Late-onset allergic reactions, including serum sickness, after insect stings. J Allerg Clin Immunol 84:331–337, 1989.
10. Sakhuja V, Bhalla A, Pereira BJG, et al: Acute renal failure following multiple hornet stings. Nephron 49:319–321, 1988.
11. Schumacher MJ, Schmidt JO, Egen NB, Lowry JE: Quantity, analysis, and lethality of European and Africanized honey bee venoms. Am J Tropical Med Hygiene 43:79–86, 1990.
12. Tumwine JK, Nkrumah FK: Acute renal failure and dermal necrosis due to bee stings: Report of a case in a child. Central African J Med 36:202–204, 1990.
13. Vetter RS, Visscher PK, Camazine S: Mass envenomations by honey bees and wasps. West J Med 170:223–227, 1999.

XV. Toxic Terrorism

64. TOXIC TERRORIST THREATS

David Tanen, M.D.

1. Why are weapons of mass destruction attractive to terrorists?

Terrorism is defined as the threat or use of violence to destabilize society in order to bring about political changes. In the past decade, the public's fear of terrorist attacks has been heightened by the bombings of the World Trade Center, the Alfred P. Murrah Federal Building, and the U.S. embassies in Tanzania and Kenya and by the nerve gas attack against civilians in the Tokyo subway system.

Weapons of mass destruction can be nuclear, biological, or chemical. These weapons may be attractive to terrorists both because of their actual destructive capacity and the mythical qualities of their potential for delayed toxic effects on the human body. Additionally, they allow terrorists to get the biggest bang for their buck. Producing mass casualties using conventional weapons costs $2000/km^2, but the production of mass casualties requires only an estimated $800/km^2 using nuclear weapons, $600/km^2 using chemical weapons, and just $1/km^2 for biological weapons.

2. What is the likelihood of nuclear terrorism occurring?

Nuclear terrorism is still considered unlikely because of the high level of technology, development, and production that is needed. However, the reported thefts of enriched uranium and plutonium from the former Soviet Union and their subsequent discoveries in Germany, Turkey, and the Czech Republic have increased the likelihood that terrorists or nations sponsoring terrorism may be able to construct nuclear weapons.

The consequences of a nuclear attack would be catastrophic. For example, the 1-day mortality after the nuclear detonation over Hiroshima was 45,000 deaths with 90,000 injuries. These numbers represent only the initial mortality and morbidity of the blast and do not include the thousands of subsequent radiation-induced injuries and deaths.

3. What is fallout?

1. **Early fallout** is radioactive material deposited within the first day of detonation. It is highly radioactive and geographically concentrated within a few hundred miles of the site of detonation (ground zero).

2. **Delayed fallout** consists of smaller particles that are deposited after the first 24 hours. These may be widely distributed and present a long-term health hazard, primarily through ingestion of radioactive particles.

4. Describe the clinical effects of acute exposure to high levels of radiation.

Damage to the human body by ionizing radiation is caused by deposition of energy. This results in reactive chemical products, including free radicals, that form further reactive species by combining with cellular components, and producing cellular damage.

Replicating cells are the most sensitive to radiation exposure. Therefore, in descending order of sensitivity, cell types most vulnerable are hematopoietic cells (e.g., lymphocytes), cells lining the gastrointestinal (GI) tract, and skin cells. Mature cells that are highly differentiated appear to be the least affected by radiation (e.g., central nervous system [CNS], muscle, and bone).

5. What is acute radiation syndrome?

Acute radiation syndrome refers to symptoms that appear soon after radiation exposure. Severity is related to the dose of radiation received. Of immediate concern are injuries to the hematopoietic and GI systems, with onset of symptoms within 1–4 weeks. Patients with bone marrow depression have increased susceptibility to infection and bleeding disorders. Treatment consists of administering blood products and preventing infection until the bone marrow recovers. The epithelial lining of the GI tract may slough, leading to excessive fluid loss and electrolyte imbalances. Intravenous fluid replacement and electrolyte correction may be necessary until the lining of the GI tract regenerates.

6. What is the most useful and rapid method of assessing a patient's degree of radiation exposure?

Serial total lymphocyte counts. Optimally, this should be done every 6 hours during the first 48 hours, or at least once every 24 hours after exposure. A 50% decrease in absolute lymphocytes within the first 24 hours followed by a second drop within 48 hours is indicative of a potentially lethal injury from penetrating ionizing radiation.

7. Name the general classifications of chemical agents.

1. **Nerve agents** (e.g., tabun, sarin, soman) are similar to organophosphates; they bind to and inhibit acetylcholinesterase, leading to the accumulation of acetylcholine and stimulation of muscarinic and nicotinic receptors. Extensive stimulation of nicotinic receptors is followed by blockade that manifests as paralysis. Treatment relies on the rapid administration of atropine to block muscarinic receptors followed by pralidoxime to treat nicotinic effects. Pralidoxime may reactivate acetylcholinesterase if aging of the complex has not already occurred. At high concentrations, death may occur within 15 minutes of absorption of a nerve agent through the skin, mucous membranes, or respiratory tract.

2. **Vesicants** (e.g., mustard compounds) consist of cytotoxic alkylating compounds such as sulfur mustard. Although clinical manifestations secondary to exposure generally do not develop for approximately 6–8 hours, cellular and biochemical damage actually occurs within minutes. Emergency responders must be aware that a patient may not exhibit clinical signs or symptoms despite a significant exposure. Immediate decontamination of the victim is the top priority. Soap and cool water is usually adequate.

3. **Cellular asphyxiants** (e.g., cyanides) are typified by cyanide, which binds to cytochrome oxidase in the electron transport chain and inhibits cellular respiration. At high concentrations, death may occur within 5 minutes of inhalation. Treatment with nitrites is aimed at inducing methemoglobinemia to which cyanide preferentially binds. Sodium thiosulfate is then given to provide sulfur and convert cyanide to thiocyanate, a compound that can be renally excreted.

4. **Pulmonary intoxicants and irritants**, such as chlorine and phosgene, cause irritation of the upper and lower respiratory tract. Dyspnea and tachypnea are the usual symptoms, but responders must be careful in their evaluation because the onset of pulmonary edema may be delayed for hours following exposure. Treatment is supportive, and most patients recover.

8. What chemical warfare agent did Aum Shinrikyo cult members use in their terrorist attack against Tokyo in 1995?

The nerve agent **sarin** was placed in five subway cars on three separate lines. The attack resulted in 12 deaths and 5000 casualties. In addition to the casualties, this event proved how easily the medical response system could be overwhelmed with widespread fear, panic, and psychological trauma. Not only were medical facilities overrun with thousands of patients with no evidence of toxicity or exposure, but emergency responders suffered an injury rate of 10% (135 out of 1354 sent to respond) secondary to gas exposure.

9. Why are biological weapons appealing to terrorists?

• They are relatively inexpensive to produce and distribute. Only an estimated $10,000 is needed for the equipment to produce sufficient quantities of biologic agents to cause massive civilian casualties.

- They require the least scientific sophistication. In fact, with a basic education in science, many students are able to master viral and bacterial culture methods.
- There is an incubation period between the dissemination and the beginning of the epidemic (typically 3–7 days for most agents), which allows time for terrorists to escape safely.
- Early symptoms associated with biological agents are nonspecific and the attack would be difficult to detect.

10. How can you recognize that a biologic attack has occurred?

During and immediately after the release of a biologic weapon, direct human health effects would be difficult to recognize. In most naturally occurring epidemics, there is a gradual rise in disease incidence, as people are progressively exposed to an increasing number of patients, fomites, or other vectors that spread the pathogen. In contrast, those exposed to a terrorist-produced biologic agent would come in contact with the agent at approximately the same time. Even taking into account varying incubation periods based on exposure dose and physiologic differences, a compressed epidemic curve with a peak in a matter of days, or even hours, would occur. Specific indicators of a biologic attack may include:

- Disease caused by exotic or nonendemic organisms
- Disease occurring in a location lacking the usual vectors for transmission
- Higher disease rate for a particular disease or atypical clinical presentation
- A cluster of patients with similar clinical syndromes
- Higher morbidity and mortality rates than normally expected for a disease
- Diseased or dead animals in the geographic location where a human epidemic is occurring

For example, in 1979, the unintended release of anthrax spores from a military compound in the former Soviet Union demonstrated some of the epidemiologic indicators of an unnatural epidemic. The location of the casualties followed a distinctive downwind pattern from the release site, and animals in the same area were affected. In addition, there was an unusual respiratory presentation of the disease rather than the more common cutaneous form. Although initially denied by the Soviet government, Boris Yeltsin admitted in 1992 that there had been an unintentional release of anthrax from a biologic warfare laboratory, confirming what epidemiologists in the West already suspected.

11. Historically, what are some examples of biological warfare or terrorism?

- In the 6th century B.C., Assyrians poisoned enemy wells with rye ergot.
- In 1346, while the Tartars were attacking the city of Kaffa, some of their troops came down with plague. To start an epidemic in the city, they catapulted the cadavers of their deceased over the city walls.
- During the French and Indian War (1754–1767), in an attempt to spread smallpox among the enemy, British troops gave blankets obtained from a smallpox hospital to the Indians who were allied with the French.
- During World War II, the infamous Japanese Unit 731 experimented on prisoners of war with biological weapons, resulting in as many as 10,000 deaths from plague, anthrax, dengue, tularemia, and other biologic agents.
- In 1978, Georgi Markov, a Bulgarian political exile, was assassinated in London with the toxalbumin ricin by subcutaneous injection. Ricin was placed in a pellet that was delivered by injection from the tip of an umbrella into Markov's leg.
- In 1984, 751 people were infected with *Salmonella enteritides* serotype typhimurium in the Dalles, Oregon, area. Followers of the Bhagwan Shree Rajneesh had contaminated salad bars at various restaurants in an effort to influence local elections.
- In 1994, Aum Shinrikyo attempted the aerial release of anthrax spores in Tokyo.

12. What is the most effective method for dissemination of biologic weapons?

Aerosol spray. An aerosol cloud would not be detectable immediately because it would be invisible, odorless, and tasteless. Furthermore, it could go undetected for days to weeks before the attack was recognized. The major limitation to aerosol spread of a biologic agent (as members of the Aum Shinrikyo cult discovered) is unpredictable meteorologic conditions such as high winds and turbulence that might disperse the cloud or divert it from the population center.

Other potential methods of dissemination include explosive munitions, food and water contamination, and percutaneous spread, but all have significant limitations. Explosive munitions destroy most of the agent during detonation, and food and water contamination requires large amounts of the agent. Percutaneous spread has been shown to be an excellent means of assassination but lacks the ability to cause mass casualties.

13. List the characteristics of an effective biologic agent.

The agent:
- Should be capable of dispersion in aerosols of particle size 1–5 µm, which can remain suspended in air for hours and, if inhaled, can penetrate into the lower respiratory system
- Should be inexpensive and relatively simple to produce
- Should be highly infective
- Should have an incubation period of days to weeks to allow the terrorist to escape

Examples of Potentially Effective Biologic Agents

AGENT	INFECTIVE DOSE	INCUBATION PERIOD (DAYS)
Bacillus anthracis	8000–50,000 spores	1–6
Coxiella burnetii	1–10 organisms	10–20
Brucella suis	10–100 organisms	5–60
Yersinia pestis	100–500 organisms	2–3
Francisella tularensis	10–50 organisms	2–10
Variola virus	10–100 organisms	7–17
Viral encephalitides	10–100 organisms	2–14
Botulinum toxin	0.01 µg/kg	1–5
Staphylococcal enterotoxin B	0.03–1.7 µg	< 1

14. How might a terrorist-initiated anthrax epidemic begin, and how might it be detected?

Of the different biological agents, *Bacillus anthracis* receives the most attention because of its long history as a warfare agent and, more recently, because of Iraq's biological warfare program that threatened U.S. troops in the Gulf War. It has been estimated that, if 100 kg of anthrax spores were released as an aerosol spray upwind of Washington, D.C., between 130,000 and 3 million people would die.

An epidemic would likely begin after the incubation period of 1–6 days, with an increased number of people coming down with flu-like syndromes. A pearl that may aid in the diagnosis of inhalational anthrax would be the finding of a widened mediastinum on the chest x-ray caused by hemorrhagic mediastinitis and lymphadenitis. Additionally, hemorrhagic meningitis may develop in 50% of cases.

Treatment of anthrax consists of intravenous penicillin plus streptomycin or ciprofloxacin. However, even with treatment, the case fatality rate from inhalational anthrax has been estimated to be as high as 80–100%, with death typically occurring 24–36 hours after the onset of severe symptoms.

In the case of an anthrax threat, prophylaxis is recommended with ciprofloxacin, 500 mg orally twice a day, continued for 4 weeks if the attack is confirmed. A vaccine is also available that is currently being given to all military members and may offer immunity from inhalational anthrax.

15. What kind of decontamination is needed for biological and chemical agent exposure?

In general, for aerosol exposure to biological agents, decontamination is not universally effective or even necessary. Patients do not have to be decontaminated at the scene and may shower at home. However, if visible contamination is apparent, victims should first wash with soap and water and then rinse with diluted bleach (0.5% sodium hypochlorite) as a bactericidal and sporicidal agent.

If there is a possibility of smallpox or plague contamination, emergency responders and medical staff should wear high-efficiency particulate air (HEPA) filter masks to reduce the risk of transmission.

In contrast, chemical agents require rapid decontamination of the skin after exposure to the liquid or aerosolized form of an agent. Decontamination of these compounds is most effective if conducted within 1 minute of exposure but should still be done to protect the patient and the emergency responders from secondary contamination.

16. What is the government doing to protect the population from terrorist use of weapons of mass destruction?

International Agreements:

- **Geneva Protocol for the Prohibition of the Use in War of Asphyxiating, Poisonous or Other Gases and of Bacteriological Methods of Warfare** (1925). This protocol was signed after the atrocities of World War I but was interpreted to be a prohibition of first use. Most countries continued their research and development of biologic and chemical warfare.
- **Convention on the Prohibition of the Development, Production and Stockpiling of Bacteriological (Biological) and Toxin Weapons and on their Destruction** (1975). This protocol prohibited development, production, and stockpiling of biologic weapons and was signed by 158 countries. There was no monitoring mechanism associated with the protocol, and, although representatives from Iraq and the Soviet Union signed this agreement, both continued researching the use of biological weapons.

United States:

- In 1989, Congress passed the **Biological Weapons Act** to protect the nation against bioterrorism. The act defined, as a federal crime, the knowing development, manufacture, transfer, or possession of any "biologic agent, toxin, or delivery system" for "use as a weapon." It enabled the federal government to intervene swiftly before a potential biological weapon could be used to cause injury or environmental harm.
- In 1995, the general framework for the response to terrorist incidents was provided by **Presidential Decision Directive (PDD) 39**. This directive assigned the Federal Bureau of Investigation (FBI) as the lead agency for crisis management and the Federal Emergency Management Agency (FEMA) as the lead agency for coordinating assistance in response to a terrorist act.
- In 1996, Congress passed the **Anti-Terrorism Act**, which authorized the Centers for Disease Control and Prevention (CDC) to create and maintain a list of biological agents having the "potential to pose a severe threat to public health and safety." The CDC was also directed to establish regulations governing the use and transfer of these restricted agents.
- In 1997, Congress enacted the **Defense against Weapons of Mass Destruction Act**, which further defined federal capabilities in handling the response to weapons of mass destruction and directed the Department of Defense to develop and implement domestic preparedness programs.

17. *Extra credit:* **In 1980, when French police and intelligence personnel raided a "safe house" at 41A Chaillot Street, Paris, they were surprised to find what toxic agent being manufactured by the German "Red Army Faction" for potential terrorist use?**

Botulinum toxin.

18. *Extra credit:* **In June 1994, in a terrorist attack, a toxic gas seeped through the open windows of homes in the Japanese city of Matsumoto, killing 8 people and seriously poisoning 200 inhabitants. What was this toxic gas?**

Sarin.

BIBLIOGRAPHY

1. Christopher GW, Cieslak TJ, Pavlin JA, et al: Biological warfare a historical perspective. JAMA 278:412–417, 1997.
2. Ferguson JR: Biological weapons and US law. JAMA 278:357–360, 1997.
3. Franz DR, Jahrling PB, Friedlander AM, et al: Clinical recognition and management of patients exposed to biological warfare agents. JAMA 278:399–411, 1997.
4. Inglesby TV, Henderson DA, Bertlett JG, et al: Anthrax as a biological weapon. JAMA 281:1735–1745, 1999.
5. Keim M, Kaufmann AF: Principles for emergency response to bioterrorism. Ann Emerg Med 34:177–182, 1999.
6. Lesho E, Dorsey D, Bunner D: Feces, dead horses, and fleas. Evolution of the hostile use of biological agents. West J Med 168:512–516, 1998.
7. Richards CF, Burstein JL, Waekerle JF, et al: Emergency physicians and biological terrorism. Ann Emerg Med 34:183–190, 1999.
8. Slater MS, Trunkey DD: Terrorism in America. An evolving threat. Arch Surg 132:1059–1066, 1997.
9. Torok TJ, Tauxe RV, Wise RP, et al: A large community outbreak of salmonellosis caused by intentional contamination of restaurant salad bars. JAMA 278:389–395, 1997.
10. U.S. Army Medical Research Institute of Infectious Diseases: Medical Management of Biologic Casualties, 2nd ed. Fort Detrick, MD, U.S. Army Medical Research Institute of Infections Diseases, 1996.

INDEX

Page numbers in **boldface type** indicate complete chapters.

1 (877) 326-5195